# Health Communication, Language, and Social Action across the Life Span

Language
as SOCIAL
ACTION

Howard Giles and David M. Markowitz
*General Editors*

Vol. 25

# Health Communication, Language, and Social Action across the Life Span

Edited by
Amber K. Worthington, Carla L. Fisher,
Janice L. Krieger, Craig Fowler, Margaret J. Pitts,
and Jon F. Nussbaum

PETER LANG
New York - Berlin - Bruxelles - Chennai - Lausanne - Oxford

Library of Congress Cataloging-in-Publication Data

Names: Worthington, Amber K.
Title: Health communication, language, and social action across the life span / Amber K. Worthington [and five others].
Description: New York : PeterLang, 2025. | Series: Language as social action, 1529-2436 ; Vol. 25 | Includes bibliographical references and index.
Identifiers: LCCN 2024018090 | ISBN 9781433197550 (paperback) | ISBN 9781433197567 (hardback) | ISBN 9781433197536 (ebook) | ISBN 9781433197543 (epub)
Subjects: LCSH: Communication in medicine. | Communication in medicine–Social aspects.
Classification: LCC R118 .H4345 2025 | DDC 610.1/4–dc23/eng/20240528
LC record available at https://lccn.loc.gov/2024018090
DOI 10.3726/b21965

Bibliographic information published by the Deutsche Nationalbibliothek.
The German National Library lists this publication in the German National Bibliography; detailed bibliographic data is available on the Internet at http://dnb.d-nb.de.

Cover design by Peter Lang Group AG

ISSN 1529-2436 (print)
ISBN 9781433197550 (paperback)
ISBN 9781433197567 (hardback)
ISBN 9781433197536 (ebook)
ISBN 9781433197543 (epub)
DOI 10.3726/b21965


Published by Peter Lang Publishing Inc., New York, USA
info@peterlang.com - www.peterlang.com



This publication has been peer reviewed.

We dedicate this book to honor the next generation in our families of origin and our families of the heart (i.e., our academic family). We further dedicate this book to Mary Ann, for supporting Jon as he supported us.

During the writing and preparation of this book, Cindy Gallois, our dear friend and internationally respected and impactful researcher within health, language, and social action, among older adults, passed away. We are all much better scholars and humans because of you, Cindy, and we will do our best to strive for your level of excellence (see also <https://www.icahdq.org/blogpost/1523657/490864/Cindy-Gallois-Remembrance-and-Legacies>)

# Table of Contents

# List of Figures

# List of Tables

# Editor Information

*Jon F. NussBaum (PhD, Purdue University, 1981)* is a Liberal Arts Professor Emeritus of Communication Arts and Sciences and Human Development and Family Studies at Penn State University. He has edited or authored 17 books and well over 150 journal articles and book chapters. He has been named a Fulbright Research Scholar to the United Kingdom, served as the president of the International Communication Association and the International Association of Language and Social Psychology, served as an editor of the Journal of Communication, has been awarded the Distinguished Scholar Award by the National Communication Association, and is a Fellow in the International Communication Association, American Psychological Association, and Gerontological Society of America. He has directed 37 dissertations.

*Carla L. Fisher (PhD, Penn State University, 2008)* is Professor of Health Outcomes and Biomedical Informatics in the College of Medicine at the University of Florida, a member of the UF Health Cancer Center, and Faculty Affiliate in the Center for Arts in Medicine. Her work focuses on helping patients, caregivers, family members, and clinicians engage in health-promoting communication at home and in clinical settings. Her primary area of expertise is in family-centered psychosocial oncology care in coping, caregiving, and risk reduction, as well as qualitative approaches to developmentally targeting and implementing interventions. Her research has been honored with national awards, and her collaborations have secured more than $15 million in funding, including from NIH, PCORI, and The Leukemia & Lymphoma Society. She has authored over 100 publications including the only evidence-based book providing mothers and daughters with developmentally tailored guidance on breast cancer coping and caregiving.

*Craig Fowler (PhD Penn State University, 2005)* is Associate Professor in the School of Communication, Journalism and Marketing at Massey University, New Zealand. His research interests focus on family communication, intergenerational relationships, and issues related to communication and successful aging.

*Janice L. Krieger (PhD, Penn State University, 2007)* is Professor of Advertising and Health Outcomes & Biomedical Informatics at the University of Florida. She is a health communication scientist who is passionate about finding innovative ways to reduce health inequities. Her work focuses on developing translational communication interventions that empower patients, families, and communities in the context of healthcare decision-making. She serves as a co-leader of the University of Florida Health Cancer Center (UFHCC) Cancer Population Sciences research program and a founding director of the STEM (*S*cience, *T*echnology, *E*ngineerin g, and *M*edicine) Translational Communication Center. Her work is funded by the National Cancer Institute and the National Institute on Aging. She was the recipient of the University of Florida Invention of Year in 2021 and Preeminence Term Professorship Award in 2015. She also won the Society for Public Health Education Technology Award in 2020. She has authored over 125 articles and book chapters.

*Margaret J. Pitts (PhD, Penn State University, 2005)* is Associate Professor of Communication (Department of Communication) and Senior Associate Dean of the Graduate College at the University of Arizona. With over 50 scholarly publications, she is recognized as an expert in positive communication with a focus on successful and satisfying communication across lifespan transitions. She approaches the study of human interactions using qualitative inquiry including grounded theory development of *communication savoring*. In her dean's role, Maggie uses principles of positive communication to lead through times of transition and trauma, most recently with COVID-19 and a campus shooting. Maggie practices applied communication with the goal of ensuring that communication research is translated and applied to the communities it serves best.

*Amber K. Worthington (PhD, Penn State University, 2017)* is Associate Professor of Communication (Department of Communication) and Department Chair at the University of Alaska Anchorage. Her research intersects communication and health sciences and focuses on behavior change theory, persuasion, and message design.

# About the Contributors

*Lindsey Anderson (PhD)* is an Associate Professor of Communication at the University of Maryland.

*Sara L. Buckingham (PhD)* is an Associate Professor of Psychology at the University of Alaska Anchorage.

*Gemme Campbell-Salome (PhD)* is an Assistant Professor of Genomic Health and Population Health Sciences at Geisinger.

*Mollie Rose Canzona (PhD)* is an Associate Professor of Communication and Social Sciences & Health Policy at the Wake Forest School of Medicine.

*Tzu-Chiao Chen (PhD)* is an Assistant Professor of Communication at the University of Alaska Anchorage.

*R. Amanda Cooper (PhD)* is an Assistant Professor of Interpersonal Communication at the University of Connecticut.

*Maria Christina Crouch (PhD)* is Deg Hit'an & Coahuiltecan and is a Postdoctoral Fellow at the Yale School of Medicine.

*Carla L. Fisher (PhD)* is a Professor of Health Outcomes & Biomedical Informatics in the College of Medicine at the University of Florida.

*Craig Fowler (PhD)* is an Associate Professor of Communication at Massey University.

*Nybony Gat (BS)* is the Peer Leader Navigator Program Director for the Alaska Literacy Program.

*Patricia Gettings (PhD)* is Associate Professor of Communication at SUNY Albany.

*Dale M. Golden (MS)* is a PhD Candidate in Clinical-Community Psychology at the University of Alaska Anchorage.

*Steven Harris, Jr.* is Alutiiq and is a PhD Student at Pacific University.

*Jake Harwood (PhD)* is a Professor of Communication at the University of Arizona.

*Britteny M. Howell (PhD, CPG, CDP)* is an Associate Professor of Population Health Sciences and Director of the Healthy Aging Research Laboratory at the University of Alaska Anchorage.

*Mary Lee Hummert (PhD)* is a Professor Emerita of Communication Studies at the University of Kansas.

*Janice L. Krieger (PhD)* is a Professor of Quantitative Health Sciences at Mayo Clinic.

*Shannon Kuhn (MPH)* is a Board Member for the Alaska Literacy Program.

*Victoria McDermott (PhD)* is an Assistant Professor of Communication and Journalism at the University of Alaska, Fairbanks.

*Allex Mahanna (BS)* is an MPH Student in Population Health Sciences at the University of Alaska Anchorage.

*Amana Mbise (PhD)* is an Assistant Professor of Social Work at the University of Alaska Anchorage.

*Julien C. Mirivel (PhD)* is a Professor of Applied Communication at the University of Arkansas at Little Rock and Founder of the Positive Communication Network.

*Jon F. NussBaum (PhD)* is a Liberal Arts Emeritus Professor of Communication Arts and Sciences & Human Development and Family Studies at Penn State University.

*Bailey M. Oliver-Blackburn (PhD)* is an Associate Professor and Graduate Coordinator of Applied Communication at the University of Arkansas at Little Rock.

*Angela L. Palmer-Wackerly (PhD)* is an Associate Professor of Communication Studies at the University of Nebraska-Lincoln.

*Margaret Jane Pitts (PhD)* is a Senior Associate Dean of the Graduate College and Associate Professor of Communication at the University of Arizona.

*Aantaki Raisa (PhD)* is a Postdoctoral Associate at Washington University, St. Louis.

*Rosellen M. Rosich, (PhD)* is a Professor Emerita of Psychology at the University of Alaska Anchorage.

*Sofia Sytniak (BS)* is a Ph.D. student in Clinical-Community Psychology at the University of Alaska Anchorage.

*Kazi Haneeya Wahed (MS)* is a doctoral student in the Department of Communication Studies at the University of Nebraska-Lincoln.

*Amber K. Worthington (PhD)* is an Associate Professor and Department Chair of Communication at the University of Alaska Anchorage.

*Kevin B. Wright (PhD)* is a Professor of Communication at George Mason University.

# Introduction: Health Communication, Language, and Social Action across the Life Span

JON F. NUSSBAUM

*We're going to make it a better life and leave it for the kids*
*It's a lovely place, a welcome home for the human race*
*We're going to make it a better life, one we can be proud of*
*So at the end of the day, we can laugh and say that we left them a better life*
– *A Better Life* (George Merrill/Graham Nash)

The Language and Social Action book series co-edited by Howie Giles and David Marcowitz presents the editors of this book with a special opportunity to come together as like-minded scholars to produce an impactful tome that encapsulates many of our core theoretical and practical beliefs within Health, Language, and Social Action across the Life Span. Three fundamental worldviews or macro-level notions serve as the foundational bedrock of this book: the centrality of Language to our understanding of human behavior and human action; the uniqueness of the Health Context as an environment that can produce impactful language associated with positive life outcomes; and the Life Span Developmental nature of human interaction. These guiding theoretical principles and the impactful behavior we have investigated move our understanding of language and social action within the healthcare context significantly beyond that which currently exists.

The editors and authors of this book place the understanding and use of language within social interaction as a necessary condition of any true attempt to grasp meaning within human behavior. George Carlin (the recently passed comedian and social commentator) spent the major portion of his illustrious career in comedy emphasizing the extreme significance of words and language that meaningfully impact every aspect of our lives. Carlin was also a staunch supporter of the significance of context that determines the appropriateness and functionality of language. While numerous scholars within the general domains of Communication, Linguistics, Social Psychology, and Language Studies have made their careers emphasizing the significance of language and language use in context, George Carlin has touched, influenced, and helped to entertain many individuals on this message and made some excellent comedy as well. In my mind, the most heinous and "fake news" saying that has ever been produced or reproduced goes something like "sticks and stones can break my bones, but names (words) can never hurt me." NO! Words are powerful, are agents of change, are the causes of all emotion, enable us to understand both the simple and complex, serve as the managerial tool for all human relationships, and can ultimately hurt as well as heal. Carlin, we think, would be proud of our scholarly attempts to scientifically confirm his act!

The general health context of interaction that contains all communicative events within both formal healthcare institutions (clinics, hospitals, continuing care facilities, etc.) and the majority of our familial and interpersonal relationships continue to be a primary focus of the editors of this book. We believe that the language constructed and utilized within these unique health communication encounters demand careful scrutiny and scientific investigation as they directly influence our physical, emotional, and spiritual well-being. The coeditors of this book have produced over 40 years of research that points to the difficulties of competent interaction within all health contexts. In many ways, the difficulties associated with efficient, effective, and competent communication within the healthcare context can be the major determinant of successful health outcomes.

We, also, place the dynamic and developmental process of language and communication into our fundamental, core notions of human behavior. While it may seem obvious that the very nature of human interaction is constantly changing as we as individuals develop throughout our lives, surprisingly few theoretical or empirical investigators within the general disciplines of Communication, Language, and Social Psychology ground their research within a life span developmental perspective. An essential ingredient to our full understanding of the possible consequences for language and social interaction within the health context is the age and relational history of the interactants. Many of the interactional contexts within health are intergenerational. These intergenerational communication encounters demand a higher level of coordination to provide possible, positive health outcomes but are often challenged by ageism and a lack of appropriate intergenerational communication skills.

Several formal theories of Intergroup and Interpersonal Communication inform and ground our thinking within this book. Communication Accommodation Theory, Socio-emotional Selectivity Theory, Intergroup Conflict Theory, and several other theoretical paradigms are highlighted and expanded upon in the sections where appropriate. We do wish to emphasize the innovative, transformative scholarship that drives this book, pointing us toward utilizing theory to help us not only better understand the communication behavior of healthcare staff and patients but ultimately also lead to pragmatic interventions and positive social action. We feel this book serves as one of the first scholarly gatherings of language/communication researchers who are moving toward pragmatic message interventions to successfully manage positive, social health outcomes across both interactive and cognitive domains.

Our book is divided into five parts. Each part is edited by one of the coeditors of the book within his/her primary area of scholarly research. Each part includes one large state-of-the-art chapter followed by several, brief research reports. Each part is meant to stand on its own as an important statement of the current state of our knowledge in the particular part focus area and to mesh within the general fundamental principles of the book to produce a coherent and rather broad-based understanding of Health Communication, Language, and Social Action across the Life Span. In addition, the parts are hierarchically ordered from more abstract concepts to much more targeted, pragmatic social actions.

I should note that each part editor completed her/his dissertation at Penn State University under my direction. Each has moved well beyond our Happy Valley home and has produced an impressive record of programmatic research. A major motivation to organize and produce this volume is to highlight the breadth and depth of impressive scholarship that continues to flow from these health researchers far removed from our graduate seminars and the very beginnings of our programmatic research efforts.

Margaret Pitts serves as part editor of the initial part of the book entitled "Positive Communication in Social Action." Positive communication is grounded in the language of potential communication and social engagement that creates opportunities for humans to flourish and thrive. Positive communication strategically and habitually uses language that promotes well-being and health across every point in the life span.

Carla Fisher edits the second part entitled "The Centrality of Interpersonal Communication to Our Health and Well-Being." Our communicative lives are as central to our health and well-being across the life span as any physical or psychological process. How we communicate and manage our language with family, friends, and health professionals has both short-term and long-term implications on our ability to cope with illness, manage, or reduce disease risk, and adjust to healthy- or aging-related transitions that most likely are characterized by extreme stress.

Craig Fowler edits the third part entitled "Social Environments Conducive to Quality of Life and Successful Aging." An individual's sense of whether he/she is aging well depends on much more than genetics or "good luck." An individual's ability to communicatively construct and then appropriately manage social environments that facilitate well-being as he/she moves through the life span is the focus of this part. How people may shape their life trajectories via communication and how the "aging spaces" we help to form and co-inhabit with others are identified as a significant key to achieving a high quality of life.

Janice Krieger edits the fourth part entitled "Translational Communication in Health." This part highlights the role of language in the social construction of health and wellness in diverse communities. The meanings associated with health messages (language) from the perspective of social group memberships (e.g., occupation, race, gender, age) are explored. This part brings together health communication, intergroup communication, and language to examine health messages from the perspective of geographic and cultural space.

Amber Worthington edits the fifth part entitled "Culturally Informed Health Communication Campaigns." The goal of this part is to examine the importance of culturally informed campaigns to promote healthy aging in diverse communities in the arctic and subarctic regions of Alaska. This part will explore culturally appropriate language choices for social action for those in Alaska, including Alaskan older adults, Alaska Native peoples, and immigrant populations within Alaska.

We are thrilled that Mary Lee Hummert has agreed to write the "Epilogue." Her highly respected and enormously impactful scholarly career has added significantly to our knowledge base within Communication and Aging focusing on age stereotypes and the language of ageism. Professor Hummert's vision for the future of "Heath Communication, Language, and Social Action across the Life Span" is enlightening and inspirational.

We invite you to read this most exhaustive and up-to-date presentation of our research programs that focus on "Health Communication, Language, and Social Action across the Life Span."

# PART ONE

# Positive Communication as Social Action

CHAPTER ONE

# Positive Communication as Social Action: Compassion and Communication Savoring

MARGARET JANE PITTS

This book opens purposively with a collection of three chapters on positive communication to focus our intention on the power of language to create space for hope within myriad contexts for social action. Positive communication is grounded in the language of potential—communication and social engagement that creates opportunities for humans to flourish and thrive. Aligned with Barbara Fredrickson's (2001, 2004) broaden and build theory of positive emotions, positive communication allows the mind to expand to take in new knowledge, to engage creativity and imagination, and to seek meaningful connections to others and to our environment. All of this is possible because of language—"our single most important tool" that allows humans to share abstract thoughts, ideas, and imagination, to collectively make meaning, to invent, and to shape the past, present, and future (Kellerman & Seligman, 2023, p. 20). Positive communication opens possibilities rather than reducing them. As such, positive communication is critical to the discursive enactments of social action—what we can achieve, what we can do, and what we can change through individual and collective action in big and small ways.

This chapter opens with an exploration of positive social science as an inclusive mode of inquiry, making a deliberate shift from a predominantly Eurocentric viewpoint to engage and integrate diverse global philosophies. Then, I provide a definition and parameters for positive communication followed by a deeper dive into two specific acts of positive communication—compassion and communication savoring—and their significant contribution to personal and social well-being across the life span. Finally, I introduce the two subsequent chapters on positive communication as social action showcasing the humanizing (Harwood & Cooper, Chapter Two, this volume) and transformative (Mirivel & Oliver-Blackburn, Chapter Three, this volume) power of positive communication. This chapter concludes with a call to action for more empirical research, theoretical development, and broad application of positive communication.

## POSITIVE SOCIAL SCIENCE

Positive social science is earning its place within psychology, organizational leadership, education, communication, and other social and behavioral disciplines. Scholarship on the bright side of human activity, human experiences, virtues, value, and potential has persisted over centuries and over continents. The cultural origins of thought, study, and practice of the highest human ethics are diverse, a point which is often obscured by a dominating Eurocentric discourse centering on Aristotelian ethics. The first part of this chapter starts by decentering Europe in order to acknowledge and give homage to the diverse streams of knowledge and human experience that have influenced contemporary thinking. Positive social science, including communication science, has been limited because of a predominant Eurocentric view. The two positive communication enactments that I address in the latter part of this chapter (compassionate communication and communication savoring) are good examples of this limitation. Roy (2016) argues that compassion has been largely overlooked and undervalued in the communication discipline due to an overemphasis of a western (Greek) rationalist paradigm in which the prevalent thinking is that compassion obscures the distance and objectivity necessary to make decisions or take an appropriate course of action. Compassion is considered a weakness. However, within many eastern paradigms of thought, compassion is considered a natural and moral response to the inherent suffering of all people (Opdebeeck & Habisch, 2011). It reflects the inseparable connection between self and other and serves as an important guide to thought and action. Similarly, western notions of savoring emphasize the "pleasure beyond pleasure" hedonic treadmill of seeking out and indulging in novel, pleasurable moments, whereas eastern ideals incorporate balance through moderating how pleasurable an experience should be and savoring the bad along with the good (Frijda & Sundararajan, 2007; Miyamoto & Ma, 2011).

Decentering Europe allows scholarship to advance and take into consideration the lived worlds, and positive communication practices, of all humankind. Centering Africa (Afrocentric scholarship) reminds us that philosophical considerations of the ethical and moral development of human goodness emerged first from Africa, hundreds of years before Europe and Asia cultivated their own (related) philosophies of thought (Asante, 2014). Indeed, Asante (2014) writes, "We know that Africans have thought about the universe longer than any other people" (np), including African teachings on values and leadership (i.e., sage Mohlomi and chief Moshoeshoe; du Preez, 2011). The African tradition is intertwined with the earliest thoughts on the essential qualities of human nature, virtue, beauty, and the afterlife inspiring Asian and European philosophers centuries later (Asante, 2014). Centering Asia (Asiacentric scholarship) reinvigorates and revalorizes Asian spiritual and philosophical guidance for human relations, behavior, aesthetics, ethics, and emotions (Miike, 2014). An Asiacentric code of positive language and communication might embrace the Buddhist ethics of *samma* vac, or right speech: (1) truthful speech (rather than false speech), (2) harmonious speech (rather than divisive speech), (3) gentle speech (rather than harsh speech), and (4) purposeful speech (rather than incessant speech; Miike, 2014).

Despite deeper and multicultural historics, many in the positive movement draw solely from classical Greek philosophy. For example, Schwartz and Sharpe (2006) draw on Aristotelian virtues to make the argument that *phronesis* (practical wisdom) is a master virtue necessary for enactment of other virtues and that *eudaimonia* (happiness) requires fulfillment and optimization of many virtues. This argument contrasts with Peterson and Seligman's (2004) preceding (and prevailing) guiding assumption that character strengths and virtues can be independently identified and developed toward fulfilling ends. Others, like Mirivel (2012), have drawn from more contemporary European philosophers such as French philosopher André Comte-Sponville to identify virtues enacted through communication.

Despite our shared roots and centuries-long studies, there appears to be little effort to harness these knowledge streams into a more comprehensive and multifaceted study of human potential. Until recently there has not been a collective effort to unify scholarship under a broader interdisciplinary, multicultural framework of positive social science. Instead, contemporary social and behavioral scientists have gotten quite good at examining, identifying, theorizing about, and ameliorating human problems, deficiencies, and pathologies to the near exclusion of an understanding what makes humans flourish and thrive (Seligman & Csikszentmihalyi, 2000). Fortunately, positive social science offers a solution to the lopsidedness of a deficit approach. While it is imperative that scholars continue to study problems, deficits, and challenges, we cannot continue to do so at the exclusion of scientific study of quality of life, health, and well-being. We must study the problems, pitfalls, and despair—the negative traits, experiences, and emotions—in conjunction with hope, glimmer, potential, and positive traits, experiences, emotions, and assets. Positive social science is a multidisciplinary framework for the scientific investigation and practical application of positively valanced and valued subjective experiences (Seligman & Csikszentmihalyi, 2000).

As a discipline, positive psychology is the clear forerunner and champion for the positive science approach. Positive psychology is built upon three pillars—positive emotions, positive traits, and positive institutions (Peterson, 2006). The core assumption of positive psychology is that "human goodness and excellence are as authentic as disease, disorder, and distress" (Peterson, 2006, p. 5). It is the study of character strengths, talents, virtues, and "the conditions and processes that contribute to the flourishing or optimal functioning of people, groups, and institutions" (Gable & Haidt, 2005, p. 104). In 2004, Peterson and Seligman published a new kind of psychological diagnostic tool designed to identify and classify character strengths and virtues in response to the widely recognized "gold standard" DSM, the *Diagnostic and Statistical Manual of Mental Disorders* (American Psychiatric Association, 2013). Peterson and Seligman argued that in addition to being able to identify, understand, treat, and predict disorders, psychologists also need tools to identify, understand, enhance, and predict human excellence and thriving. They identified 24 character strengths that are recognized and valued across cultures. The 24 strengths are classified under six core virtues: Wisdom (creativity, curiosity, judgment, love of learning, and perspective), courage (bravery, honesty, perseverance, and zest), humanity (kindness, love, and social intelligence), justice (fairness, leadership, and teamwork), temperance (forgiveness, humility, prudence, and self-regulation), and transcendence (appreciation of beauty and excellence, gratitude, hope, humor, and spirituality). Having classified these strengths, scholars can assess their presence and measure their impact through empirical tests and interventions. Indeed, positive psychological interventions (PPIs) are one way in which positive social and behavioral sciences are contributing to a better understanding of how to cultivate higher quality of life through optimizing positive affect and engaging strengths and virtues (Klibert et al., 2022). Communication has much to learn from this approach, but also much to offer.

## POSITIVE COMMUNICATION

Like positive psychology, positive communication scholarship centers on conditions and (communication) processes that cultivate human flourishing and resilience. Positive communication serves to (1) *E*nhance positive experiences and emotions, (2) *F*acilitate positive institutions, including families and contexts for living, and (3) *G*enerate positive traits and behaviors—what I call the EFGs of positive communication. Although positive communication has a shorter disciplinary history than positive psychology, the field has started to take shape. In 2012 Socha and Pitts published the first edited volume on positive interpersonal communication. At the time, we described positive interpersonal communication as "relational communication facilitative of happiness, health, and wellness" (Socha & Pitts, 2012, p. 1). The first volume included key concepts such as aesthetic relating (Baxter et al., 2012), synchrony in positive intercultural encounters (Kim, 2012), and excellent and virtuous communication (Miczo, 2012; Mirivel, 2012). It included chapters on fundamental processes of positive communication including listening (Bodie, 2012), affection (Floyd & Deiss, 2012), play (Aune & Wong, 2012), and forgiveness and relational justice (Kelley, 2012). A second volume quickly followed with a focus on flourishing in domains of personal health and wellness, interpersonal relationships, and institutions and organizations (Pitts & Socha, 2013b). In the second volume, we took the stance that positive communication is not merely the absence of negative, diminishing, or hurtful messages but the presence of words, messages, and gestures that enhance and facilitate relationships, individual growth, and human connection (Pitts & Socha, 2013a). It is the difference between what my mother told me, "If you can't say anything nice, don't say anything at all," and what I tell my own children, "When you have the opportunity to communicate for positive impact—do it!" Positive communication holds the power to "inspire people to achieve higher moments, greater good, and to act selflessly" (Pitts & Socha, 2013a, p. 3).

Other books and collections dedicated to the advancement of positive communication followed, expanding its development and impact. These include Mirivel's (2014) *The Art of Positive Communication*, Beck and Socha's (2015a) edited volume, *Communicating Hope and Resilience across the Lifespan*, and Muñiz-Velázquez and Pulido's (2019) edited volume, *The Routledge Handbook of Positive Communication: Contributions of an Emerging Community of Research on Communication for Happiness and Social Change*. Variations on the theme have also emerged at scholarly meetings including a positive communication workshop and preconference at the 2016 National Communication Association Convention (co-convened by Socha, Mirivel, Pitts, and Beck). "Positive Communication" was the theme of the 2010 annual convention of the Southern States Communication Association with Socha presiding as Vice President and convention planner. "Accentuate the Positive" was the Western States Communication Association (WSCA) convention theme in 2015 and "Mindfulness and Communication" was the theme in 2018. WSCA returned to the theme in 2023 with "Communication and Well-Being." The 2014 theme of the International Communication Association convention was "Communication and the Good Life." This was followed by the 2015 theme, "Communication across the Lifespan" about which Nussbaum wrote in his presidential address, "Communication across the life span is at the very heart of any reasonable notion of quality of life" (Nussbaum, 2007, p. 2).

The establishment of the Positive Communication Network reflects continued dedication among positive communication scholars to shape and direct communication research, theory, and practice to improve the human condition (<www.positi vecommunication.net>). Julian Mirivel founded the Positive Communication Network in 2022. I am happy to be among the co-founders, a list which includes Tom Socha, Phillip Glenn, Amy Young, Kristen Christman, and Ryan Fuller. Together, we argue that positive communication holds great potential to (1) enhance individuals' health, well-being, and happiness, (2) create meaningful and authentic relationships, (3) facilitate mindful, compassionate communication in daily living, (4) inspire and contribute to resilient, flourishing organizations and communities, and (5) create better social worlds that cultivate individual and collective virtues (<www.positivecommunication.net>).

Though the concerted collaboration and framing around positive communication theory and research is relatively new, there is already a history of significant work in our and related fields that advance positive communication and social science. Theories such as Fredrickson's (2001, 2004) broaden and build theory on positive emotions, Afifi's theory of resilience and relational load (Afifi et al., 2016), Floyd's (2019) affection exchange theory, and Snyder's hope theory (Snyder et al., 1991) demonstrate that positive emotions and positive communication are not just momentary bursts of happiness but instead contribute to a sustainable toolkit we can routinely invest in so that we can meet unexpected and difficult experiences when they arise *with strength and support.* In other words, positive communication not only holds the potential to make a difference in the moment but also creates the mental and social structures that allow individuals to capitalize on those accumulative benefits again and again—upward spirals. Eliminating or mitigating negative affect and experiences does not promise positive affect or achievements. Rather, individuals must build positive skills to optimize potential for positive outcomes. While eliminating the negative does not necessarily result in increasing the positive, positive communication and psychological practices can both mitigate the negative while bolstering the positive.

Finally, while positive social science must intentionally focus on identifying, measuring, and reporting on human activity that contributes to quality of life, it does not have to do so at the exclusion of conflict, challenge, or difficulty. More recently, positive psychology scholars have moved beyond a sole focus on positive phenomena to acknowledge that human flourishing and fulfillment necessarily means experiencing and managing the negative alongside the positive (Lomas et al.,

2021) reminiscent of guiding Asiacentric philosophies (Miike, 2014; Miyamoto & Ma, 2011). Thus, positive communication is not only measured by behaviors "that reflect our best, that produce personal and relational happiness and satisfaction" but also "those that challenge our self to move in the direction of others and to act ethically" (Mirivel, 2014, p. 7). Positive communication can also be a force for social action through disruption. Anti-racist, anti-ageist, and humanizing communication are forms of positive communication that disrupt harmful patterns of social interaction—just as joyful communication and play within contexts of human rights and human tragedy can disrupt cycles of despair (see Simmons, 2019). After all, as Beck and Socha (2015b) argue in the writing about hope and resilience across the life span, "the experience of when things 'go wrong' is not exclusively negative" (p. 2).

## POSITIVE COMMUNICATION AS SOCIAL ACTION

Language and communication are critical means of social action as Howie Giles' edited series on *Language as Social Action* (Peter Lang) has shown with more than two dozen books devoted to exploring and exposing the constitutive and reflective nature of communication in shaping and mirroring social realities. For example, we may draw from Kinney and Pörhölä's (2009) contribution to the series, *Anti and Pro-social Communication*, to understand positive communication as a specific form of *prosocial communication* that functions to actively assist, help, or support others (versus antisocial communication which serves to hurt, disadvantage, or diminish others). More recently, Villarejo-Carballido et al. (2019) argued that theorizing about positive communication needs to advance from descriptive phenomenon toward purposive social action to meet larger societal goals. With an eye toward the 17 sustainable development goals set by the United Nations, they argued for the need to "collect evidence of the social impact of positive communication strategies for addressing behavior change" (Villarejo-Carballido et al., 2019, p. 17). Specifically, they called for work that can demonstrate measurable improvements in meaningful global contexts including climate action, the development of just societies, gender equality and educational equity, and the generation of health and well-being for people of all ages and stages, and so forth. Indeed, as Muñiz-Velázquez and Pulido (2019) argued, perhaps by "focus[ing] our research on positive communication effects, maybe we can help to increase them" (p. 3).

One form of prosocial communication generative of positive social action is the communicative enactment of virtues. To exemplify this notion, Mirivel (2012) drew from the works of French philosopher André Comte-Sponville to identify five virtues that can be enacted through communication: Gentleness, generosity, courage, justice, and compassion. When embodied as communicative acts, each of these virtues exemplifies mindful attention toward self and other creating space not only for individual flourishing but also social structures for community flourishing. Communicating with *gentleness* considers the other when crafting a message that will attend to one another's face (identity) *especially* in difficult and highly charged communication encounters. Communicating with a *generous* spirit allows us to listen and speak with humility. Mirivel (2012) offers three forms of generous communication: (1) to interpret the messages and the acts of others positively, (2) to offer one's own best communication move in each encounter, and (3) to closely attend to how one's communicative actions are being met. The final communicative acts identified by Mirivel move toward more engaged forms of positive communication relevant to social action. *Courageous* communication is bold, defiant in the face of injustice, and vulnerable—"Courage is to reveal information when there are risks or consequences" (Mirivel, 2012, p. 62). Courageous communication is a requirement for social action—speaking truth, invoking the goodness in others, calling out injustices, humanizing others, and stopping harmful talk. *Justice* is embodied in communication when we create structures that empower individuals to make well-reasoned and well-informed decisions without coercion. Justice is also embodied in communication when we refuse to participate in the dehumanization of others. Finally, Mirivel identifies *compassionate* communication as that which responds to, eases, and shares the burden of others' suffering, such as deep listening, sitting in active/attentive silence with another, and turning toward another's suffering through body orientation, touch, or nearness rather than turning away from it. Compassion also compels people to engage the other virtues—to communicate with gentleness to reduce the suffering of and minimize harm toward the other, to communicate with a generous spirit, assuming the best in others and offering our best to others, to communicate courageously to expel untruths, to connect with others through the practice of disclosure, to verbally praise and recognize others, as well as to halt harmful talk, and to communicate for justice because we see and we feel our inherent humanity. When we feel compassion, we communicate in ways that humanize. When we use language that humanizes, we open opportunities to act with compassion (see Harwood & Cooper, Chapter Two, this volume).

There are many acts of positive communication—kindness, gratitude, microaffirmations, celebrations, forgiveness. Some acts are grand while others are small and mundane, but all matter and serve a collective purpose to bind humanity and organize social encounters for optimal outcomes. Many of our daily social engagements are habitual enactments of positive communication. Mirivel (2014) identified six fundamental acts of communication in his theoretical model of positive communication: greeting, asking, complimenting, disclosing, encouraging, and listening (see also Mirivel & Oliver-Blackburn, Chapter Three, this volume). Those six acts work together to form the seventh act—to inspire. From those acts and outcomes of positive communication, Mirivel derived seven principles that undergird the model. Greeting creates contact and allows relationships to develop and sustain. Asking discovers the unknown. Complimenting contributes to the positive development of self and others. Disclosing deepens relationships. Encouraging gives support. Listening transcends human separateness. Inspiring influences others. Each of these acts of positive communication contributes to the fundamental processes of social action—to recognize, value, assert, and inspire the humanity in others—our collective humanity. While these practices of positive communication form the foundation of many of our daily encounters, I turn now to two specific acts of positive communication that can cultivate and inspire social action.

## Compassionate Communication as Social Action

Compassionate communication, though overlooked and understudied in the communication discipline, may be the most critical starting point to engage positive social action. Roy (2016) believed so:

> [Cultivating compassion] will help transform the hard realities of suffering by exploring ways to create more sustainable and empowering forms of relationality for all people regardless of whether we are at the center or on the margins. In short, it is not enough to have a social justice focus. We, as Communication Studies scholars, need to put compassion at the center of engagement in our discipline. (p. 85)

Compassion impels us to communicate to relieve the suffering of others or to share their burden. Compassionate speech (interpersonal and intergroup communication) and compassionate thoughts (intrapersonal communication and self-compassion) are behavioral enactments of compassion (Ozawa-de Silva et al., 2012), as is compassionate listening (Kimble & Bamford-Wade, 2013). Compassionate communication allows speakers to shape appropriate messages that respond to the relationship, the context, and the event in ways that care for the other. In describing the Dalai Lama as a champion of compassionate communication, Ozawa-de Silva et al. (2012) point toward his teachings that compassion is the basis for ethical thought and action and the foundation for a meaningful life in which we should strive to benefit others. They argue that compassion and warm-heartedness can ease communication with others and enhance our connectivity with them as part of our community of friends and fellow human beings.

Thus, compassion is not just a fundamental requirement for our psychological and physical health, but it is an essential quality of the human character that connects humanity (Ozawa-de Silva et al., 2012) and indeed all sentient beings (Roy, 2016).

Despite its importance and potential for social action and connectedness, compassion has been largely overlooked in the communication discipline (Roy, 2016) or considered synonymously with empathy and related concepts. Of the many virtuous needs, Hariman (2009) argued the "emotion that is most in need of cultivation is compassion" (p. 200). Compassion is active. Compassion can also be fierce, "taking a strong and resolute stand against harm" and offering "resilience in difficult circumstances" (Neff, 2023, p. 7.10). Experiencing compassion compels us to engage in social activity to relieve the suffering of others. This is distinct from empathy which, although it may prompt compassion, is primarily emotional resonance with another person. Empathy allows us to share in another's experience, while compassion moves us to act to reduce their suffering. Roy (2016) urged scholars to consider that the essence of being human is not only found in a rational and logical mind, but it is also in the heart, the soul, and the spirit. Cultivating a "compassionate vision," argued Hariman (2009), is

> essential to bridging the gap between self and other...an intentional act—more to the point, an act of seeing the world from the position of the other's pain—and of adjusting one's place in the world accordingly...Suffering is part of the shared human experience—so is the compulsion to relieve the suffering of others—drawing us together as one common humanity. (p. 202)

In his Presidential Address delivered to the Western States Communication Association Convention in 2019, Brian Heisterkamp argued that mindfulness and self-reflection are important tools in the cultivation of compassion and social justice. It is through the practice of mindful living that one can better understand the self and its relationship and interconnectedness with others. The compassion engendered by the recognition of human suffering can promote social justice and social action. Whereas the lack of self-awareness and lack of compassion obscures and obfuscates our intimate, fragile, but resilient and fierce connection to all humanity. Heisterkamp (2019) argued that only through mindfulness and self-reflection can we see how we may contribute to social structures that perpetuate injustices and ways in which we may be able to use positive communication to disrupt those structures.

We share in common with all humans a desire for happiness and well-being for ourselves and those we hold dear. We also hold in common the desire to be free from suffering, want, and harm (Ozawa-de Silva et al., 2012). And yet, we also share the human experience of suffering. We need only to bring to mind the tremendous grief, anger, anxiety, and uncertainty experienced by *all humanity* because of COVID-19. Moreover, by recognizing the suffering within oneself, accepting it, tending to it, holding it in gratitude because it reminds us that we are human, fragile yet resilient, we allow ourselves to be open to the suffering of others and cultivate compassion.

Likewise, we can connect to others through deep communicative acts of self-compassion. Kristin Neff, the foremost scholar in self-compassion, as the productive act of communicating kindness, support, tenderness, and understanding to the self when experiencing suffering or pain. Like compassion, self-compassion can also be fierce and powerful. Self-compassion is a means of approaching and dispelling negative and distressing thoughts and emotions to foster well-being (Neff, 2023). Individuals can engage in self-compassion by communicating inwardly (intrapersonal communication) messages of warmth, caring, and support in response to feelings of failure, unworthiness, and psychological and psychological suffering. Neff (2023) describes compassion as an inherently relational activity with self-compassion directed toward enhancing the relationship with oneself but that also has broader relational benefits. "The sense of common humanity that is inherent to self-compassion helps us to feel connected to, rather than separate from, others" (Neff, 2023, p. 7.4). It is turning toward, rather than away from, those who are suffering. In their research on nursing care, Kimble and Bamford-Wade (2013) describe the connection as *embodied knowing* achieved through "humanness, patience, an acknowledgement of one's own vulnerability, and a willingness to interact with a person in a meaningful way and so alleviate some of his or her suffering" (p. 285). Similarly, Huffman (2017) described *embodied aboutness* as an act of compassion in which individuals use their physical bodies to increase immediacy by turning toward each other even when (especially when) that turn is toward a suffering other such as homeless youth (or an aging adult living with dementia).

## Communication Savoring as Social Action

Communication savoring is a second act of positive communication that has the potential to promote social action and human flourishing across the life span (Pitts, 2019). *Savoring* is a psychological process of emotion regulation that allows individuals to recognize and then enhance or prolong positive emotions and pleasurable experiences through mindful attention (Bryant, 2003; Bryant & Veroff, 2007). *Communication savoring* directs the focus of savoring on social encounters; it is the practice of "mindfully attending to pleasurable or meaningful social interaction in real, remembered, or anticipated/imagined encounters and enhancing or prolonging the positive affect" (Pitts, 2019, p. 254). Communication savoring necessarily connects us to others and strengthens our shared bonds with humanity and capacity for social action. By savoring, or deeply attending to meaningful communication moments, we may be compelled to act toward ourselves or others with compassion, to draw others into and raise their awareness of a critical or powerful communication moment, to intensely experience and recall communication moments, and to connect across intergroup and intergenerational boundaries. Communication savoring has already shown potential for building individual and relational resilience (Pitts et al., 2023; Pitts et al., 2019) and enhancing subjective well-being (Jiao et al., 2021).

Generalized savoring may be an especially beneficial practice in later life as older adults can draw upon their wealth of lived experiences to recall treasured memories and generate and profoundly experience positive affect connected with that memory. For example, research on psychological savoring has demonstrated that older adults who savor have greater well-being and fewer depressive symptoms (Smith & Hanni, 2019), greater resilience (Smith & Hollinger-Smith, 2015), greater life satisfaction (Smith & Bryant, 2016), and more positive perceptions of aging (Smith & Bryant, 2019) than older adults who score lower on savoring. Julian (2022) found that older adults who scored high on communication savoring also scored high on subjective well-being. It may be that as a life span developmental practice, people can strengthen and capitalize on the benefits of communication savoring from childhood to older adulthood (Pitts et al., 2023).

Research on communication savoring is still in the early days, but I believe it is promising. Inspired by Bryant and Veroff's (2007) model of psychological savoring, Pitts and Socha (2013a) first posed the questions, "Can we savor communication? Can we savor relationships and social connections? And if we can, does savoring…increase our quality of life" (p. 8). In my initial work on the grounded model of communication savoring (Pitts, 2019), I began to answer those questions. The first goal of the original study was to determine whether people savored communication encounters and if so what types of communication experiences do people savor. Second, I sought to ascertain whether communication savoring had boundary conditions and unique features that distinguished it from the broader construct of psychological savoring. Third, I sought to define and describe communication savoring from a phenomenological point of view.

To answer these questions, I examined the written narratives of 68 college students. Participants were asked to write in as much detail as possible about a time they *savored* communication and to fully describe their experience of savoring so that the reader could almost feel it. The rich and detailed narratives provided by participants unequivocally showed that people do savor communication as a unique experience. Participants were not only able to recount communication moments they savored, but they also provided rich details about how they experienced savoring. Communication savoring was manifested in physical, metaphysical, and temporal sensations. For example, participants described a heightened consciousness of the present moment where time seemed to slow down. Some experienced this heightened sensation as an out of body experience (being completely at ease at watching oneself from the outside), while others experienced it as an enhanced embodied experience (a whole-body experience of exaggerated physical and/or emotional arousal). Participants also described *knowing* they were experiencing communication savoring because they actively employed intrapersonal messages to enhance their present-moment awareness through self-talk (i.e., instructing the self to savor a moment by soaking in all the details). Participants not only savored to intensify their present-moment experience, but they also savored with intent to bank positive affect for the future. Participants described a desire to savor meaningful communication encounters in the moment to recall and relish them in the future. Participants also experienced retrospective communication savoring through vivid recall, reflection, and replay of meaningful communication moments.

The initial study not only established how people *experience* communication savoring but also the common types of communication moments that they savor. The study revealed seven types of communication savoring. This was later validated and refined in a follow-up study comparing a new sample of emerging adults to a sample of mature and older adults (Pitts et al., 2023). The validation study confirmed the robustness of the original typology with one exception—we expanded the extraordinary communication category to include both rare and quotidian events resulting in the new label, (extra)ordinary communication. The common types of communication savoring are described below.

### Aesthetic Communication

Aesthetic communication refers to savoring communication moments that delight a person because of the beauty, playfulness, impact, perfect timing, or rich quality of the spoken word. Poetry, a moving speech, a pretty turn of a phrase, an unfamiliar accent, or deep resonate tones, might prompt one to savor the aesthetic features in a communication encounter.

### Communication Presence

Communication presence refers to savoring moments in which the individuals involved are so deeply and meaningfully engaged that everything seems to recede in the background. People describe this experience as losing awareness of time and having an intense focus on the other person—feeling as though one was being appreciated and communicated with as a whole person with undivided attention.

### Nonverbal Communication

Nonverbal communication refers to savoring communication elements beyond the actual words in an encounter. People describe this type of savoring as heightening a positive or meaningful communication experience through nonverbal signs including touch (holding hands and good hugs), soft speech in difficult conversations, and authentic and spontaneous facial expressions (surprise, joy). People also savor the natural environment surrounding some communication encounters—perfect settings for specific speech acts.

### Recognition and Acknowledgment

Recognition and acknowledgment refer to savoring communication moments in which a person either gives or receives praise, appreciation, and respect. People savor being commended for their achievements in public and in private, but also being able to authentically compliment or praise another person. Speech acts that honor an individual, group, event, achievement, or process fall under this communication-savoring category.

### Relational Communication

Relational communication refers to savoring communication moments that move a relationship closer or perhaps provide more clarity about the nature of a relationship. Intimate disclosures, like confessions of love, are particularly prominent in this category, but so too are smaller, more implicit disclosures that reveal future intent such as talking about "we," "us," and "our" in the future tense. Savoring relational communication often centers on turning points in a relationship.

### (Extra)Ordinary Communication

Initially focused only on extraordinary communicative events, savoring (extra) ordinary communication has been expanded to also include savoring ordinary (routine, ritualized) communication encounters that when habitually and mindfully enacted result in extraordinary moments. These moments include communication at the end of life and communication surrounding injury and illness, but also serendipitous encounters with strangers and daily, routine chats with family members. It is a recognition and appreciation for big and small communication moments that matter.

### Implicitly Shared Communication

Implicitly shared communication is unique in that it refers to savoring communication moments that are not articulated. Instead, there is an individual or shared sense that one is experiencing a special moment, either with another person or in a group, but that talking about it might ruin the moment. Savoring implicitly shared communication is more of an intuitive experience that individuals describe as just knowing they are sharing the same meaningful experience and deriving pleasure from that unspoken mutual experience.

Since the initial work, there has been steady progress in testing and refining the grounded model of communication savoring (Pitts, 2019). This includes recent and forthcoming papers on the validation of the typology and application to generational cohorts (Pitts et al., 2023) and an examination of communication savoring within military families as it pertains to relational resilience surrounding deployment (Beck et al., 2023). Jiao et al. (2021) conducted the first communication-savoring intervention demonstrating its correlation to subjective well-being among college students. Julian (2022) developed and tested the first Communication Savoring Index to be used in future empirical studies. A promising next direction for communication-savoring interventions includes difficult communication contexts, such as caring for a person living with dementia or speech aphasia. Communication savoring may be a way for patients, their families, and caregivers to infuse and strengthen positive communication in end-of-life encounters (Terrill et al., 2018).

## LIMITATIONS OF POSITIVE COMMUNICATION

Positive communication is a complementary approach to the more familiar, deeply rooted research and scholarship traditions in communication. It seeks to extend post-positivistic, interpretivist, and critical paradigms by including measures, questions, and criticism purposively designed to identify and address the fuller potential of human character and capacity. Our questions and instruments must begin to measure predispositions, experiences, relationships, contexts, and outcomes that relate to human flourishing. While it is important, for example, to know that savoring interventions can reduce depression and mitigate negative experiences, it is also important to acknowledge that savoring is an especially powerful tool to elevate the positive emotions of healthy, happy people. We need to ask the questions, build the instruments, and explore the lived experiences of people who flourish. We need to add positive social science tools to move beyond a deficit and limiting approach to the study of human communication.

Applying a positive social scientific frame to communication research can enhance our understanding of how to help individuals, families, and communities create communication structures to promote quality of life across the span of life. However, it is certainly not the only answer. Not even positive communication is always positive. Gaps between the intention behind a message and the interpretation of that message can result in misunderstanding or misconstrued meanings. A message that is intended to be kind or supportive by the sender may not be interpreted as such by the receiver. We need only look at "positive" speech acts such as giving compliments or asking for/offering forgiveness, both of which obligate the receiver to respond in certain ways, to recognize the inherent complexity of studying and promoting positive communication.

Finally, there is still a significant lack of evidence and programmatic evaluation of the impact of positive communication (Villarejo-Carballido et al., 2019). How do we know it is working? This again is where measurement comes into play, but also systematic reviews and evaluations of interventions. We are not yet in the scientific habit of measuring things that are going well and have spent little enough time struggling with how to meaningfully measure tops of scales (ceiling effects) or, better yet, develop scales with taller ceilings that allow us to see just how high we can go.

## CONCLUDING THOUGHTS AND CALL TO ACTION

I hope this chapter inspires readers to heed Socha's (2019) call to study and enact the "higher purposes" (p. 31) of the communication discipline, to achieve our higher selves and higher societies through language and social action that holds greatest potential to impact health, well-being, and quality of life. Moreover, we must attend to the accumulated wisdom of all peoples and draw upon the many ways of knowing and of being that are deeply rooted in our shared ancestry to engage in positive social action for humanity (Miike, 2014). For my part, I will continue to study and practice the language and communication acts of compassion and savoring with a determination to make our lived worlds better. The two chapters that follow provide an equally deep look at positive communication in social action—the power to humanize and the power to transform.

Harwood and Cooper (Chapter Two, this volume) address the importance of engaging humanizing language in the provision of care for people living with Alzheimer's disease and other dementias. Humanizing language is powerful positive communication that confirms our collective humanity and promotes social action toward a greater good *and better care*. We can act with compassion toward others when we see that we are one humanity. Indeed, Roy (2016) writes that "the Buddhist teachings on compassion require that we turn our face toward the suffering of others and resist all temptation to dehumanize those who suffer by reducing their sufferings to abstract academic problems or challenges rather than engaging in their suffering" (p. 92). We cannot act toward others with compassion if we dehumanize, demean, and devalue them.

Mirivel and Oliver-Blackburn (Chapter Three, this volume) showcase the importance of language and communication experiences as they contribute to a life well-lived. Drawing from in-depth interviews, Mirivel and Oliver-Blackburn demonstrate the power of language in creating peak communication experiences and the transformative potential of those memorable moments. They advance theorizing on positive communication in their chapter by distinguishing peak communication moments from other similar positive communication constructs (memorable messages and communication savoring) and linking findings back to Mirivel's (2014) theoretical model of positive communication.

Positive communication strategically and habitually uses language that promotes well-being and health across the life span. It is a "choice that keeps important ways of speaking and doing alive in the culture of which we are part" (Mirivel, 2014, p. 7). When considered the fundamental aspect of social action, positive communication enables us to cultivate the world in which we wish to live. It is part of the solution for building a future that is not about just "making it" or "surviving," but it is about fighting for and creating a future for people to live with purpose, to live their highest potential, and to flourish, not merely in their own life span, but across generations and in the life span of humanity (Beck & Socha, 2015b; Seligman, 2011). By examining acts of positive communication, especially as they relate to well-being outcomes and positive social action, scholars and practitioners can achieve a better understanding of strategies and communication acts that make bad things better, better things good, and good things great. The study and practice of positive communication can move scientific inquiry beyond the limited scope of the taken-for-granted assumption that well-being is the natural outcome of eliminating difficulties. The absence of ill-being is not the presence of well-being, but until scholars begin to examine seriously the presence of good health, positive emotions, thriving relationships, and other positive traits, enactments, and institutions, scholarship will continue to be limited by a deficit approach to the study of human activity. A deeper understanding of acts of communication that contribute to the good life is warranted.

## REFERENCES

Afifi, T. D., Merrill, A. F., & Davis, S. (2016). The theory of resilience and relational load. *Personal Relationships*, *23*(4), 663–683. doi: 10.1111/pere.12159

American Psychiatric Association (2013). *Diagnostic and statistical manual of mental disorders* (5th ed.). doi: oi.org/10.1176/appi.books.

Asante, M. K. (2014). Afrocentricity: Toward a new understanding of African thought in the world. In M. K. Asante, Y. Miike, & J. Yin (Eds.), *The global intercultural communication reader* (2nd ed.). Routledge.

Aune, K. S., & Wong, N. C. H. (2012). Fun with friends, pranks with partners: How we play in our closest relationships. In T. J. Socha & M. J. Pitts (Eds.), *The positive side of interpersonal communication* (pp. 143–159). Peter Lang.

Baxter, L. A., Norwood, K. M., & Nebel, S. (2012). Aesthetic relating. In T. J. Socha & M. J. Pitts (Eds.), *The positive side of interpersonal communication* (pp. 19–38). Peter Lang.

Beck, G., Fanari, A., Cooper, R. A., & Pitts, M. J. (2023, November). Bolstering military couple relational resilience through savoring: Applying the theory of resilience and relational load. National Communication Association (NCA) Conference, National Harbor, MD, USA.

Beck, G. A., & Socha, T. J. (Eds.) (2015a). *Communicating hope and resilience across the lifespan.* Peter Lang.

Beck, G. A., & Socha, T. J. (2015b). Embracing the insights of "Murphy": New frontiers of communication, hope and resilience across the lifespan. In G. A. Beck & T. J. Socha (Eds.), *Communicating hope and resilience across the life-span* (pp. xi–xv). Peter Lang.

Bodie, G. D. (2012). Listening as positive communication. In T. J. Socha & M. J. Pitts (Eds.), *The positive side of interpersonal communication* (pp. 109–125). Peter Lang.

Bryant, F. B. (2003). Savoring beliefs inventory (SBI): A scale for measuring beliefs about savouring. *Journal of Mental Health, 12*(2), 175–196. 10.1080/0963823031000103489

Bryant, F. B., & Veroff, J. (2007). *Savoring: A new model of positive experience.* Lawrence Erlbaum.

du Preez, M. (2011). The Socrates of Africa and his student: A case study of pre-colonial African leadership. *Leadership, 8*(1), 7–15. doi: 10.1177/1742715011426955

Floyd, K. (2019). *Affectionate communication in close relationships.* Cambridge University Press.

Floyd, K., & Deiss, D. M. (2012). Better health, better lives: The bright side of affection. In T. J. Socha & M. J. Pitts (Eds.), *The positive side of interpersonal communication* (pp. 127–142). Peter Lang.

Fredrickson, B. L. (2001). The role of positive emotions in positive psychology. *American Psychologist, 56*(3), 218–226. doi: 10.1O37//0OO3-O66X.56.3.218

Fredrickson, B. L. (2004). The broaden-and-build theory of positive emotions. *Philosophical Transactions of the Royal Society B, 359*(1449), 1367–1377. doi: 10.1098/rstb.2004.1512

Frijda, N. H., & Sundararajan, L. (2007). Emotion refinement: A theory inspired by Chinese poetics. *Perspectives on Psychological Science, 2*(3), 227–241. doi: 10.1111/j.1745-6916.2007.00042.x

Gable, S. L., & Haidt, J. (2005). What (and why) is positive psychology? *Review of General Psychology, 9*(2), 103–110. doi: 10.1037/1089-2680.9.2.103

Hariman, R. (2009). Cultivating compassion as a way of seeing. *Communication and Critical/Cultural Studies, 6*(2), 199–203. doi: 10.1080/14791420902867971

Heisterkamp, B. (2019). Self-reflection and communication: Experiences in social justice and compassion. *Western Journal of Communication, 83*(5), 537–541, doi: 10.1080/10570314.2019.1600010

Huffman, T. P. (2017). Compassionate communication, embodied aboutness, and homeless young adults. *Western Journal of Communication, 81*(2), 149–167. doi: 10.1080/10570314.2016.1239272

Jiao, J., Kim, S., & Pitts, M. J. (2021). Promoting subjective well-being through communication savoring. *Communication Quarterly, 69*(2), 152–171. doi: 10.1080/01463373.2021.1901758
Julian, R. (2022). *The art of conversation: Does the degree or nature of communication savouring differ with age.* [Unpublished Honours Psychology Thesis]. Southern Cross University, Australia.
Kellerman, G. R., & Seligman, M. (2023). *Tomorrowmind: Thriving at work with resilience, creativity, and connection – now and in an uncertain future.* Atria.
Kelley, D. L. (2012). Forgiveness as restoration: The search for well-being, reconciliation, and relational justice. In T. J. Socha & M. J. Pitts (Eds.), *The positive side of interpersonal communication* (pp. 193–209). Peter Lang.
Kim, Y. Y. (2012). Being in concert. In T. J. Socha & M. J. Pitts (Eds.), *The positive side of interpersonal communication* (pp. 39–56). Peter Lang.
Kimble, P., & Bamford-Wade, A. (2013). The journey of discovering compassionate listening. *Journal of Holistic Nursing, 31*(4). 285–290. doi: 10.1177/0898010113489376
Kinney, T. A., & Pörhölä, M. (Eds.) (2009). *Anti and pro-social communication: Theories, methods, and applications.* Peter Lang.
Klibert, J. J., Sturz, B. R., LeLeux-LaBarge, K., Hatton, A., Smalley, K. B., & Warren, J. C. (2022). Savoring interventions increase positive emotions after a social-evaluative hassle. *Frontiers in Psychology,* 13(Art. 791040), 1–13. doi: 10.3389/fpsyg.2022.791040
Lomas, T., Waters, L., Williams, P., Oades, L. G., & Kern, M. L. (2021). Third wave positive psychology: Broadening towards complexity. *The Journal of Positive Psychology, 16*(5), 660–674. doi: 10.1080/17439760.2020.1805501
Miczo, N. (2012). Reflective conversation as a foundation for communicative virtue. In T. J. Socha & M. J. Pitts (Eds.), *The positive side of interpersonal communication* (pp. 73–89). Peter Lang.
Miike, Y. (2014). The Asiacentric turn in Asian communication studies: Shifting paradigms and changing perspectives. In M. K. Asante, Y. Miike, & J. Yin (Eds.), *The global intercultural communication reader* (2nd ed.). Routledge.
Mirivel, J. (2012). Communication excellence: Embodying virtues in interpersonal communication. In T. Socha & M. J. Pitts (Eds.), *The positive side of interpersonal communication* (pp. 57–72). Peter Lang.
Mirivel, J. (2014). *The art of positive communication: Theory and practice.* Peter Lang.
Miyamoto, Y., & Ma, X. (2011). Dampening or savoring positive emotions: A dialectical cultural script guides emotion regulation. *Emotion, 11*(6), 1346–1357. doi: 10.1037/a0025135
Muñiz-Velázquez, J. A., & Pulido, C. M. (Eds.). (2019). *The Routledge handbook of positive communication: Contributions of an emerging community of research on communication for happiness and social change.* Routledge.
Neff, K. D. (2023). Self-compassion: Theory, method, research, and intervention. *Annual Review of Psychology, 74,* 7.1–7.26. doi: 10.1146/annurev-psych-032420-031047
Nussbaum, J. F. (2007). Presidential address: Lifespan communication and quality of life. *Journal of Communication, 57*(1), 1–7. doi: 10.1111/j.1460-2466.2006.00325.x
Opdebeeck, H., & Habisch, A. (2011). Compassion: Chinese and western perspectives on practical wisdom in management. *Journal of Management Development, 30*(7/8), 778–788. doi: 10.1108/02621711111150272
Ozawa-de Silva, B. R., Dodson-Lavelle, B., Raison, C. L., & Negi, L. T. (2012). Compassion and ethics: Scientific and practical approaches to the cultivation of compassion as a foundation for ethical subjectivity and well-being. *Journal of Healthcare, Science and the Humanities, 2*(1), 145–161.

Peterson, C. (2006). *A primer in positive psychology*. Oxford.

Peterson, C. & Seligman, M.E.P. (2004). *Character strengths and virtues: A handbook and classification*. Oxford University Press.

Pitts, M. J. (2019). The language and social psychology of savoring: Advancing the communication savoring model. *Journal of Language and Social Psychology, 38*(2), 237–259. doi: 10.1177/0261927X18821404

Pitts, M. J., Fanari, A., Cooper, R. A., Jiao, J., & Kim, S. (2023). The grounded model of communication savoring: Theory development and age cohort study. *American Journal of Qualitative Research, 7*(3), 139–159. doi: 10.29333/ajqr/13399

Pitts, M. J., Kim, S., Meyerhoffer, H., & Jiao, J. (2019). Savoring as positive communication. In J. A Muñiz-Velázquez & C. M. Pulido (Eds.), *The Routledge handbook of positive communication: Contributions of an emerging community of research on communication for happiness and social change* (pp. 98–107). Routledge.

Pitts, M. J., & Socha, T. (2013a). Positive communication in creating healthy lives, healthy relationships, and healthy institutions. In M. J. Pitts & T. J. Socha (Eds.), *Positive communication in health and wellness* (pp. 1–42). Peter Lang.

Pitts, M. J., & Socha, T. J. (Eds.). (2013b). *Positive communication in health and wellness*. Peter Lang.

Roy, A. (2016). Cultivating compassion in communication studies. *Journal of Communication and Religion, 39*(1), 84–96.

Schwartz, B., & Sharpe, K. E. (2006). Practical wisdom: Aristotle meets positive psychology. *Journal of Happiness Studies, 7*, 377–395. doi: 10.1007/s10902-005-3651-y

Seligman, M. E. P. (2011). *Flourish: A visionary new understanding of happiness and well-being*. Atria.

Seligman, M. E. P., & Csikszentmihalyi, M. (2000). Positive psychology: An introduction. *The American Psychologist, 55*(1), 5–14. doi: 10.1037/0003-066X.55.1.5.

Simmons, W. P. (2019). *Joyful human rights*. University of Pennsylvania Press.

Smith, J. L., & Bryant, F. B. (2016). The benefits of savoring life: Savoring as a moderator of life satisfaction in older adults. *International Journal of Aging & Human Development, 84*(1), 3–23. doi: 10.1177/0091415016669

Smith, J. L., & Bryant, F. B. (2019). Enhancing positive perceptions of aging by savoring life lessons. *Aging & Mental Health, 23*(6), 762–770. doi: 10.1080/13607863.2018.1450840

Smith, J. L., & Hanni, A. A. (2019). Effects of a savoring intervention on resilience and well-being of older adults. *Journal of Applied Gerontology, 38*(1), 137–152. doi:10.1177/0733464817693375

Smith, J. L., & Hollinger-Smith, L. (2015). Savoring, resilience, and psychological well-being in older adults. *Aging and Mental Health, 19*(3), 192–200. 10.1080/13607863.2014.986647

Snyder, C. R., Harris, C., Anderson, J. R., Holleran, S. A., Irving, L. M., Sigmon, S. T., et al. (1991). The will and the ways: Development and validation of an individual-differences measure of hope. *Journal of Personal and Social Psychology, 60*(4), 570–585. doi: 10.1037//0022-3514.60.4.570

Socha, T. J. (2019). The future of positive interpersonal communication research. In J. A. Muñiz-Velázquez & C. M. Pulido (Eds.), *The Routledge handbook of positive communication: Contributions of an emerging community of research on communication for happiness and social change* (pp. 31–49). Routledge.

Socha, T. J., & Pitts, M. J. (Eds.). (2012). *The positive side of interpersonal communication*. Peter Lang.

Terrill, A. L., Ellington, L., John, K. K., Latimer, S., Xu, J., Reblin, M., & Clayton, M. (2018). Positive emotion communication: Fostering wellbeing at the end of life. *Patient Education and Counseling, 101*(4), 631–638. doi: 10.1016/j.pec.2017.11.018

Villarejo-Carballido, B., Pulido, C. M., & Ramis, M. (2019). Research on positive communication and social impact. In J. A. Muñiz-Velázquez & C. M. Pulido (Eds.), *The Routledge handbook of positive communication: Contributions of an emerging community of research on communication for happiness and social change* (pp. 14–19). Routledge.

CHAPTER TWO

# Humanization as Positive Communication: (De)Humanization, Personhood, and Dementia

JAKE HARWOOD AND R. AMANDA COOPER

A prerequisite for allowing humans to flourish and thrive is treating them... like humans. Granting people their full human status allows them to engage in social actions that provide fulfillment, growth, intimacy, and self-knowledge. On the other hand, denying full humanity constrains people's worlds, limits their freedom and the depth of their experiences, and can result in social, even physical, death. It also constrains societies, rendering the collective less productive and less humane. To be fully human, we must mindfully communicate in ways that recognize others' full humanity, and actively challenge discourses that deny the humanness of individuals and groups.

In this chapter, we have four main goals. First, we will discuss the role of communication in the processes of humanization and recognizing personhood. We will discuss humanization as a communicative accomplishment—something that is constructed in conversation. Second, we apply these ideas in the context of dementia. People with dementia (e.g., Alzheimer's disease) are often targets of dehumanizing communication. Interventions for dementia caregivers often focus on acknowledging the "personhood" of the person with dementia, but this literature on personhood often operates somewhat independently of the literature on humanization and dehumanization. We will provide some initial integration of these literatures. Third, we examine how these processes unfold in close personal relationships (e.g., with spousal caregivers of dementia patients). Fourth, we explore the extent to which the insights we provide extend to other contexts of intergroup communication (e.g., ethnic, religious, and other areas of prejudice and discrimination) and present a preliminary model of intersections between forms of dehumanization, rehumanization, stereotype content, and patronizing communication.

## DEHUMANIZATION AND COMMUNICATION

To understand what it means to treat someone as human, it is useful to understand what it means to dehumanize someone. Dehumanization can be explicit and radical, as in the moral disengagement and denial of identity often necessary to engage in mass killing (e.g., during war: Kelman, 1976). More often, though, we dehumanize in subtle ways. Infrahumanization processes (Leyens et al., 2000) occur when we attribute fewer attributes that appear to be uniquely human to others (especially members of outgroups) than to ourselves (or members of our ingroup). So, for instance, we might acknowledge that outgroup members can experience happiness or sadness but see ingroup members as more capable of experiencing complex or secondary ("human") emotions such as embarrassment or regret. By viewing someone as less capable of full human experiences, we treat them as less human.

Haslam (2006) built on these conceptualizations of dehumanization to develop a dual-model approach. According to Haslam, we can dehumanize others in two, fairly distinct, ways. First, we can treat others like robots/objects. When we do this, we deny people characteristics like *warmth* and other emotions (*human nature* in Haslam's terms). Denial of human nature is common for groups that are stereotyped as less warm and perhaps threatening to "our" interests—the rich, Jewish people, Asian people, and political elites, for instance. Second, we can treat others like animals via infrahumanization that treats people as being driven by relatively simple and basic emotional urges. This is the denial, in Haslam's terms, of *human uniqueness* (civility, refinement). Denial of human uniqueness often occurs with groups that are stereotyped as *less competent* than "us" (whoever "we" happen to be)—in contemporary US society, older adults, people with disabilities, and young children are often targets of this form of dehumanization. People who are denied *both* warmth and competence (e.g., homeless people) may suffer both forms of dehumanization (see Cuddy et al., 2007; Fiske et al., 2002).

Theorizing around dehumanization often mentions language and communication (e.g., describing other groups as *vermin, animals, zombies,* etc.). However, systematic empirical examinations of the communicative dimensions of dehumanization are rare. Where it occurs, research tends to examine talk about immigrants and more broadly ethnic groups. Markowitz and Slovic (2020) demonstrate that people who dehumanize immigrants are more likely to describe them negatively, and in *impersonal* terms (e.g., *it, whoever*), and in terms that emphasize power (e.g., *judge, punish*). Interestingly, their work shows that such language use is associated with desiring to impose stiffer punishments (e.g., jail term) on people attempting to immigrate without documentation. Similar discourses are apparent in van Dijk's (1987) discussions of racist communication by Dutch and American nationals concerning immigrant groups, and Tileagă's (2007) rich examples of dehumanizing language in ethnic Romanians' (the dominant group) descriptions and stories of Romanies (a marginalized minority). Such descriptions often characterize Romanies as uncivilized, lazy, and not conforming to standard moral codes. Solomon (1985) examines rhetorics in scientific reports of the Tuskegee syphilis studies. The reports focus on the *disease* as the agent, thus rendering "invisible" the people who had the disease. The patients become simply the "scene" in which the disease operates.

Stereotyping is a major driver of dehumanization-related language and communication. There is insufficient space here to describe all the ways in which this occurs. To provide one example, the communication predicament model (Ryan et al., 1986) outlines how stereotype-driven patronizing speech to older people constrains their communicative environments and impacts their well-being. Media discourses provide similar examples—Montagut and Moragas-Fernández (2020) discuss how Spanish news media use *metaphors* that dehumanize migrants (e.g., describing "floods" of migrants, or discussing migrants as "goods" being traded).

Our focus here has been on language, but dehumanization is also apparent in visual communication. For example, Cassesse (2020) demonstrates how political candidates are dehumanized in online material such as cartoons, and other forms of political satire. At times, these descriptions provide clear connections to the psychological literature on dehumanization. For example, Cassesse provides illustrations of both Hilary Clinton and Donald Trump being portrayed as animals (e.g., Trump portrayed as a chimpanzee) and robots (e.g., Clinton shown being operated by a remote control). Thus, visual portrayals reflect Haslam's (2006) dual-model approach.

The consequences of dehumanization are, perhaps obviously, negative. As noted above, dehumanizing is associated with the desire to punish the other; in its most extreme form, dehumanization is commonly seen among people practicing genocide. Dehumanization and other forms of social exclusion can also result in self-dehumanization: denying *oneself* specific traits associated with being a unique and full human being (e.g., Bastian & Haslam, 2010). Murray et al. (2022) provide illuminating examples of the *humiliating* effects of dehumanizing treatment of domestic workers in South Africa. The consequences of such dehumanizing communication reveal one other fact—clearly apparent to communication scholars, but perhaps less so to psychologists working in this area. Dehumanization is not "just" a psychological belief or orientation. Dehumanization is something that gets *done* in communication—it is an active process whereby we use language and other symbols to systematically deny people the essential qualities that make them people. Likewise, we use communication to transmit our vision of others' (lack of) humanity to our social networks, thus perpetuating and propagating shared visions of what types of people are more (or less) human.

With good reason, the vast majority of research on dehumanization considers its negative intent and consequences. However, while rare, there are specific situations in which degrees of dehumanization might be functional. For medical personnel, for instance, some degree of dehumanization of patients can aid in rational decision-making and reduce burnout for staff (Capozza et al., 2016; Molero Jurado et al., 2021). Similarly, there are elements of dehumanization in pro-diversity initiatives such as anonymous interviewing or "blind" auditions, wherein judges aim to assess people based on a specific talent or ability, while removing human qualities that might otherwise lead to bias (Goldin & Rouse, 2000). These "positive dehumanization" situations are rare but merit attention to understand fully the trade-offs and complexities involved. Does anonymity inevitably lead to dehumanization? What strategies can we use to maintain a sense of the *humanity* of a target while simultaneously maintaining anonymity? As academics, anonymous peer review represents a familiar context where a positive intent (judgment of the content, independent of the person) can sometimes result in negative consequences (hostile and humiliating comments) that might perhaps be driven by anonymity-driven dehumanization (Comer & Schwartz, 2014).

## HUMANIZATION AS POSITIVE COMMUNICATION

In the spirit of a positive communication focus, the prior discussion of dehumanization raises the obvious question of what "humanizing" communication might look like. If we can construct others in ways that deny their humanity, then we should also be able to proactively communicate in ways that construct, reinforce, and transmit their fundamental humanness.

At a minimum such communication would, of course, avoid the things discussed thus far. Clearly, explicitly equating people to animals or robots is demeaning and humiliating, and is typically done with harmful intent. In medical contexts, talking to patients instead of talking "over" them, respecting their privacy, and explaining procedures before doing them are simple strategies to avoid dehumanizing (Basile et al., 2021). Building from the earlier discussions of warmth and competence, communicating with people in ways that respect and emphasize their warmth and competence is humanizing. Similarly, communicating *about* people and groups in ways that emphasize their warmth and competence qualities will counteract prevailing dehumanizing narratives and myths. In a dementia care context, for instance, talking about a person's occupational and family history works to resist treating them as "just another resident." As noted in models such as the communication enhancement model (Ryan et al., 1995), communicating in ways that acknowledge individuals' unique capacities, strengths, and limitations is key to acknowledging them as a person. Understanding specific ways that specific groups might be dehumanized is also important here. For a group that is often stereotyped as lacking warmth (Asian people, for instance), communication that emphasizes warmth is probably more effective in humanizing the group than communication emphasizing competence (a trait that may be already assumed). On the other hand, settings and activities that provide opportunities for demonstrating competence (task-based activities, discussions on status-loaded topics such as politics or science) should lead to more positive outcomes for groups stereotyped as lacking competence. Such considerations apply to interpersonal contexts, but also to media portrayals. While the intergroup media literature focuses heavily on valence of group portrayals (positive and negative), the degree of counterstereotypicality, and the extent to which characters are humanized in ways that counteract prevailing perceptions, is also critical (Ramasubramanian & Oliver, 2007).

The choice of communication medium bears on this discussion—different media reflect more of our personal richness and hence our humanity. Schroeder and Epley (2016; Schroeder et al., 2017) demonstrate the humanizing properties of the human voice, thus illuminating the ways that choosing a richer medium for communication (Daft & Lengel, 1986) reduces dehumanization and increases the chances for humanizing outgroups. Telephone and Zoom are thus likely to be more humanizing media than email. Indeed, many recommendations surrounding the use of voice and video feedback for students suggest that it humanizes the instructor, hence building a better interpersonal connection which allows the student to focus on the content of the feedback without "demonizing" the person providing it (Fiock & Garcia, 2022). Data support the notion that high richness media can facilitate positive intergroup communication (Cao & Lin, 2017). However, the literature also suggests that the use of low(er) richness media can be effective in reducing intergroup anxiety, for instance (Amichai-Hamburger & McKenna, 2006; Imperato et al., 2021). This last point suggests connections to the earlier discussion of phenomena such as blind auditions and anonymous peer review. Anonymity and depersonalization carry benefits in terms of equal participation and bias-reduction, but they also open doorways to dehumanization and incivility. We suspect that there are strategies to maintain a sense of humanity, even when individual identities are obscured—perhaps "baby on board" stickers on cars are effective in combatting road rage, for instance, by reminding surrounding drivers that "a human" occupies the metal box in front.

We regard humanizing communication as a tool to build interpersonal relationships and demonstrate individual tolerance and allophilia (liking the "other"). It is a form of social action that moves us toward constructing a more equitable society, helping to demarginalize groups that have been dehumanized. Accompanying the use of humanizing communication is, of course, the rejecting of dehumanizing talk. That involves assertively *challenging* it when we hear it—a radical act of positive communication. In the next section, we examine humanizing communication in Alzheimer's disease and other dementias, a context where dehumanizing and depersonalizing communication is all too common.

## CONNECTING (DE)HUMANIZATION, PERSONHOOD, AND DEMENTIA

Dementia is one of the most common health problems experienced by older adults. Current estimates suggest that approximately 1 in 9 Americans over the age of 65 are living with dementia, and rates of dementia are expected to increase significantly over the next 25 years (Alzheimer's Association, 2022). Dementia refers to symptoms of cognitive impairment including memory loss, difficulty with language processing and conversation, confusion, hallucination, and behavior change. Alzheimer's disease is the most common cause of dementia, accounting for 60–80% of cases (Alzheimer's Association, 2022). Other causes include vascular disease, Lewy body disease, and Parkinson's disease. Regardless of the cause, people experiencing the cognitive impairments and symptoms of dementia are often vulnerable to subtle and blatant mistreatment. This has raised concerns about the treatment of these individuals in both scholarly and public spheres.

The dementia literature has focused on recognizing *personhood* (akin to humanization) and *depersonalization* (akin to dehumanization) in the treatment and care of people with dementia. Personhood acknowledges that individual humanity is central to dementia care (Kitwood & Bredin, 1992), while depersonalization refers to an indifferent, impersonal approach to interacting with people living with dementia. Although the term "dehumanization" has not been widely used in dementia research, and theoretical perspectives driving dementia work rarely reference (de) humanization, dehumanization and depersonalization represent complementary category errors. Depersonalization involves *over*-categorizing: treating humans as interchangeable. Dehumanization involves *mis*-categorizing: treating a human as if they were non-human. Both the dehumanization and dementia literatures focus on ways that human characteristics (including human individuality) are denied and how they might be preserved. Thus, considering these two literatures together might provide rich insight into the communication behaviors that serve to support humanness and maintain personhood, particularly for individuals in vulnerable conditions such as those living with dementia.

Depersonalized communication directed *to* people with dementia is well documented. In medical consultations, people with dementia are often ignored, with questions and instructions directed to a companion or another healthcare provider rather than the patient (Branson et al., 2019; Miron et al., 2017). The individual characteristics and humanity of dementia patients often go unrecognized (Boddington & Featherstone, 2018). Similar themes are apparent in how people with dementia are talked *about*. Kitwood (1997) and Brooker (2003), among others, bemoan the application of a biomedical model to dementia, noting how it results in treatment of the disease rather than the person, and that it can negate the idea of "care" for cases where death is inevitable (Alzheimer's disease, for instance, is fatal). Behuniak (2011) draws similarities between the language used to describe people with Alzheimer's disease and language used to describe zombies (the "walking dead"; bodies without minds).

These depersonalized and dehumanized views of people with dementia might help us understand and explain communication in abusive relationships involving them (Giles & Helmle, 2011; Lin & Giles, 2013). Low competence (animalistic) perceptions have been associated with passive harm (neglect) orientations in the intergroup literature (Cuddy et al., 2007). Active harm derives from low warmth perceptions. Abuse of older people, and particularly dementia patients, covers the range of these forms of treatment, with neglect being common, and actual physical and other forms of material harm (e.g., predatory financial relationships) also prevalent. Indeed, while older people in general are often viewed as high in warmth but low in competence, people with dementia are often viewed as low in both—an unpromising recipe for humanizing communication.

What can be done to combat the negative consequences of dehumanization, and build toward more human(e) care for people living with dementia? A fully person-centered approach to care has been advocated for and adopted in recent decades, driven in large part by the pioneering work of Kitwood (1997) and Brooker (2003; Brooker & Latham, 2015). Such care involves four key components, each representing a positive form of communication, and explicitly laid out by Brooker as a VIPS model:

- Value for people with dementia and their caregivers: Valuing means continuing to treat a person as a whole and complete self, even when they do not conform to the behaviors that we conceive of as normative.
- Treating the individual: People with dementia share some characteristics, but they are also unique individuals, with real preferences, values, histories, skills, and family relationships. Attending to those factors drives positive, person-centered communication, and renders dehumanization less likely.
- Taking the perspective of the person with dementia: Part of valuing a person is attempting to see the world through their eyes. Hence, for instance, while people with dementia may believe things that are untrue, valuing their personhood involves attempting to take their perspective(s) on their social and physical environment, and work within that reality.
- Constructing a positive social environment for the person with dementia: Kitwood's approach places meaningful personal relationships at the center of what it means to be a person—we are defined by our networks. Hence, care that is grounded in positive relationships and that works to maintain existing relationships is critical. The social environment also encompasses environmental elements that maximize the potential for growth and independence. Offering freedom of choice, for instance, wherever possible is one way to maximize such potential and to humanize the care recipient.

This person-centered approach to dementia care and communication, along with others that have similar goals and sometimes more in the way of concrete communication recommendations (e.g., Savundranayagam et al., 2020; Young et al., 2011), clearly illustrates a promising and liberating approach to humanizing communication. This approach requires mindful attention to the personal and relational needs of individuals with dementia and the ways communication impacts them. Although person-centered humanizing communication requires ongoing intentional effort, promoting this approach to care and communication has the potential to transform not only the lives of individuals with dementia but also of those that care for them.

## (DE)HUMANIZATION / PERSONHOOD, CLOSE RELATIONSHIPS, AND DEMENTIA

Although (de)humanization is often studied in intergroup contexts and personhood and depersonalization have been studied in medical care contexts, matters of (de)humanization and personhood are relevant in close relationships as well. Recently, dehumanization research has begun to extend into interpersonal contexts. This work focuses on social exclusion (a lack of social connection) as a form of dehumanization (Haslam, 2022). Social connection is an innate need for human beings, and it is strongly associated with the dimension of human nature in Haslam's (2006) dual model of dehumanization. Bastian and Haslam (2010) show that individuals recalling an experience of social exclusion attributed fewer traits of human nature (e.g., warmth) to themselves *and* to the people who excluded them. Being socially excluded is, therefore, a form of dehumanization that occurs within personal relationships. Social exclusion is a common experience for people with dementia who often experience social distance from friends and family as the disease progresses. This phenomenon is referred to as "social death" (Sweeting & Gilhooly, 1997), a phrase that is strongly reminiscent of the idea of dehumanization by denying an individual's human nature.

Recent work on dehumanization within social and interpersonal relationships reveals *how* dehumanization occurs in intimate partnerships. Building on the dual model of dehumanization, Karantzas et al. (2022) proposed that dehumanization in close relationships occurs through the denial of both human uniqueness and human nature. Denial of human uniqueness occurs in romantic relationships through behaviors reflecting contempt or hostility toward the partner. Relevant to dementia relationships, human uniqueness is also denied through insensitive, controlling caregiving that denies the persons' agency (Karantzas et al., 2022). Human nature is denied in close relationships through behaviors of disassociation such as rejecting, ostracizing, or ignoring. Relational behaviors such as contempt and criticism deny both human uniqueness and human nature (Karantzas et al., 2022). This work shows that dehumanization is not only restricted to intergroup relationships but also occurs within close personal relationships.

The cognitive and social losses associated with dementia contribute to a unique loss of personhood/humanness in close relationships for people with dementia. This is evident in the ways that family caregivers describe dementia as a loss of the person they knew prior to the onset of the disease. Language like "he is just like a shell of his former self" (Walters et al., 2010, p. 174), or dementia is "death a little at a time" (Cooper et al., 2022, p. 228) represents loss of personhood, by alluding to the idea that the person is dead or gone long before they physically die. People who are thought of as "dead" or "gone" are at risk of dehumanizing or depersonalizing treatment from caregivers who no longer "see" the person they once knew.

Acknowledgment that the person with dementia remains a *person* despite the changes of the disease is an important step in combatting this tendency toward depersonalization. The person is not *gone* but rather *changed.* A focus on change rather than loss might enable continued humanizing treatment of people with dementia; humanization might be enhanced further by looking for the *continuities* in the person in addition to acknowledging change. As noted by Ryan et al. (2005), the person is still there but may be buried or hard to access. For example, one of Walters et al.'s (2010) spousal caregiver respondents said, "Thank goodness he's kept... his quirky sense of humor... he's there if I look for him" (p. 175). Moments of lucidity which can occur across the disease trajectory (Gilmore-Bykovskyi et al., 2023) may help dementia caregivers recognize the continued presence of their loved one, and their continued personhood. Seeking interventions and strategies to increase the chances of such moments is a concrete step that caregivers can take. For example, music enhances memory recall for people with dementia (García et al., 2012; Irish et al., 2006) and may be one method for helping family caregivers appreciate the continued personhood of their loved one with dementia.

Family members and friends of people who have dementia play an important role in sustaining personhood and preventing dehumanizing treatment of their loved ones. For instance, Cooper et al. (2022) found that caregiving spouses strategically avoided drawing attention to the symptoms of dementia as a means of protecting their partners from embarrassment or shame. One way these spouses did this was by giving written reports to the doctor, rather than talking about their partner's symptoms and behaviors in front of them. Other means of supporting personhood and preventing dehumanization within personal relationships include encouraging agency by finding activities the person with dementia can complete on their own, listening closely to what they have to say, and giving them choices (Young et al., 2011). These communication strategies and other behaviors that treat the person with dementia as an individual are important in combating dehumanization and loss of personhood.

## EXTENSIONS TO OTHER GROUPS AND INTERGROUP CONTEXTS

Examining the context of dementia reveals intersections between dehumanization, depersonalization, and communication. The chapter has demonstrated forms of communication that construct and perpetuate both the internal homogenization of the group and the separation of the group from the broader category of "humanity." People with dementia evoke complex patterns of warmth and competence evaluations, involving at times high warmth perceptions (e.g., as revealed by the "pity" emotion often associated with older people in general, and people with dementia in particular), but also evaluations that are low on both warmth and competence (e.g., in terms of disgust perceptions associated with nursing homes, for instance: Behuniak, 2011). These thoughts, in turn, lead us to consider the broader intergroup landscape and the ways that group perceptions, dehumanization, and various forms of patronizing talk might intersect. We summarize our broad (and very preliminary) ideas in Table 2.1. The table incorporates perceptions of groups seen as high in competence but low in warmth, providing a comparison for dehumanization of people with dementia against other forms of dehumanization. We address three key considerations emerging from the table in the following paragraphs.

First, understanding the warmth-competence stereotype profiles of groups is important in understanding how they are likely to be depersonalized and dehumanized. High competence and low warmth stereotyped groups (e.g., Asians: Fiske et al., 2002) are likely to be dehumanized as "robots." As such, they are often the target of passive helping ("going along with") but are denied human nature, and hence may be treated with a lack of politeness and communicative cooperation. High warmth and low competence groups are likely to be associated with overly nurturing depersonalization, excessive politeness, and simplified speech. Interestingly, while these groups are at times depersonalized as "animal-like," we note subtle differences between true "animalistic" dehumanization and "child-like" dehumanization. In a sense, "child-like" versus "animalistic" dehumanization reflects our differing orientations to different types of animals: our pets versus wild animals. Hummert et al.'s (1998) work on age stereotypes provides clear guidance here. She notes two distinct, but related forms of age-adapted speech, based on different forms of stereotyping. Overly nurturing patronizing speech is directed toward older adults who are perceived to be frail and dependent (high warmth, low competence). Overly directive and controlling speech is directed to those perceived as angry or confused (low warmth, low competence). We encourage more examination of these differences. The communication patterns in the table are not "merely" communicative effects of dehumanization but rather *the means by which* dehumanization is established and maintained (Murray et al., 2022). More work should explore how communicatively robbing someone of their individuality (depersonalization) is accomplished in ways that also rob the target of their humanity and the specific forms this takes depending on the prevailing stereotypes of their group.

Second, and taking a more positive approach, our chapter and Table 2.1 illustrate numerous ways in which communication can build a personalized and humanized other. Strategies rooted in the VIPS model (Brooker, 2003) clearly show this in practice in the context of dementia care. In other contexts, research on forms of person-centered communication across contexts suggests ways to

Table 2.1: Preliminary schematic of connections between stereotype content, patronizing communication, dehumanization, and rehumanization

| Dimension | Group Types | | |
|---|---|---|---|
| Example groups | *Asian People, Jewish People* | *Older People* | *People who are Homeless; People with Dementia* |
| Stereotype content model evaluations | *Low Warmth, High Competence* | *High Warmth, Low Competence* | *Low Competence, Low Warmth* |
| BIAS map behavioral orientation | *Passive Helping* | *Passive Harm (e.g., neglect)* | *Active Harm (e.g., physical/financial abuse)* |
| Emotional responses | *Envy* | *Pity* | *Disgust* |
| Dehumanization | *Robot-like* | *[Child-like?]* | *Animal-like* |
| Denial of… | *Human Nature* | *Human Uniqueness* | *Human Uniqueness and Human Nature* |
| Patronizing speech | *[Overly obsequious?]* | *Overly nurturing* | *Overly controlling* |
| Potential for abusive behaviors | *[Sabotage?]* | *Neglect* | *Active harm (e.g., physical abuse)* |
| Humanizing communication emphasis | *Warmth-reinforcing* | *Competence-reinforcing* | *Warmth- and competence-reinforcing* |
| Personalizing communication emphasis | *Individualized communication emphasizing unique personal characteristics* | | |

*Note.* Entries in square brackets are entirely speculative and represent apparent gaps in the literature.

acknowledge individuality and respect personhood (e.g., Barker et al., 2008; Jones, 2004; Savundranayagam et al., 2020; Soliz, 2010). Implicit here is the idea that contact between groups has the potential to reduce dehumanization—an idea for which there is considerable evidence (Capozza et al., 2012). But *intra*group discourse *about* groups is also important (Harwood & Gim, 2023), and an area in which challenging dehumanizing discourses is an important goal, particularly for members of privileged groups.

Third, the table notes at least one potentially new area for the study of patronizing speech. While that literature has typically focused on either controlling or nurturing speech styles, we argue that patronizing might also be present in talk addressed to groups seen as low warmth and high competence. In such settings (e.g., a service worker and a wealthy client), an overly obsequious, excessively (insincerely) courteous style might be apparent, reflecting awareness of the power dynamics at play. Whereas the abusive potential for relationships with others perceived as low competence is somewhat obvious (see our earlier discussion), high competence perceptions represent a novel context for "abuse," but one where it can occur (e.g., via sabotage, collective action, asymmetrical strategies).

## CONCLUSIONS

Dehumanization is a communicative process by which communication to and about other people denies them some form of humanity: culture, interpersonal warmth, individuality, or agency, for instance. Dehumanizing communication can take many forms, but all forms operate not merely to deny individual humanity but also to reify the dehumanizing assumptions on which that communication is based. However, just as communication provides the constitutive basis for dehumanization, so it can be used to challenge dehumanizing perceptions and construct more humanized social environments. Humanizing is a social act—a practice of positive communication that contributes to individual, relational, and societal flourishing. We hope that this chapter provides some directions for more human, humane, and humanized communication in interpersonal and intergroup relations.

## REFERENCES

Alzheimer's Association. (2022). *2022 Alzheimer's disease facts and figures.* <https://www.alz.org/media/documents/alzheimers-facts-and-figures.pdf>

Amichai-Hamburger, Y., & McKenna, K. Y. (2006). The contact hypothesis reconsidered: Interacting via the Internet. *Journal of Computer-Mediated Communication, 11*(3), 825–843. <https://doi.org/10.1111/j.1083-6101.2006.00037.x>

Basile, M. J., Rubin, E., Wilson, M. E., Polo, J., Jacome, S. N., Brown, S. M., … & Hajizadeh, N. (2021). Humanizing the ICU patient: A qualitative exploration of behaviors experienced by patients, caregivers, and ICU staff. *Critical Care Explorations, 3*(6), Article e0463. <https://doi.org/10.1097/cce.0000000000000463>

Barker, V., Giles, H., Hajek, C., Ota, H., Noels, K., Lim, T. S., & Somera, L. (2008). Police-civilian interaction, compliance, accommodation, and trust in an intergroup context: International data. *Journal of International and Intercultural Communication, 1*(2), 93–112. <https://doi.org/10.1080/17513050801891986>

Bastian, B., & Haslam, N. (2010). Excluded from humanity: The dehumanizing effects of social ostracism. *Journal of Experimental Social Psychology, 46*(1), 107–113. <https://doi.org/10.1016/j.jesp.2009.06.022>

Behuniak, S. M. (2011). The living dead? The construction of people with Alzheimer's disease as zombies. *Ageing & Society, 31*(1), 70–92. <https://doi.org/10.1017/S0144686X10000693>

Boddington, P., & Featherstone, K. (2018). The canary in the coal mine: Continence care for people with dementia in acute hospital wards as a crisis of dehumanization. *Bioethics*, *32*(4), 251–260. <https://doi.org/10.1111%2Fbioe.12446>

Branson, C. F., Houseworth, J., & Chipman, J. G. (2019). Communication deficits among surgical residents during difficult patient family conversations. *Journal of Surgical Education*, *76*(1), 158–164. <https://doi.org/10.1016/j.jsurg.2018.05.014>

Brooker, D. (2003). What is person-centered care in dementia? *Reviews in Clinical Gerontology, 13*(3), 215–222. <https://doi.org/10.1017/S095925980400108X>

Brooker, D., & Latham, I. (2015). *Person-centered dementia care: Making services better with the VIPS framework.* Jessica Kingsley Publishers.

Cao, B., & Lin, W. Y. (2017). Revisiting the contact hypothesis: Effects of different modes of computer-mediated communication on intergroup relationships. *International Journal of Intercultural Relations*, *58*, 23–30. <https://doi.org/10.1016/j.ijintrel.2017.03.003>

Capozza, D., Falvo, R., Boin, J., & Colledani, D. (2016). Dehumanization in medical contexts: An expanding research field. *TPM: Testing, Psychometrics, Methodology in Applied Psychology*, *23*(4), 545–559. <https://doi.org/10.4473/TPM23.4.8>

Capozza, D., Trifiletti, E., Vezzali, L., & Favara, I. (2012). Can intergroup contact improve humanity attributions? *International Journal of Psychology, 48*(4), 527–541. <https://doi.org/10.1080/00207594.2012.688132>

Cassese, E. C. (2020). Dehumanization of the opposition in political campaigns. *Social Science Quarterly*, *101*(1), 107–120. <https://doi.org/10.1111/ssqu.12745>

Comer, D. R., & Schwartz, M. (2014). The problem of humiliation in peer review. *Ethics and Education, 9*(2), 141–156. <https://doi.org/10.1080/17449642.2014.913341>

Cooper, R. A., Pitts, M. J., & Harwood, J. (2022). "That's when the relationship shifted": Relational and communicative turning points in Alzheimer's disease and related dementias. *Personal Relationships, 29*(1), 217–235. <https://doi.org/10.1111/pere.12412>

Cuddy, A. J., Fiske, S. T., & Glick, P. (2007). The BIAS map: Behaviors from intergroup affect and stereotypes. *Journal of Personality and Social Psychology*, *92*(4), 631–648. <https://doi.org/10.1037/0022-3514.92.4.631>

Daft, R. L., & Lengel, R. H. (1986). Organizational information requirements, media richness and structural design. *Management Science,* 32(5), 554–571.

Fiock, H., & Garcia, H. (2022). How to give your students better feedback with technology. *Chronicle of Higher Education*, July 7. <https://www.chronicle.com/article/how-to-give-your-students-better-feedback-with-technology/>

Fiske, S. T., Cuddy, A. J., Glick, P., & Xu, J. (2002). A model of (often mixed) stereotype content: Competence and warmth respectively follow from perceived status and competition. *Journal of Personality and Social Psychology*, *82*(6), 878–902. <https://doi.org/10.1037/0022-3514.82.6.878>

García, J. J. M., Iodice, R., Carro, J., Sánchez, J. A., Palmero, F., & Mateos, A. M. (2012). Improvement of autobiographic memory recovery by means of sad music in Alzheimer's disease type dementia. *Aging Clinical and Experimental Research, 24*(3), 227–232. <https://doi.org/10.3275/7874>

Giles, H., & Helmle, J. (2011). Elder abuse and neglect: A communication framework. In A. Duszak & U. Okulska (Eds.), *Language, culture, and the dynamics of age* (pp. 223–252). De Gruyter Mouton.

Gilmore-Bykovskyi, A., Block, L., Benson, C., Fehland, J., Botsch, M., Mueller, K. D., … & Shah, M. J. (2023). "It's you": Caregiver and clinician perspectives on lucidity in people living with dementia. *The Gerontologist, 63(1),* 13–27. <https://doi.org/10.1093/geront/gnac095>

Goldin, C., & Rouse, C. (2000). Orchestrating impartiality: The impact of "blind" auditions on female musicians. *American Economic Review, 90*(4), 715–741. <https://doi.org/10.1257%2Faer.90.4.715>

Harwood, J., & Gim, H. (2023). The process and domain of intergroup communication: Mapping the field. *Psychology of Language and Communication, 27*(1), 199–207. <https://doi.org/10.58734/plc-2023-0010>

Haslam, N. (2006). Dehumanization: An integrative review. *Personality and Social Psychology Review, 10*(3), 252–264. <https://doi.org/10.1207/s15327957pspr1003_4>

Haslam, N. (2022). Dehumanization and the lack of social connection. *Current Opinion in Psychology, 43*, 312–316. <https://doi.org/10.1016/j.copsyc.2021.08.013>

Hummert, M. L., Shaner, J. L., Garstka, T. A., & Henry, C. (1998). Communication with older adults: The influence of age stereotypes, context, and communicator age. *Human Communication Research, 25*(1), 124–151. <https://doi.org/10.1111/j.1468-2958.1998.tb00439.x>

Imperato, C., Schneider, B. H., Caricati, L., Amichai-Hamburger, Y., & Mancini, T. (2021). Allport meets internet: A meta-analytical investigation of online intergroup contact and prejudice reduction. *International Journal of Intercultural Relations, 81*, 131–141. <https://doi.org/10.1016/j.ijintrel.2021.01.006>

Irish, M., Cunningham, C. J., Walsh, J. B., Coakley, D., Lawlor, B. A., Robertson, I. H., & Coen, R. F. (2006). Investigating the enhancing effect of music on autobiographical memory in mild Alzheimer's disease. *Dementia and Geriatric Cognitive Disorders, 22*(1), 108–120. <https://doi.org/10.1159/000093487>

Jones, S. (2004). Putting the person into person-centered and immediate emotional support: Emotional change and perceived helper competence as outcomes of comforting in helping situations. *Communication Research, 31*(3), 338–360. <https://doi.org/10.1177/0093650204263436>

Karantzas, G. C., Simpson, J. A., & Pizzirani, B. (2022). The loss of humanness in close relationships: An interpersonal model of dehumanization. *Current Opinion in Psychology, 46*, Article 101317. <https://doi.org/10.1016/j.copsyc.2022.101317>

Kelman, H. (1976). Violence without restraint: Reflections on the dehumanization of victims and victimizers. In G. M. Kren, & L. H. Rappoport (Eds.), *Varieties of psychohistory* (pp. 282–314). Springer.

Kitwood, T. (1997). *Dementia reconsidered: The person comes first.* Open University Press.

Kitwood, T., & Bredin, K. (1992). Towards a theory of dementia care: Personhood and well-being. *Ageing & Society, 12*(3), 269–287. <https://doi.org/10.1017/S0144686X0000502X>

Leyens, J. P., Paladino, P. M., Rodriguez-Torres, R., Vaes, J., Demoulin, S., Rodriguez-Perez, A., & Gaunt, R. (2000). The emotional side of prejudice: The attribution of secondary emotions to ingroups and outgroups. *Personality and Social Psychology Review, 4*(2), 186–197. <https://doi.org/10.1207/S15327957PSPR0402_06>

Lin, M. C., & Giles, H. (2013). The dark side of family communication: A communication model of elder abuse and neglect. *International Psychogeriatrics, 25*(8), 1275–1290. <https://doi.org/10.1017/s1041610212002347>

Markowitz, D. M., & Slovic, P. (2020). Social, psychological, and demographic characteristics of dehumanization toward immigrants. *Proceedings of the National Academy of Sciences, 117*(17), 9260–9269. <https://doi.org/10.1073/pnas.1921790117>

Miron, A. M., McFadden, S. H., Nazario, A. S., & Buelow, J. (2017). Perspective taking, empathic concern, and perceived humanness of people with dementia. *Educational Gerontology, 43*(9), 468–479. <https://doi.org/10.1080/03601277.2017.1333788>

Molero Jurado, M. D. M., Herrera-Peco, I., Pérez-Fuentes, M. D. C., Oropesa Ruiz, N. F., Martos Martínez, Á., Ayuso-Murillo, D., & Gázquez Linares, J. J. (2021). Communication and humanization of care: Effects over burnout on nurses. *PLoS One, 16*(6), e0251936. <https://doi.org/10.1371/journal.pone.0251936>

Montagut, M., & Moragas-Fernández, C., M. (2020). The European refugee crisis discourse in the Spanish press: Mapping humanization and dehumanization frames through metaphors. *International Journal of Communication, 14,* 69–91. <https://ijoc.org/index.php/ijoc/article/view/10626/2898>

Murray, A. J., Durrheim, K., & Dixon, J. (2022). Everyday dehumanization: Negative contact, humiliation, and the lived experience of being treated as "less than human". *British Journal of Social Psychology, 61*(3), 1050–1066. <https://doi.org/10.1111/bjso.12524>

Ramasubramanian, S., & Oliver, M. B. (2007). Activating and suppressing hostile and benevolent racism: Evidence for comparative media stereotyping. *Media Psychology, 9*(3), 623–646. <https://doi.org/10.1080/15213260701283244>

Ryan, E. B., Byrne, K., Spykerman, H., & Orange, J. B. (2005). Evidencing Kitwood's personhood strategies: Conversation as care in dementia. In B. H. Davis (Ed.), *Alzheimer Talk, Text and Context* (pp. 190–198). Palgrave Macmillan.

Ryan, E. B., Giles, H., Bartolucci, G., & Henwood, K. (1986). Psycholinguistic and social psychological components of communication by and with the elderly. *Language & Communication, 6*(1–2), 1–24. <https://doi.org/10.1016/0271-5309(86)90002-9>

Ryan, E. B., Meredith, S. D., MacLean, M. J., & Orange, J. B. (1995). Changing the way we talk with elders: Promoting health using the communication enhancement model. *The International Journal of Aging and Human Development, 41*(2), 89–107. <https://doi.org/10.2190/fp05-fm8v-0y9f-53fx>

Savundranayagam, M. Y., Basque, S. R., & Johnson, K. (2020). Feasibility of a dementia-focused person-centered communication intervention for home care workers. *Clinical Gerontologist, 43*(2), 181–192. <https://doi.org/10.1080/07317115.2019.1694116>

Schroeder, J., & Epley, N. (2016). Mistaking minds and machines: How speech affects dehumanization and anthropomorphism. *Journal of Experimental Psychology: General, 145*(11), 1427. <https://doi.org/10.1037/xge0000214>

Schroeder, J., Kardas, M., & Epley, N. (2017). The humanizing voice: Speech reveals, and text conceals, a more thoughtful mind in the midst of disagreement. *Psychological Science, 28*(12), 1745–1762. <https://doi.org/10.1177%2F0956797617713798>

Soliz, J. (2010). Family as an intergroup domain. In H. Giles, S. Reid, & J. Harwood (Eds.), *The dynamics of intergroup communication* (pp. 181–193). Peter Lang.

Solomon, M. (1985). The rhetoric of dehumanization: An analysis of medical reports of the Tuskegee syphilis project. *Western Journal of Speech Communication, 49*(4), 233–247. <https://doi.org/10.1080/10570318509374200>

Sweeting, H., & Gilhooly, M. (1997). Dementia and the phenomenon of social death. *Sociology of Health & Illness, 19*(1), 93–117. <https://doi.org/10.1111/j.1467-9566.1997.tb00017.x>

Tileagă, C. (2007). Ideologies of moral exclusion: A critical discursive reframing of depersonalization, delegitimization and dehumanization. *British Journal of Social Psychology, 46*(4), 717–737. <https://doi.org/10.1348/014466607X186894>

van Dijk, T. A. (1987). *Communicating racism: Ethnic prejudice in thought and talk.* Sage.

Walters, A. H., Oyebode, J. R., & Riley, G. A. (2010). The dynamics of continuity and discontinuity for women caring for a spouse with dementia. *Dementia, 9*(2), 169–189. <https://doi.org/10.1177/1471301209354027>

Young, T. J., Manthorp, C., Howells, D., & Tullo, E. (2011). Developing a carer communication intervention to support personhood and quality of life in dementia. *Ageing & Society, 31*(6), 1003–1025. <https://doi.org/10.1017/S0144686X10001182>

CHAPTER THREE

# How Positive Communication Creates Peak Communication Moments: A Qualitative Study of Adults' Peak Experiences

JULIEN C. MIRIVEL AND BAILEY M. OLIVER-BLACKBURN

One of our academic advisors once disclosed that she had stumbled into academia, sharing that a failed attempt in a former profession led her to question what she truly wanted to do with a career. This advisor's revelation, that she only learned her career path after failing in another, ended with a charge for her advisee to do the same: think deeply and reflectively on what kind of impact you want to make on the world, and choose a career that reflects that intent. This communication exchange was pivotal, as it encouraged the young advisee to pursue their dreams and change their own career path, despite being just a few weeks shy of undergraduate graduation. Such wise advice from this mentor echoed in the mind of the advisee as they went on to pursue a graduate degree, doctoral degree, and ultimately a career they only once dreamed of. In short, this was a memorable peak communication moment.

Scholars know well that communication is fraught with dilemmas, tensions, and problems (e.g., Craig & Tracy, 1995), yet there are also communicative moments in people's lives when the spoken word has a positive impact on the individual and/or their relationship. Unfortunately, those positive experiences remain largely undocumented in the field of communication and are greatly understudied across all disciplines (see Socha & Beck, 2015). In this chapter, we explore the nature of peak communication to understand what critical behaviors shape and inform those experiences for everyday communicators. Drawing on dozens of in-depth interviews with adults, we show that peak experiences are created by three dominant positive communication behaviors: disclosing, encouraging, and complimenting.

To support this central finding, we first offer a review of literature, defining three key concepts to frame our work: the concepts of memorable messages, communication savoring, and peak communication. We then describe our theoretical framework, Mirivel's (2014, 2017) model of positive communication, and follow with our methodological approach. The heart of our paper provides a thematic analysis of 27 interviews and 94 coded peak communication narratives, and we conclude with reflections on our findings and consider this study's practical and theoretical implications.

## REVIEW OF LITERATURE

As Pitts (Chapter One, this volume) described in the opening of this part on positive communication as social action, there is a burgeoning body of work in the field of communication that focuses on the positive side of communication (for a review, see Socha & Beck, 2015). We label this body of work *Positive Communication Scholarship* (PCS).

Positive Communication Scholarship is the rigorous and systematic inquiry into the acts, mechanisms, antecedents, and outcomes of social interaction that promote life-sustaining systems (see Mirivel & Fuller, 2024). This field of inquiry first seeks to identify and measure communication practices and experiences that contribute to *human flourishing*. At its core, PCS investigates both processes of communication as well as outcomes (Mirivel & Fuller, 2024). In studying "process," scholars attend to communicative acts, sequences, and episodes, situated contextually, that reflect, embody, and constitute "best practices" for human communication and connection. Such practices might include active listening (e.g., Weger et al., 2014), communicating with compassion (e.g., Way & Tracy, 2012), supportive communication (e.g., High & Dillard, 2012), dialogic communication (e.g., Cissna & Anderson, 1998), and communication that embodies virtues (Mirivel, 2012).

Second, PCS scholarship takes an affirmative stance toward *inquiry* (Mirivel & Fuller, 2024). PCS focuses "on strengths and capabilities, and on affirming human potential" (Cameron, 2012, p. 13). Rather than focusing on problems, dilemmas, or challenges, PCS documents and makes visible the nature of positive, generative communication across contexts and celebrates capacity and potentiality.

Finally, PCS is designed to cultivate communication *praxis* (applied practice), as this type of scholarship contributes to the metatheoretical stance that the communication field is and should be thought about as a practical discipline (Craig, 1999, 2018). As Craig (2018) explained, "a practical discipline cultivates critical, creative, and well-informed deliberation on normative and technical aspects of practical conduct; it cultivates phronesis (practical wisdom), as well as techne (productive skill) in a culture's communication *praxis*" (p. 298). "To cultivate a social practice," Craig adds, "means to improve it" (p. 290). PCS embraces this metatheoretical stance, which is inherently applied and seeks to improve our social worlds (see Mirivel et al., 2024).

The study introduced in this chapter contributes to Positive Communication Scholarship by exploring the nature of peak communication experiences and the role that positive communication plays in those interactions. We draw on three key concepts to ground our research. The first concept, which has been extensively studied, is the concept of memorable messages (Knapp et al., 1981). The second concept is communication savoring (Pitts, 2019). The last concept, which is the focus of this study, is peak communication (Gordon, 1985).

## Memorable Messages

Developed by Knapp et al. (1981), the concept of memorable messages came out of a desire to explore how messages could have a profound impact on a person's life. A memorable message, for instance, might include a conversation from a father encouraging his daughter to not worry about the future and to "focus on what you can control." Or, it could be the final words spoken at the end of life.

According to Stohl (1986), "there are only two necessary characteristics of a memorable message—an individual remembers the message for a long period of time and perceives the message had a major influence on the course of his or her life" (p. 232). Since the publication of Knapp et al.'s (1981) article on memorable messages, scholars have explored the construct across various areas of study. In a recent review of the literature between 2017 and 2021, Cooke-Jackson and Rubinsky (2022) found that 34 peer-reviewed articles had been published in over 20 distinctive communication-related scholarly journals. Over half of those publications are connected to issues of health and well-being.

In their original research, Knapp et al. (1981) found that "messages perceived as memorable are most often brief oral injunctions that prescribe rules of conduct for solving a personal problem" (p. 36). In other words, memorable messages are short messages that people remember in part because the main function of the message is to help the individual solve a problem. For example, a supervisor might share tangible advice to an employee: "You're like a sign holder when giving feedback, sharp and direct. You've got to learn how to soften your edges." In fact, Knapp and his colleagues found that 72 % of memorable messages are action-based and that 42 % offer advice that is designed to improve another person's sense of self. In short, "memorable messages are a rich source of information about ourselves, our society, and our ways of communicating" (p. 40).

The concept of memorable messages has been applied in a number of contexts. First, researchers have explored this construct within the workplace. For example, Stohl (1986) revealed the role of memorable messages in the process of organizational socialization, showing how messages could help facilitate or hinder a process of integration. Memorable messages, she showed, can help new individuals manage a new culture more effectively and learn more quickly how to adapt. Barge and Schuetler (2004) and others (see Steimel, 2013) extended this research to show that memorable messages help co-construct interpersonal and organizational relationships. In particular, Barge and Schuetler showed that memorable messages in the early stages of joining an organization serve positive functions for assimilation. A second dominant context is connected to education. Here, scholars have explored a variety of topics, including high school coaches' memorable messages (Kassing & Pappas, 2007), messages that helped students navigate college life (Nazione et al., 2011), and parental communication about college (Kranstuber et al., 2012). A third area is connected to health communication, including the relationship of memorable messages with resilience and mental health (Kuang et al., 2021), memorable messages from parents about diet and exercise (Dorrance Hall et al., 2016), and messages during the grieving process following the death of a loved one (Droser & Seurer, 2022). Together, these studies document that verbal messages are consequential, impactful, and are critical milestones across the lifespan.

In this study, we build on this body of work focusing on memorable messages, realizing that the concept has benefits and limitations. For example, memorable messages can either reflect a positive or a negative experience. Another useful construct to study positive moments of communication, therefore, is the concept of communication savoring (Pitts, 2019).

## Communication Savoring

Savoring is both a psychological and communicative experience. From a psychological perspective, savoring is the "capacity to attend to, appreciate, and enhance the positive experiences in one's life" (Bryant & Veroff, 2007, p. 87). Viewed from a communication perspective, communication savoring is a "unique form of positive communication that allows people to enhance, prolong, and build positive experiences by attending to the social and relational dimensions of savoring" (Pitts, 2019, p. 239).

In one study, which is based on personal narratives, Pitts (2019) found that there are at least seven types of communication experiences connected to the experience of savoring. For example, one type is *aesthetic communication* or the "appreciation of the beauty and playfulness of language" (p. 244). Another is *relational communication*, which is about finding pleasure in moments of deeper connection with another person (most often through disclosure). A third is *extraordinary communication*, which often takes place around landmark events such as a wedding, the birth of a child, a marriage proposal, a conversation at the end of life, and so forth. Across all the types of communication experiences, savoring a moment of communication carries positive effects (Jiao et al., 2021) and in that way it's similar to our third construct: peak communication.

## Peak Communication

Originally introduced by Gordon (1985), and extending the work of Maslow (1968), peak communication experiences refer to "our 'greatest moments' in interpersonal communication, our moments of highest mutual understanding, happiness, and fulfillment deriving from the process of communicating with other human beings" (Gordon, 1985, p. 824). Surprisingly, and unlike the construct of memorable messages, peak communication experiences have largely not been applied in communication research (for an exception, see Beals Hopkins, 2011; Mirivel, 2019).

In his original work, Gordon (1985) collected quantitative data to reveal the major factors constituting peak communicative experiences. Four factors were especially salient: loving acceptance, open-minded insight, spontaneity, and pleasant fear. In a study based on qualitative interviews, Beals Hopkins (2011) found that in the context of friendship, peak communication experiences reflected a difficult experience, moments of companionship, and instances of helpfulness. Notably, aside from these studies, researchers have yet to identify what behaviors, messages, or speech acts constitute peak communication experiences. Moreover, researchers have not studied the memorable messages that might be part of these peak communication experiences, or what the relationship is between the three concepts.

All three concepts offer an interesting frame through which to study human experience. The concept of memorable messages focuses participants on recalling events that are easily accessible to memory. The concept of communication savoring asks participants to reflect on instances in which they paid attention to the details of an interaction. We chose the concept of peak communication because it is understudied and focuses on a unique aspect of human communicative experience: moments in which people experience happiness and joy. Specifically, our purpose is to explore peak communication experiences to identify what positive communication behaviors help to co-construct those experiences. To achieve this goal and to guide our analysis, we draw on Mirivel's (2014) model of positive communication.

## THEORETICAL FRAMEWORK

The theoretical framework grounding this study is Mirivel's (2014, 2019; Mirivel & Lyon, 2023) practical model of positive communication. Developed in 2014, the model provides a theoretically grounded, heuristic framework for describing the nature of positive communication in interpersonal and group contexts and thus the model is both descriptive and normative. As a descriptive framework, the model synthesizes academic literature and theory across areas of study to reveal core behaviors that function positively in human interaction. As a normative model, the model serves as a call to ethical action, calling laypersons and professionals alike to practice positive communication in their own lives. Mirivel proposed six core principles of communication, each tied to a significant behavior that should guide practice.

The behaviors illustrate concrete communication actions, or speech acts (Tracy & Robles, 2013), that individuals can draw on to communicate more positively in their own lives. Those behaviors, which are designed to create a language of possibility and hope, include greeting, asking, complimenting, disclosing, encouraging, and listening. Each behavior centers on a corresponding principle. The principles include the following:

1. *Greeting creates human connection.* This first principle highlights a constitutive view of communication (see Craig, 1999; 2018) in that it sees communication as the process by which our social realities are brought to life. Our relationships are co-constructed in and through the process of communication. Greeting, the first behavior in the model, calls attention to the fact that the opening to relationships and our ability to establish connection is through the act of greeting.
2. *Asking discovers the unknown.* This second principle is grounded in the Coordinated Management of Meaning theory (Pearce & Pearce, 2000) and Conversation Analysis (Hutchby & Wooffitt, 2008), especially the notion

that utterances are both context-shaped and context-renewing. When we say something, we respond to a previous utterance (what was said before) and we shape what the next utterance will be about. This is especially critical in the way that questions function. Some questions narrow and control interaction while others open up dialogue. When we ask open-ended questions, the model suggests, we can place ourselves in a position of humility and discover others.

3. *Complimenting affects a person's sense of self.* Drawing on symbolic interactionism (see Littlejohn, 1977), the third principle suggests that communication has consequences. Communication affects both who people are in the moment, as well as who they might become. For instance, if a teacher tells a young student that they have natural talent in public speaking, the student will not only view themselves as a public speaker, but they might even embrace speaking in public as a profession. Viewed through the lens of symbolic interactionism, Mirivel (2014) argues that complimenting is an essential behavior through which we can strengthen personal and professional identities.
4. *Disclosing deepens relationships.* The fourth principle draws on social penetration theory (see Carpenter & Greene, 2015) to emphasize the positive functions of the act of disclosure. By definition, disclosure is the process of revealing information about who we are. Disclosure serves multiple purposes and is often dilemmatic, but one crucial function is to deepen the connection that people experience in a relationship. Disclosing is vital to the development and maintenance of personal and professional relationships.
5. *Encouraging gives support.* The literature on social support grounds the fifth principle (see Burleson et al., 1994). Although there are many specific behaviors that give support to others (instrumental support, emotional support, esteem support, etc.), the model focuses on the act of encouraging, which denotes the ability to help a person overcome a challenge, difficulty, or crisis. When we encourage others, Mirivel (2014) argues, we give social support.
6. *Listening transcends human difference.* The last principle is grounded in the work of Buber (1970), Rogers (1995), and a larger body of work on the importance and effectiveness of deep listening in human relationships. Whether it is at home or at work, listening is a skill we can all develop to overcome conflict, difficult interactions, and meet one another more fully.

When individuals practice positive communication, Mirivel (2014) argues that they place themselves in a position to influence and inspire others. If individuals create a significant change in their communication, they can ultimately help to co-create a change in their relationships.

Mirivel's model of positive communication has been well-received in both practice and scholarly endeavors. In a recent study, for example, Biganeh and Young (2021) used the model to develop a positive communication behavior scale to assess leadership qualities and impact. The authors added that the model has "wide-reaching applicability in a diverse workforce; specifically, it may benefit leadership training curricula through development of actionable training methods designed to guide the ways in which leaders engage with employees, foster and strengthen relationships, and create cohesion in diverse work groups" (p. 13). In another study, Ahmed (2022) applied the model to a quasi-experimental study and found that positive communication programming grounded in the model is "effective in transforming interpersonal and intergroup relationships and resolving difficulties associated with such connections" (p. 78).

Although useful in the studies and professional environments discussed above, the model still needs to be tested in a variety of contexts. For example, we do not know whether these six communication behaviors have a long-term impact on individual, group, or organizational outcomes. Similarly, we do not know whether practicing positive communication has any effect on well-being and relational closeness. In his work, Socha (Socha & Beck, 2015; Socha & Pitts, 2012) argued that positive communication should be connected to personal happiness and well-being, but we have little empirical evidence to support this connection. In this chapter, we draw upon Mirivel's (2014) model of positive communication to determine if positive communication behaviors are at the heart of peak communicative experiences and if so how. Our study was guided by the following research questions:

RQ1: What communication behaviors are central to peak communicative experiences?
RQ2: What positive communication behaviors in Mirivel's model help to co-create peak communicative experiences?

## METHODS

To answer our research questions, our research team held semi-structured interviews with 27 participants. Interviews, instead of surveys, were used to elicit detailed responses from participants, to best understand their lived experiences and meaning-making from their point of view (Miles et al., 2014). Each interview asked participants to detail examples of times in their lives that they self-identified as "peak communication moments."

## Participants and Recruitment

The research team recruited participants through network (Baxter & Babbie, 2004) and snowball sampling techniques (Lindlof & Taylor, 2011). First, an initial, small number of participants were recruited through the professional networks of the research team, including undergraduate and graduate students, instructors, and professors at a mid-sized South-Central university in the United States. Additional participants were recruited through snowball sampling, where researchers used the network links of the initial participants to locate additional participants (Parker et al., 2019). In order to reach a wide range of participants, the only requirement to participate was to be at least 18 years old at the time of the interview. Participants included 19 females and 8 males ($n$ = 27). No additional demographic information was collected; however, participants represented a wide age group ranging from their early 20s to their mid-60s.

## Data Collection and Analysis

Interviews were conducted in person in a secure conference room on the same university campus in which recruitment took place. Informed consent was collected prior to the start of each interview. Interviews ranged from 15 to 45 minutes in length, with an average of 25 minutes. Once interviews were completed, audio recordings of the interviews were downloaded and then transcribed by the research team. Transcripts were compared to the audio recordings to confirm accuracy and then audio files were promptly deleted. Participants' identifying information was changed in the transcripts to ensure participant confidentiality, including assigning each participant a pseudonym.

We defined peak communicative moments as "moments of communication shared with others that have brought a great sense of satisfaction, happiness, and fulfillment." We briefed participants on the meaning of this term at the start of each interview, adding that "in this interview, we would like to talk with you about peak communication that you have experienced at home or at work. Our goal is to capture examples of peak communication in your life." Participants were encouraged to share each example in turn, detailing the full story of the peak communication moment before moving on to the next. On average, participants reported at least three examples of peak communicative moments during the interview (average = 3.48; range = 1– 6 examples). Additional questions asked participants to describe the impact each peak communication moment had on their lives, and if needed, interviewers probed for more detail on what occurred (such as what words were exchanged or communicated) during each moment.

Our data included 173 single-spaced pages of interview transcripts. We collected 94 examples or stories of peak communicative moments from participants. We analyzed these stories across five stages, with two research team members working together as a coding team and meeting frequently to refine and discuss the analysis. First, each coder read through all of the transcripts holistically to get acquainted with the data. Second, an initial codebook was created using Mirivel's (2014, 2019) model of positive communication. The six practices within this model served as the initial codes (Codes 1–6), with code "7" referring to any new or emerging codes that could not be accounted for within the current model. Initially, coders were encouraged to assign only one code or practice for each story.

Third, both coders used the initial codebook to code the same six interviews (22 % of the data) to validate the use of the model. The coding team then met to compare codes, and determined agreement on over 83 % of the codes, validating the use of the model and convergence on coding practices. During this first coding meeting, the team also determined that the same story could be coded with more than one code, as long as the participant described two separate behaviors within the same story with equal emphasis. For example, if a participant equally described the importance of both disclosing (code 4) and encouraging (code 5) within the same story, the coder applied both codes to the same story.

Fourth, the two coders each individually coded the remaining interviews (78 % of the data), with one coding 10 interviews, and the other coding 11. Fifth, the research team held a data conference (Braithwaite et al., 2017), where frequency of codes, overall findings, and examples of each code were discussed. This session focused on collaborative sensemaking of the data and reaching an agreement on the coded data. Through this process, 118 codes were assigned to the 94 stories (see Table 3.1).

## RESULTS

In response to our research question concerning what positive communication behaviors help to co-create peak communicative experiences, we identified the presence of each practice from Mirivel's model of positive communication across participant interviews. We discuss the six practices in order of frequency (see Table 3.1), ending with a discussion of three codes ($n$ = 3) that were not reflected within the model (identified as "other" below).

Table 3.1: Positive communication praxis

| Code | Frequency | % of Total Codes |
|---|---|---|
| *Disclosing* | 44 | 37.29 |
| *Encouraging* | 28 | 23.73 |
| *Complimenting* | 17 | 14.40 |
| *Asking* | 13 | 11.02 |
| *Listening* | 9 | 7.63 |
| *Greeting* | 4 | 3.39 |
| *Other* | 3 | 2.54 |
| Total | 118 | 100 % |

## Disclosing

*Disclosing* involved participants recalling a significant or memorable time where they, or someone else, shared information about themselves. This practice represented 37.29 % of all codes ($n$ = 44) and was the most frequently identified code. Peak communicative moments that involved disclosing were often memorable for participants because they included the opportunity to reveal information about themselves and their feelings, which led to deeper, more intimate relationships.

Many peak communicative moments coded for disclosure included verbalized affectionate communication. For example, one participant discussed the significance of him and his partner both disclosing that they love each other for the first time, "Telling another person 'I think I'm in love with you' and it's reciprocated. It's nice.... To have the courage to say to someone 'hey, I'm in love with you' and they say 'I'm in love with you too'" (Participant L; participants identified by assigned pseudonym initials). Another participant echoed the significance of affectionate disclosure, recalling when her husband proposed, "He said something to the effect of 'you knew we would be here before I knew we would be, but I'm here now and I want to spend forever with you.' He [said] he loved me and got on his knee!" (Participant A). Affection was not only within romantic disclosure but among friends and family relationships as well. For example, one participant revealed a peak moment with her father after she told him she had filed for divorce from her husband.

> He is a stoic, hardcore [northerner] who doesn't talk. He sat next to me, not looking at me, and he said "I just want you to be happy." And that's all he said... he just sat down next to me and said "I just want you to be happy, it doesn't matter." (Participant N)

Another common type of disclosure referenced by participants included the participant or someone else revealing previously unknown information. One participant mentioned a moment when she revealed a family secret to her sister for the first time:

> I'll never forget the first time I [told] my sister about my daughter being an alcoholic. I just wanted to crawl under a rock ... I thought, "why did I say that? Why did I reveal that?"... But it felt good, actually, to get it off my chest. (Participant E)

The significance of this disclosure not only impacted this participant's relationship with her sister but also her own relief of revealing information she had long kept secret.

Another participant mentioned the significance of hearing her father share previously unknown stories about his past, and how this disclosure helped her not only better understand him and his background but also made her feel more connected to him than ever before:

> [It's him] reminiscing and me listening to his stories. I really love it. It makes me feel closer to him. I'm getting to know him through his past experiences. My dad isn't very talkative but when I can get him on something like that, telling a story, he really gets into the conversation... I appreciate him sharing those things with me. (Participant NA)

Similarly, one participant, a mother whose young son was going to camp for the first time, detailed how her son's disclosure helped her understand not only his affection for her but his new maturity and empathy toward others. After she told her son that he did not have to bunk with her but could instead spend his time with his friends, she revealed, "He said it was important to him that he come stay one night with me, possibly two ... It just made me feel good because I know how important this week was to him. It was almost like he was concerned about me as well, that I didn't feel left out" (Participant I). Overall, memorable peak communicative moments often involved disclosure as this practice allowed participants to reveal previously unknown feelings or information to someone, and had a positive effect both on their relationships and their own self-understanding.

## Encouraging

Participants also detailed moments where they were offered or gave encouragement. *Encouraging* made up 23.73 % of all codes ($n$ = 28) and was the second most frequently identified positive communication practice across participant disclosure. Peak communicative moments identified as encouraging often included participants receiving social or esteem support in a time of need. These moments appeared significant to participants as the support was either unexpected, or pivotal in them getting through or adapting to a personal hardship or crisis.

Encouragement was often communicated in two unique ways. First, participants detailed stories of encouragement to make a change. For example, one participant recalled a time where her former boss encouraged her to take the leap and change careers after years in the same industry, "he said, 'This is one of those life-changing decisions, particularly in this stage in your life… You have to do it. You have to explore and find out what could be.' That brought me comfort, relief, and joy knowing that I was supported by someone I worked with" (Participant NN). Another participant echoed this theme of encouragement to make a change:

> A friend of mine said, "I want to see you post a positive post at least once a day on Facebook." I was like, "Are you kidding me? I'm not that kind of person" [but] I did that for about two weeks… and then I realized it really started changing my attitude, making me a more positive person, because by nature, I am a pessimist. So, it really I think helped. (Participant E)

Second, participants revealed peak communication moments where encouragement was used to reiterate their identity and to reaffirm who they are and what they are capable of. One participant, who was struggling as a new teacher, recalled the encouragement she received from her principal:

> The principal was basically like, "the kids really just need you to be you…. You don't need to, like, put on a character or think about the teachers that you are trying to be exactly like… you just need to be who you are. With these children, be authentic and genuine and real, and you will start seeing the positive things that are happening around you…" [that made me] think, you know, like, I'm going to try this. I'm just going to be me! (Participant EL)

Another participant recalled a memorable time where she encouraged her daughter to achieve her dream of becoming a video game creator:

> [My daughter] said, "well there's not a lot of girls doing it, so maybe I shouldn't". And I was like, "you're gonna do it! This is not a man's world, it's everybody's world, you do what you want to do. You're not gonna give up because you don't see people like you in that field. That just makes you want to do it even more. You do what you love!" (Participant DA)

Overall, these moments were identified by participants as peak communicative moments because encouragement signaled the potential someone had to overcome a circumstance, or affirmed their overall identity.

## Complimenting

The third most frequent positive communication behavior was complimenting (14.4 % of all codes; $n$ = 17). *Complimenting* referred to communicative moments that involved verbalized compliments, such as positively complimenting a behavior, accomplishment, or personality trait. For example, one participant discussed how his parents showered him with compliments after being the first in the family to graduate from college, "[My parents said] 'we are really proud of you, you are the first one to graduate. It's a big deal and we are really happy. We are honored you are our son'" (Participant IE). Another participant discussed the significance of a manager complimenting his work effort, "[He said] 'there's something special about you. You have a drive that I think will take you far in the company... I didn't know you wanted to be a leader, but I can see you as a leader.' And that's when I went down that road" (Participant AN). Complimenting was powerful, as we see how in this example it led the participant not only to feel more confident in his abilities, but to seek out a new role within the company. Complimenting created peak experiences when these moments positively affected how the participant felt about themselves or their attributes.

## Asking

*Asking* represented 11.02 % of all codes ($n$ = 13) and involved participants or others asking pertinent questions to investigate the unknown. Participants described asking as peak experiences when these moments showed another person taking interest in understanding their thoughts, desires, or overall ideas. One participant recalled when a professor asked him to make professional goals for himself:

> I'd never had that question asked of me... when [my professor] asked, "What do you want to do?" I was like, "I don't know!" ... What I realized is that when you don't have any goals, you don't have anything to work for in that moment... that [conversation] was something that was pivotal to my success growth. Not only in school, but in my corporate job as well. (Participant AN)

Another participant detailed the significance asking had on rectifying a previously distant or strained relationship with a friend. After the friend posted about her recent engagement, the participant reached out and asked:

> "Who are you getting married to?" and so she told me, "Oh, it's this guy." And I was like, "Who?" [Turns out] it's a whole complete other guy... I said "I thought you were getting married to your ex and I wasn't going to let you marry him cause he's no good". She was like really happy that I was going to do that, like, talk her out of that type of situation. So, she surprised me and was like, "Be my bridesmaid!" And I was like, "Okay!" ... it was just surprising, because we had barely talked between that time, and now she's like the one person who I still talk to from high school. (Participant E)

As seen in this example, asking may also serve as a reciprocal process, where this practice opens up the opportunity for further communication and connection, thereby facilitating the co-creation of a peak experience.

## Listening

*Listening* referred to peak experiences when participants felt heard or listened to, or when they were able to offer a listening ear to someone else. Listening represented 7.63 % of all codes ($n$ = 9). Peak communicative moments coded as listening involved paying attention to others, both verbally (e.g., paraphrasing back for clarity) and/or nonverbally (e.g., showing attentive nonverbal behaviors including sustained eye contact, body posture, head nods, or simply being present). For example, one participant shared how he listened to his mother who was suffering from late stage dementia as she sang a hymn, "She paused, looked at me, smiled, and started singing… she'd just never done that… [what I learned from that moment was] the significance of presence and being there. That the point isn't really the talk, or the information exchange… it's being there" (Participant D). For some participants, listening did not come easy, but allowed them to put themselves in another's shoes and understand a different perspective than their own. As one participant noted,

> I was able to give this person a chance. By actively listening and saying "ok, I'm going to let you tell me, and I'm going to take my opinions and my preconceived ideas about what I think you think, and I'm really just going to listen to you." It was really the first time I actually listened to her and I let her tell me what she felt. (Participant RE)

This was a peak experience for the participant because their strained relationship was healed in some way, and it allowed the participant to let go of negative energy. As she put it, "From that time, forward, our relationship has really changed and evolved and I don't feel that anger and bitterness anymore. It's gone. It feels so good not to be carrying that around, not to have that on my shoulders anymore." Listening functioned as a peak experience when participants were truly able to listen or inherently felt heard.

## Greeting

The final practice from the positive communication model, *greeting*, was identified in 3.39 % of all codes ($n$ = 4). Participants referenced greetings mostly as verbalized and noted the significance of addressing terms. For example, one participant shared this story after receiving her PhD, "Whenever you finish one of [my professor's] classes, when you get your final assignments she'll call you 'Dr.' so and so. It was really sweet… made me feel a lot of positive emotions, made me feel better about myself and my own abilities" (Participant KR). Another participant shared the significance of his son greeting him by his chosen familial addressing term, "he puts his head on my cheek and says 'papa are you sleeping?' It's this little moment. He will joke with me and say 'daddy daddy' because he knows I don't like it… [but when] he calls my name and says 'Papa papa'… that kind of moment, I think is really cool" (Participant L). Overall, these greetings invited the participant and another to connect and served as an initial act to establish further human connection. Greetings can produce peak communicative experiences when they are associated with feelings of joy or happiness as a result of the encounter.

### Other

There were three codes (2.54 % of all codes) that could not be placed within Mirivel's model of positive communication. Each of these codes referred to a memorable moment described by a participant, but included stories where participants discussed a purely cognitive or intrapersonal experience or revelation, and thus was not codable using the model which focuses more so on verbalized, interpersonal communication practices. In one story, a participant described an intrapersonal communication moment when she realized that she had made the right decision in ending a relationship. Another participant described a moment when he realized the nonverbal behaviors between him and his stepson constituted affection. The third instance was a moment of communication savoring, which typically denotes "individuals' tendency and capacity to mindfully appreciate, immerse in, and prolong their positive feelings about life experiences that occur in the past, present, or future" (Jiao et al., 2021, p. 153).

## DISCUSSION

Drawing on a constitutive view of communication, the data shows that peak communication experiences are *constituted* by six primary positive communication behaviors, with three behaviors being especially consequential: disclosing, encouraging, and complimenting. Our findings contribute to both theory and practice and are significant in four distinct ways.

First, the findings strongly support Mirivel's model of positive communication. In fact, 97.46 % of peak communication experiences in our data set featured one or more of the six critical communication behaviors that Mirivel put forth in his practical model. In addition, we found 100 % representation of all of the positive communication behaviors across the data set. The model, of course, does not account for all of the practices that lead to peak experiences. As discussed above, more subtle, cognitive, or nonverbal practices such as laughing, hugging, or moments of interpersonal transcendence (Geiman & Greene, 2019) and savoring (Jiao et al., 2021) can also be part of peak communication experiences but are currently not represented within the model. Importantly though, they only represented a small fraction of stories participants recalled as peak communicative moments and participants appeared more primed to identify interpersonal or verbalized communicative moments that brought them joy or happiness. This study, then, echoes Biganeh and Young (2021) who found that the "model of positive communication provides basic behavioral building blocks which can both inform theory and point to specific interventions for practice" (p. 13). In addition to this theoretical implication, we found that the model has methodological usefulness as well as it can serve as an easy-to-use tool for coding qualitative and textual data.

Second, this study adds value and understanding to the concepts of memorable messages and peak communication, specifically in how they are related. Memorable messages, by definition, can include moments of problematic or dark communication. The concept of peak communication, however, brings emphasis to the positive side—to moments that bring joy, happiness, and/or lead to positive emotions. Frequently though, as we showed in the data, peak experiences are grounded in a memorable message and the meaningfulness of the experience was often supported by the spoken word. This finding emphasizes the pivotal role communication plays in human interaction and connection, as the communication practices within this model, disclosing, encouraging, and complimenting specifically, were not only considered memorable for their impact on a relationship, but often our participants benefited personally from the experience. Peak conversations offered a self-boost and helped participants understand more deeply who they are and who they might become. They are not simply, to quote Knapp et al., "oral injunctions that prescribe rules of conduct for solving a personal problem" (1981, p. 36).

Third, this chapter makes a significant contribution to our understanding of the relationship between communication and happiness, and to Positive Communication Scholarship more broadly. In their review of literature, Socha and Beck (2015) argued that "among the 'new' and important areas of future inquiry, the topic of peak communication, or how good can communication get, is important to address" (p. 191). As they explained, communication scholars have been "shy about seeking to understand 'peak experiences' or the 'upper bounds' of relating and have yet to fully consider the role of communication not only in needs-satisfaction of lower levels of needs but also in the development of human potentialities" (pp. 191–192). This study shows that there are simple and practical communication behaviors that can help to produce peak experiences for the self, but also for others. It shows that there is an intricate relationship between the experience of joy and happiness and human communication.

Finally, in her introduction to this section, Pitts (Chapter One, this volume) wrote that "positive communication is critical to the discursive enactments of social action—what we can achieve, what we can do, what we can change through individual and collective action and in big and small ways." The stories featured in this chapter illustrate what positive communication can accomplish as a social action. When we greet and invite dialogue, we can create new relationships but also heal existing ones. When we compliment, we can give joy and happiness, but also solidify a person's sense of self. When we disclose and reveal who we are in an authentic way, we can deepen our connections with others. Positive communication is a choice: a choice that can enable each of us to (a) enhance our health and well-being and those of others, (b) foster mindfulness and compassion in our personal and professional relationships, (c) make possible more resilient and flourishing organizations, and ultimately co-create better social worlds through all.

## CONCLUSION

This chapter featured a qualitative study of peak communication experiences. Drawing on 27 in-depth interviews with adults from all walks of life and a total of 94 stories, the data shows that three key positive communication behaviors help to co-create peak experiences. Those behaviors include disclosing, encouraging, and complimenting. In developing the model of positive communication, Mirivel (2014) hoped to inform communication *praxis* and inspire everyday communicators to use the spoken word to make a positive difference in the life of others. This study shows that anyone—a parent, a boss, or even an academic advisor sharing about their past career failures—can create peak experiences by using the power of positive communication.

## REFERENCES

Ahmed, A. H. (2022). *The effect of positive communication on Ethiopian university students' interpersonal and intergroup relationships: The case of Jigjiga University* [unpublished doctoral dissertation]. Anadolu University.

Barge, J. K., & Schlueter, D. W. (2004). Memorable messages and newcomer socialization. *Western Journal of Communication*, *68*(3), 233–256. <https://doi.org/10.1080/10570310409374800>

Baxter, L. A., & Babbie, E. (2004). *The basics of communication research.* Wadsworth.

Beals Hopkins, M. E. (2011). *An exploratory study of peak communication experiences between friends.* Unpublished Master's Thesis. Western Michigan University.

Biganeh, M., & Young, S. L. (2021). Followers' perceptions of positive communication practices in leadership: What matters and surprisingly what does not. *International Journal of Business Communication.* <https://doi.org/10.1177/2329488420987277>

Braithwaite, D. O., Allen, J., & Moore, J. (2017). Data conferencing. In J. P. Matthes, C. S. Davis, & R. F. Potter (Eds.), *The International Encyclopedia of Communication Research Methods.* Wiley-Blackwell. <https://doi.org/10.1002/9781118901731.iecrm0057\>

Bryant, F. B., & Veroff, J. (2007). *Savoring: A new model of positive experience.* Lawrence Erlbaum.

Buber, M. (1970). *I and Thou* (Vol. 243). Simon and Schuster.

Burleson, B. R., Albrecht, T. L., & Sarason, I. G. (1994). *Communication of Social Support: Messages, Interactions, Relationships, and Community.* Sage.

Cameron, K. (2012). *Positive leadership: Strategies for extraordinary performance.* Berrett-Koehler.

Carpenter, A., & Greene, K. (2015). Social penetration theory. In C. R. Berger & M. E. Roloff (Eds.,), *The International Encyclopedia of Interpersonal Communication* (pp. 1–4). Wiley-Blackwell. <https://doi.org/10.1002/9781118540190.wbeic0160>

Cissna, K. N., & Anderson, R. (1998). Theorizing about dialogic moments: The Buber-Rogers position and postmodern themes. *Communication Theory, 8*(1), 63–104. <https://doi.org/10.1111/j.1468-2885.1998.tb00211.x>

Cooke Jackson, A., & Rubinsky, V. (2022). Extending the roots of memorable messages: A comprehensive review and forecast of memorable message literature and theory. *Health Communication,* 1–11. <https://doi.org/10.1080/10410236.2022.2105620>

Craig, R. T. (1999). Communication theory as a field. *Communication Theory, 9*(2), 119–161. <https://doi.org/10.1111/j.1468-2885.1999.tb00355.x>

Craig, R. T. (2018). For a practical discipline. *Journal of Communication, 68*(2), 289–297. doi:10.1093/joc/jqx013

Craig, R. T., & Tracy, K. (1995). Grounded practical theory: The case of intellectual discussion. *Communication Theory, 5*(3), 248–272. <https://doi.org/10.1111/j.1468-2885.1995.tb00108.x>

Dorrance Hall, E., Ruth-McSwain, A., & Ferrara, M. (2016). Models of health: Exploring memorable messages received from parents about diet and exercise. *Journal of Communication in Healthcare, 9*(4), 247–255. <https://doi.org/10.1080/17538068.2016.1187892>

Droser, V. A., & Seurer, L. (2022). "God doesn't make mistakes": Memorable messages, adjustment, and grief following family death. *Health Communication, 37*(4), 498–507. <https://doi.org/10.1080/10410236.2020.1853328>

Geiman, K. L., & Greene, J. O. (2018). Listening and experiences of interpersonal transcendence. *Communication Studies, 70*(1), 114–128. <https://doi.org/10.1080/10510974.2018.1492946>

Gordon, R. D. (1985). Dimensions of peak communication experiences: An exploratory study. *Psychological Reports, 57*(3), 824–826. <https://doi.org/10.2466/pr0.1985.57.3.824>

High, A. C., & Dillard, J. P. (2012). A review and meta-analysis of person-centered messages and social support outcomes. *Communication Studies, 63*(1), 99–118. <https://doi.org/10.1080/10510974.2011.598208>

Hutchby, I., & Wooffitt, R. (2008). *Conversation analysis.* Polity.

Jiao, J., Kim, S., & Pitts, M. J. (2021). Promoting subjective well-being through communication savoring. *Communication Quarterly, 69*(2), 152–171. <https://doi.org/10.1080/01463373.2021.1901758>

Kassing, J. W., & Pappas, M. E. (2007). "Champions are built in the off season": An exploration of high school coaches' memorable messages. *Human Communication, 10*(4), 537–546. <https://doi.org/10.1177/2167479516641934>

Knapp, M. L., Stohl, C., & Reardon, K. K. (1981). "Memorable" messages. *Journal of Communication, 31*(4), 27–41. <https://doi.org/10.1111/j.1460-2466.1981.tb00448.x>

Kranstuber, H., Carr, K., & Hosek, A. M. (2012). "If you can dream it, you can achieve it." Parent memorable messages as indicators of college student success. *Communication Education, 61*(1), 44–66. <https://doi.org/10.1080/03634523.2011.620617>

Kuang, K., Tian, Z., Wilson, S. R., & Buzzanell, P. M. (2021). Memorable messages as anticipatory resilience: Examining associations among memorable messages, communication resilience processes, and mental health. *Health Communication, 38*(6), 1136–1145. <https://doi.org/10.1080/10410236.2021.1993585>

Lindlof, T. R., & Taylor, B. C. (2011). *Qualitative communication research methods* (3rd ed.). Sage.

Littlejohn, S. W. (1977). Symbolic interactionism as an approach to the study of human communication. *Quarterly Journal of Speech, 63*(1), 84–91. <https://doi.org/10.1080/00335637709383369>

Maslow, A. H. (1968). *Toward a psychology of being*. Van Nostranr Company.

Miles, M. B., Huberman, A. M., & Saldaña, J. (2014). *Qualitative data analysis: A methods sourcebook* (3rd ed.). Sage.

Mirivel, J. C. (2012). Communication excellence: Embodying virtues in interpersonal communication. In T. J. Socha & M. J. Pitts (Eds.), *The positive side of interpersonal communication* (pp. 55–72). Peter Lang.

Mirivel, J. C. (2014). *The art of positive communication: Theory and practice*. Peter Lang.

Mirivel, J. C. (2017). *How communication scholars think and act: A lifespan perspective*. Peter Lang.

Mirivel, J. (2019). On the nature of peak communication: Communication behaviors that make a difference on well-being and happiness. In J. A. M. Velázquez & C. Pulido (Eds.), *The Routledge handbook of positive communication: Contributions of an emerging community of research on communication for happiness and social change* (pp. 50–59). Routledge.

Mirivel, J. C., & Fuller, R. P. (2024). A world of possibilities: Introducing positive communication scholarship to inspire better business and organizational communication research. International Journal of Business Communication, 61, 743–759. <https://doi.org/10.1177/23294884241264268>

Mirivel, J. C. & Lyon, A. (2023). *Positive communication for leaders. Proven strategies for inspiring unity and effecting change*. Rowman & Littlefield.

Nazione, S., Laplante, C., Smith, S. W., Cornacchione, J., Russell, J., & Stohl, C. (2011). Memorable messages for navigating college life. *Journal of Applied Communication Research, 39*(2), 123–143. <https://doi.org/10.1080/00909882.2011.556138>

Parker, C., Scott, S., & Geddes, A. (2019). Snowball sampling. *SAGE research methods foundations*. Sage.

Pearce, W. B., & Pearce, K. A. (2000). Extending the theory of the coordinated management of meaning (CMM) through a community dialogue process. *Communication Theory, 10*(4), 405–423. <https://doi.org/10.1111/j.1468-2885.2000.tb00200.x>

Pitts, M. J. (2019). The language and social psychology of savoring: Advancing the communication savoring model. *Journal of Language and Social Psychology, 38*(2), 237–259. doi: 10.1177/0261927X18821404

Rogers, C. R. (1995). *On becoming a person: A therapist's view of psychotherapy*. Houghton Mifflin Harcourt.

Socha, T. J., & Beck, G. A. (2015). Positive communication and human needs: A review and proposed organizing conceptual framework. *Review of Communication*, *15*(3), 173–199. <https://doi.org/10.1080/15358593.2015.1080290>

Socha, T. J., & Pitts, M. J. (Eds.). (2012). *The positive side of interpersonal communication*. Peter Lang.

Steimel, S. (2013). Connecting with volunteers: Memorable messages and volunteer identification. *Communication Research Reports*, *30*(1), 12–21. <https://doi.org/10.1080/08824096.2012.746220>

Stohl, C. (1986). The role of memorable messages in the process of organizational socialization. *Communication Quarterly*, *34*(3), 231–249. <https://doi.org/10.1080/01463378609369638>

Tracy, K., & Robles, J. S. (2013). *Everyday talk: Building and reflecting identities* (2nd ed.). Guilford Press.

Way, D., & Tracy, S. J. (2012). Conceptualizing compassion as recognizing, relating and (re) acting: A qualitative study of compassionate communication at hospice. *Communication Monographs*, *79*(3), 292–315. <https://doi.org/10.1080/03637751.2012.697630>

Weger Jr., H., Castle Bell, G., Minei, E. M., & Robinson, M. C. (2014). The relative effectiveness of active listening in initial interactions. *International Journal of Listening*, *28*(1), 13–31. <https://doi.org/10.1080/10904018.2013.813234>

PART TWO

# The Centrality of Interpersonal Communication to Our Health and Well-Being

CHAPTER FOUR

# Interpersonal Communication as Central to Health across the Lifespan: A Family-Centered Approach to Psychosocial Oncology Care

CARLA L. FISHER

> The interpersonal communication that fuels our social world is as essential to our survival as any biological or physical process that keeps us alive.
>
> – [Hummert, Nussbaum, & Wiemann, 1994]

These simple yet profound words have been the anchor of my work since I was a graduate student under the mentorship of our esteemed "father" of lifespan communication, Jon F. Nussbaum, PhD. Co-authored with his colleagues—interpersonal and lifespan communication pioneers Mary Lee Hummert, PhD and John M. Wiemann, PhD—they eloquently declare that our *interpersonal communication is as critical to our health as are biomedical components.* What and how we communicate with others, through our language and behavior, contributes to short- and long-term health outcomes. At the same time, interpersonal communication is behavior and, therefore, a means of adapting to (i.e., coping with) any health-related experience, be it an acute or chronic illness or facing health challenges like inherited disease risk or aging-related changes. Quite simply and indisputably, at the root of health is how we communicate—our interpersonal lives.

Our social behavior must be recognized as a key element in our adaptability, wellness, resilience, and survival across the lifespan. In doing so, we must also appreciate that our behavior can function in both health-promoting and health-inhibiting ways. As such, *individuals and families need help learning how to communicate in ways that contribute to healthy relational, mental, and physical health outcomes.* Interpersonal health communication research is essential to promoting healthier behavior in both clinical and family settings and, thus, key to advancing healthcare practice, augmenting psychosocial care, and promoting healthier outcomes in our society.

Communication scientists conducting research in the subdiscipline of interpersonal health communication greatly value interdisciplinary, collaborative scholarship, sometimes called team science. We concurrently prioritize applied or translational research, also referred to as *social action-focused research—scholarship that can be (or is) put (i.e., implemented) into action.* Social action research has been defined as the "systematic gathering of information by people who are both affected by a problem and want to solve that problem" (Rubin & Rubin, 1986). While the scientific approach may vary, translational or social action-focused scientists work together to solve social problems impacting our society while generating new knowledge critical to solving these problems (Herr, 1995; Reason, 1994; Wagner, 1991).

*Interpersonal health communication research is central to solving health-related problems.* Our scholarship provides evidence on how we can enrich our interpersonal communication to promote better individual, relational, and family health outcomes. Through interpersonal health communication research, we can enhance clinicians' healthcare practice and patients' engagement, help families and patients communicate in health-promoting ways during health crises, identify behavior critical to reducing disease risk for individuals and generations of families, and elucidate communication patterns that promote better long-term mental, physical, and relational health outcomes. Even though interpersonal health communication research is a central element to solving health-related problems, healthcare practice and even how we approach health in society still largely ignores the role of interpersonal communication.

In this chapter, I use my work to illustrate how interpersonal health communication scholarship can also be critical to engaging in social action to improve healthcare and health-related outcomes. To do so, I'll highlight the overarching social action goal driving my own research. Ultimately, I aim to flip the script on how we approach and think about healthcare practice by bringing family communication to the forefront of care, thereby advocating for a *family-centered healthcare approach.* I will also share the biopsychosocial lens and foundation that informs my social action goal. In doing so, I'll specifically focus on research from my primary area of expertise—family-centered psychosocial oncology care—to provide examples of social action research informed by this lens in pursuit of my goal toward shifting to a more family-centered healthcare model. Finally, I will demonstrate how interpersonal health communication research becomes social action by providing an in-depth exploration of an online communication skills program called the *Healthy Communication Practice*™, an intervention targeting family blood cancer caregivers that I co-developed in partnership with my long-time collaborator (Carma L. Bylund, PhD, FACH) and our invaluable community partner, The Leukemia & Lymphoma Society (LLS). I will then turn it over to the next two chapters of this part, led by three rockstar family-health-lifespan scholars (Kevin B. Wright, PhD; Mollie R. Canzona, PhD; Gemme Campbell-Salome, PhD). They collectively extend the conversation further by illustrating both the centrality of interpersonal/family communication to health across the lifespan and how their research in this realm functions as social action in improving the health of society.

## BLENDING FAMILY SYSTEMS, RESILIENCE, AND LIFESPAN FRAMEWORKS

It wasn't until the late 1970s that the medical field began to recognize behavior as a central component of health with the emergence of subfields like behavioral medicine, biobehavioral health, and health psychology (Matarazzo, 1980; Schwartz & Weiss, 1978). By the mid-1990s, the United States government had also integrated a formal prioritization of behavioral-focused health research with Congress' establishment of the Office of Behavioral and Social Sciences Research (OBSSR) within the realm of the National Institutes of Health (NIH). At the same time, clinician-researchers predominantly in the fields of medical family therapy, health psychology, and psychiatry introduced a new way of thinking about health and clinical intervention—a biopsychosocial approach. This lens was instrumental in elevating behavior as an equally important component of health as biomedical factors.

With this shift, we also saw a move from biomedical models of health to ecological and systems approaches. Traditionally, much of the focus in healthcare practice and research had been centered on attending to the patient's individual, physically focused needs. Ecological and systems approaches to health recognize that patients' needs and experiences are embedded within their social environment—an environment that involves multiples "systems," one of which is their family system (McDaniel et al., 1992). As clinicians and researchers expanded their thinking about health to be inclusive of the bidirectional influence of a patient's social environment, family-focused models of behavior and health emerged, thereby recognizing the family as an important "resource" in a patient's ability to adapt to illness and emerge strengthened or resilient (Rolland & Walsh, 2006). As Kathleen Galvin, PhD, a founder of the Family Communication Division of the National Communication Association, explained, "All illness influences, and is influenced by, the family members who interpret and manage interactions about the illness" (Galvin & Young, 2010, p. 104).

With this in mind then, a family's behavior becomes front and center in health. *How a family behaves or responds to the health/illness challenge is critical and informs their adaptability or resilience.* According to theorists John Rolland, MD and Froma Walsh, PhD:

> *Resilience* can be defined as the ability to withstand and rebound from disruptive life challenges, becoming strengthened and more resourceful. Not simply general strengths, resilience involves dynamic processes that foster positive adaptation in the context of significant adversity. It is a misconception that resilience means innate hardiness, invulnerability, or simply bouncing back. It rather involves *struggling well, effectively working through and learning from adversity, and integrating the experience into the fabric of individual and shared lives.*

Walsh's family resilience framework includes a conceptual map to inform both clinical practice and intervention development. She identifies the key processes in patients' and families' ability to "struggle well, effectively working through it," in other words, their ability to cope, adapt and emerge resilient. These processes include finding meaning in their experience and addressing how the family is communicating to help them strengthen their family bond(s). *Families need help learning how to cope with illness together, to engage in adaptive behavior or as I like to call it, engaging in "healthy communication practice."* Healthy communication practice helps them strengthen family ties and cultivate resilience. Since Walsh's ground-breaking work, the concept of resilience has become an important clinical outcome to consider in both practice and intervention development, and it has expanded traditional thinking about stress, coping, and adaptation.

Rolland's Family System Genetic Illness Model (FSGI), initially named Family Systems-Illness Model (FSI), extends the notion of a family-centered, biopsychosocial approach to health further. Based on his clinical experience with over 1,000 families at the Center for Illness in Families at Yale University and the Center for Family Health at the University of Chicago, Rolland's model is grounded in the argument that families are both partners and resources to patients coping with acute and chronic illness and how they respond to such challenges has implications on their ability to both adapt but also emerge resilient—to grow together as a family. He extends this further by establishing the importance of customizing this psychosocial support to families' unique developmental needs by incorporating a multigenerational life cycle approach—ultimately the consideration of *lifespan factors*. He integrates time into our understanding of how families cope with illness.

Very much in line with lifespan communication theorizing, time impacts so many things—our communication competence or skill development, our developmentally grounded needs, as well as the communication dynamics and tensions that characterize our intergenerational relationships (Pecchioni et al., 2005). Rolland's integration of a lifespan lens elevates clinicians' understanding of the importance of meeting families where they are in the lifespan or developmentally to best attend to their needs. According to Rolland (1994),

> The impact of chronic conditions on the patient, well family members, and key caregivers differs, and *depends on when an illness strikes in the family and in each member's individual development*. … Most families enter the world of illness and disability without a psychosocial map to navigate the normative (i.e. common and expectable) strains. … Families are better able to master the challenges when clinicians help them to gain an understanding of their illness experience—a bridge between the biomedical and psychosocial worlds. … Clinicians can help families to gain relational resilience by pulling together as a functional family unit.

Rolland also makes a direct call to clinicians to "bridge" the biomedical world of illness with a patient's psychosocial environment and provides a blueprint of various behavioral, relational, and lifespan factors that should be considered in developing clinical interventions, i.e., the "psychosocial map" that can guide families through the unchartered waters of disease and illness. The FSGI model highlights three dimensions (which are inherently communication contexts) that should be considered to personalize families' psychosocial support needs.

We must consider (1) the type of illness/disease or disability, with a focus on the psychosocial nature of the health challenge (i.e., the health context); (2) developmental factors like each person's phase of the lifespan, multigenerational differences, or the illness trajectory (i.e., the developmental context); and (3) family system variables like the relationships type, relational roles, and relational connection or intimacy (e.g., the relational context). The model also stresses the importance of time in relation to a family's history or how they have functioned together (and within each bond) across the lifespan—both typical behavioral patterns and relational dynamics as well as their "multigenerational history of coping with illness, loss and adversity." Thus, again, the illness experience cannot be considered in a vacuum. It must be understood within the family environment and history as well as within the healthcare system.

One of the most beautiful, empowering notions of these lifespan, biopsychosocial, and resilience approaches is the awareness that when a family faces a traumatic illness, the crisis itself is an opportunity for families to grow—to become strengthened individually, relationally, and collectively. Illness doesn't have to be the event that knocks them down catastrophically. Rather, the health challenge itself can be a catalyst to cultivate their resilience by "pulling together" and learning how to engage in adaptive behavior (i.e., healthy communication practice). As Rolland and Walsh (2006) describe it, it's about "bringing out the best in the worst of times." At the same time, families shouldn't be given a false sense that they should innately know how to respond to an illness and "struggle effectively." Rather they need our expertise and support. Here is where interpersonal health communication scientists can serve by helping families foster resilience by bringing their best communication practices to center stage.

## FAMILY-CENTERED ONCOLOGY CARE: PROVIDING FAMILIES WITH A PSYCHOSOCIAL MAP

Nearly 20 years ago, Rolland advocated at the National Cancer Institute (NCI) and American Cancer Society (ACS) bi-annual meeting on survivorship that families direly need a *psychosocial map t*o learn healthy communication central to cancer coping and reducing disease risk (Rolland, 2005). While the biopsychosocial and family-focused shift in health models has contributed to more psychosocial oncology research as well as more patient-centered approaches to oncology care, families facing cancer still typically do not encounter family-focused approaches to care. The "psychosocial map" gap persists today, with patients, caregivers, and their families frequently disclosing that they struggle to cope together, to understand one another, and that they encounter unhelpful or painful interactions within the family system. They admit wanting help learning to communicate in ways that help the family bind together. Even in healthcare settings that offer patients and families access to clinical psychological services or social services, they are often suggested as an "as needed" or "add-on" service, sometimes informing them of its existence or ensuring patients "you won't need this but...," as if unmet psychosocial needs are a sign of weakness or atypical.

We need to flip the script on oncology care by making it both psychosocial in focus, integrated alongside the biomedical treatment, *and* family-centered. By integrating family-focused resources and psychosocial services, we recognize not only that "cancer is a disease of the entire family" but also that families do not innately have the communication knowledge and skills needed to psychosocially cope with cancer in health-promoting ways (Surbone et al., 2010).

## Linking Health Outcomes to Family Communication Patterns

Two goals drive my social action goal of making healthcare more family-centered in psychosocial oncology care. First, is the importance of heightening clinicians,' patients,' and families' appreciation and awareness that *how* we communicate is inevitably contributing to our health outcomes. The idea that our communicative behaviors or patterns contribute to physical, social, and mental health outcomes is new to many—clinicians and patients alike. It is also a striking reality that gets the attention of patients, families, and clinicians. I've used a well-known communication theory (Family Communication Patterns Theory or FCP) to generate evidence of this fact in my work focused on mothers and daughters coping with breast cancer as well as adult children caring for a parent with a blood cancer.

Studies informed by an FCP lens illustrate that families develop norms about how to communicate, which include patterns of openness (in topic and frequency) and interdependence (how much they expect each other to conform to each other's ideas or beliefs). These patterns characterize a family system (i.e., their environment) and persist or remain stable across the lifespan. As such, a family's communication environment informs how they communicate during strenuous experiences as well as what they come to expect (and accept) as typical behavior by family members. With this in mind then, these communication patterns will inform how willing (and comfortable) caregivers, patients, and family members are to openly talk about cancer. These communication patterns inform how they are coping and may, in turn, contribute to healthy or unhealthy outcomes.

I conducted one of the first applications of FCP in a cancer context with mothers and daughters facing breast cancer. My colleagues and I found that when women diagnosed with breast cancer are coping within a mother–daughter bond that has a history of communicating more openly with one another, regardless of when they were diagnosed in the lifespan (e.g., young adulthood to later life), they also exhibited better health outcomes. They had less cancer-related pain and fatigue as well as better relational well-being with their mother/daughter (Fisher et al., 2017). I found similar results and extended this finding in another cancer context, with adult children caring for an aging parent living with a blood cancer. Those adult child caregivers with more open parent–child bonds also exhibited less debilitating caregiving burden. At the same time, they described feeling more socially supported in their caregiving role in comparison to caregivers with less open dynamics in their parent–child bond (Campbell-Salome et al., 2022). Other more recently published cancer-related studies framed by FCP further show that social support and family openness are interrelated—when families communicate more openly they ultimately open the door for more opportunities for receiving (or exchanging) social support. Not only are family members' perceptions of social support tied to how openly the family communicates, but this extends to their perceptions of healthcare encounters, as caregivers' perceptions of support are positively associated with their perceptions of receiving quality care (Bevan et al., 2022).

With these findings in mind then, we also need to recognize that our interpersonal communication dynamics or long-standing patterns within the family inform how we communicate in other settings, like clinical interactions. Studies utilizing FCP demonstrate that families' open communication patterns inform how involved (or not) they are during clinical interactions as well as their preferences for the clinician's communication style (e.g., authoritative vs. shared decision-making) (Rauscher et al., 2020). Such findings indicate that strongly rooted family communication patterns transfer to how individuals communicate in clinical settings. In my recent work in blood cancer caregiving, we found evidence supporting this notion in that adult child caregivers with a more open family communication environment also reported better perceptions of their ability to communicate with their parents' clinicians (Campbell-Salome et al., 2022).

These findings collectively suggest that two specific interpersonal communication processes—openness and support—may be especially impactful for families as they provide care for a loved one with cancer and cope with the disease together. Moreover, families who tend to be less open or supportive may need help developing such communication skills to promote effective family *and* clinical communication. We also need to extend this revelation further by identifying communication approaches, strategies, or behaviors family can engage in to facilitate openness and support or quality clinical interactions to promote healthier outcomes.

## Providing Targeted Communication Guidance to Families on How to Communicate

If we want to provide families with a psychosocial map, we need to capture what this communication looks like –the quality of our behaviors or *how* we can communicate in healthy ways in familial and clinical settings. My second prioritized goal focuses on this by illustrating for families how they can cope together in adaptive ways to strengthen their ties and promote resilience. In this work I also prioritize two approaches to developing a psychosocial map: (1) the importance of providing targeted guidance and (2) harnessing the power of narrative.

Several reviews in the last 15 years demonstrate that psychosocial oncology interventions need to be developed based on *theoretically grounded targeted approaches* to be efficacious in meeting families' needs. The reviews illustrate that interventions have mostly ignored diversity in needs related to disease specifics (e.g., type of cancer), relational considerations (e.g., even considering family members), and time (e.g., phase of the disease) (Lambert et al., 2012; Samuelsson et al., 2021; Ussher et al., 2009). Using a blended metatheoretical approach informed by family systems and lifespan communication concepts (Galvin & Young, 2010; Nussbaum, 1989, 2014; Pecchioni et al., 2005; Rolland, 2005), I target my family-focused psychosocial oncology research based on (1) the cancer context (e.g., disease type and cancer-related topic like talking about end of life or future risk); (2) the developmental context (e.g., phase of the lifespan of family members; disease trajectory like diagnosis versus the transition to survivorship); and (3) the relational context (e.g., bond type like mother–daughter; role of patient or caregiver or daughter or mother; intergenerational dynamics).

For instance, much of my early work was based specifically on the experiences of one type of cancer (breast cancer), one intergenerational family bond (mothers and daughters—as patient and healthy partner), and understanding their experiences at various phases of the lifespan. This meant including multiple stakeholders, patients and their mothers/daughters, who were diagnosed (or providing care) at various phases of life (ranging from emerging/young adulthood to later life) to fully understand their variant needs/experiences as they were informed by their relational role (mother/daughter), health status (patient/caregiver or family member), and phase of the lifespan or developmental maturity. By capturing multiple perspectives, we can identify overlapping and divergent needs to better target our guidance to mothers and daughters on how to facilitate healthy communication and adjustment (Fisher, 2010, 2011, 2014; Fisher et al., 2012; Fisher et al., 2017; Fisher & Nussbaum, 2015).

I also prioritize narrative approaches across the research process—from theory to data to analysis to translation. Narrative-driven interventions are shown to be more efficacious than information-based interventions alone (Mcqueen & Kreuter, 2010), as narratives function as tools to "facilitate the mental simulation of unknown, difficult, or frightening procedures (e.g., screening) and provide role models for behavior change" (Green, 2006). Drawing on social cognitive theory (Bandura, 1977) or transportation theories (e.g., Green & Brock, 2000), narratives are critical behavioral modeling tools that help motivate individuals to enact certain behaviors and build their self-efficacy. Moreover, narratives have incredible "healing power" both for those participating in research by sharing their lived experiences and for those who learn from them (Harter et al., 2005; Sunwolf et al., 2005). As Beach et al., 2013 advocated in their narrative-focused cancer research, the "power of the arts as an exceptional learning tool for extending empirical research" (p. 1).

By capturing targeted narratives, I can provide a psychosocial map of cancer for families that is tailored to their unique needs, thereby giving them a sense of what to expect across the cancer trajectory and how to communicate in ways that help them cope or reduce disease risk. For instance, I published the only evidence-based book on mother–daughter breast cancer communication written to be accessible for researchers, clinicians, and families alike based on nearly 100 women's experiences captured in surveys, interviews, and diaries (Fisher, 2014). Inspired by narrative medicine translational goals, I structured the book around mothers'/daughters' storied accounts of disease coping across the lifespan to depict the complicated nature of learning to cope together and the challenges they face talking (or not) about cancer, how they share the disease experience, and how they provide emotional support to one another. Their stories provide models of how to cope together in healthier ways with targeted communication guidance based on their developmental phase in life (e.g., young versus later adulthood) and relational role (e.g., patient or caregiver; mother or daughter).

In partnership with Mayo Clinic, I later extended this work to focus primarily on the needs of the most distressed and vulnerable group: adolescent and young adult (AYA) daughters of diagnosed women. AYA daughters not only are increasingly serving as their mothers' caregivers, but they also are the most distressed caregiver type and family member, which impacts them psychologically, socially, developmentally, and physiologically (Cohen & Pollack, 2005; Fenton et al., 2020; Fisher, 2010, 2014; Spira & Kenemore, 2000; Stiffler et al., 2008; Wellisch et al., 2012). In interviews with both diagnosed mothers and their AYA daughters, we captured topics they find challenging (Fisher et al., 2022a) as well as strategies that they both perceive as helpful to use when navigating these distressing conversations (e.g., talking about physical changes) (Fisher et al., 2022b). We also identified strategies preferred by each relational partner (mother versus daughter) to give targeted guidance (Fisher et al., 2022b).

I've also prioritized the needs of another group of mothers and daughters encountering ongoing or chronic psychological distress and risk: mothers and daughters living with hereditary breast and ovarian cancer (HBOC) and/or a genetic mutation (BRCA 1/2). In collaboration with Memorial Sloan Kettering, we analyzed genetic counseling sessions capturing the interactions between high-risk mothers with adolescent daughters and genomic practitioners. We sought to identify ways to enhance both family and clinical communication, as well as how to help mothers and daughters manage their distressing uncertainty. Using uncertainty management theory (UMT) as a sensitizing lens, we identified mothers' sources of uncertainty about their AYA daughters' risk that emerge during genetic counseling sessions (Bylund et al., 2012). We also captured communication strategies clinicians can engage in and use to help these mothers and daughters manage their distressing uncertainty (Fisher et al., 2019). We also extended this with focus group interviews to identify strategies mothers can use to talk to their AYA daughters about risk (Fisher et al., 2014).

I later advanced this guidance with an interview study with "previvors" (women who have tested positive for a BRCA mutation) in collaboration with Marleah Dean, PhD, a well-known interpersonal health communication scholar and previvor herself. We again used UMT to show how a previvor's ongoing risk management decisions (e.g., surveillance) are characterized by chronic uncertainty and informed by evolving lifespan factors (e.g., family planning, the mother's cancer history, age). We created a lifespan, uncertainty decision-making model clinicians can use to consider lifespan factors as they help previvors manage their uncertainty, re-assess their risk management needs and decisions, and facilitate family decision-making discussions (Dean & Fisher, 2019).

Targeted studies and implementing that knowledge into social action (e.g., interventions, practice, resources) take time, funding, and multidisciplinary collaboration. To provide a more in-depth look at how we can move research into social action and elevate family-centered oncology care, I share one psychosocial cancer resource that I've co-developed using the same targeted family systems-lifespan, narrative-driven approach in conjunction with a team that bridged multiple disciplines and community partners to develop a psychosocial map for families facing blood cancer.

## INTERPERSONAL HEALTH COMMUNICATION RESEARCH IN ACTION: THE *HEALTHY COMMUNICATION PRACTICE* INTERVENTION

The *Healthy Communication Practice* is an intervention I recently co-developed with my long-standing colleague, Carma L. Bylund, PhD, who I've had the honor of collaborating with for more than 15 years. Bylund is one of the most renowned scholars in patient–provider communication and one of the first "boundary spanners" of our disciplines. She put interpersonal health communication scholarship into social action by being one of the first communication scholars to become embedded within a healthcare institution when she became part of Memorial Sloan Kettering Cancer Center's Division of Psychological and Behavioral Services two decades ago. There she created ComSkills—a program to teach clinicians how to communicate with individuals living with cancer—which is also the first formal communication initiative integrated in a cancer center in the nation. Still thriving in existence 20 years later, MSK staff in the program train more than 100 clinicians annually. She later launched the same initiative in Doha, Qatar, tailoring it to their healthcare system.

In recent years, we've been privileged to collaborate with one of the most invaluable non-profit, advocacy organizations serving the needs of families facing cancer: The Leukemia and Lymphoma Society (LLS). In partnership with LLS, we developed a broad program of research focused on building family caregiver resources, a foundational program that became the bedrock of the *Healthy Communication Practice* intervention: <https://healthycommunicationpractice.org/>.

This intervention was also an opportunity for us to fuse together our distinct areas of expertise and prior research programs, merging a focus on developing family caregivers' communication skills in both clinical and family settings.

To illustrate how we put our interpersonal health communication scholarship into social action, I unpack the social action goal informing the Healthy Communication Practice intervention. I then share our formative research that we conducted to inform its development, followed by an overview of how our work was implemented into the intervention—highlighting the major components. I'll also share some initial pilot study findings and where we are going next in our mission to provide more family-centered psychosocial resources in oncology care and healthcare at large.

## Social Action Goal

In 2009, a systematic review of psychosocial oncology resources highlighted how family caregivers' needs were virtually ignored (Ussher et al., 2009). Yet, evidence informing the Cancer Family Caregiving Experience Model and the Dyadic Cancer Outcomes Framework shows that caregivers' and patients' behavior and health outcomes are interrelated and, as such, a diagnosed family member and caregiver should be approached as "unit of care" not separately or the patient alone (Badr et al., 2019; Fletcher et al., 2012; Magsamen-Conrad et al., 2015; Regan et al., 2015; Thompson et al., 2021; Yuen et al., 2016). Family caregivers of individuals diagnosed with cancer face a multitude of emotional, financial, and physical challenges as they integrate caregiving into their current complicated, demanding roles and responsibilities (Fenton et al., 2022; Hunt et al., 2016).

It is also noteworthy that blood cancers are less often studied, particularly from a family lens. Resources supporting blood cancer caregivers' needs are scant, which is especially concerning, given families who face blood cancer are also at a higher risk for psychological distress compared to those coping with other types of cancers (Dionne-Odom et al., 2019; Pailler et al., 2016). This is in part due to distinct traumatic stressors across the disease trajectory ranging from extended years of heightened uncertainty during "watch and wait" to at times needing immediate in-patient treatment on the day of diagnosis, to repeated emergency department visits, and to life-threatening treatment complications (Berterö et al., 1997a, 1997b; Bryant et al., 2015; Dionne-Odom et al., 2019; Pailler et al., 2016; Zimmermann et al., 2013).

Given the median age at diagnosis for the most common types of blood cancer (leukemia and non-Hodgkin lymphoma) is 67 (American Cancer Society, 2019; Howlander et al., 2019), adult children in midlife often become their aging parent's blood cancer caregiver after diagnosis. They ultimately experience caregiving in the midst of their lifespan, a time period characterized as a complex juggling act when we encounter the most demands personally and professionally consecutively (Bachner et al., 2009). Midlife caregivers report significant stress and burden related to family functioning, as they manage this juggling act of multiple roles while they take on caring for their parent in conjunction with managing the demands within their own families, homes, and professional lives (Teixeira & Pereira, 2014).

## Formative Research

In partnership with LLS, we sought to build families a psychosocial map for coping with blood cancers by targeting the needs of family caregivers. To do so, we developed a multidisciplinary team spanning multiple institutions and disciplines, including clinical psychology, sociology, interpersonal health communication, and instructional design. As a first step, we began our intervention development with two formative studies that enabled us to ultimately target the intervention to the unique needs of adult children caring for their diagnosed aging parent. First, we conducted an interview study comparing 39 different family caregivers' experiences, prioritizing the importance of context in understanding patients', caregivers', and family members' coping needs. We compared these family caregivers' experiences (and thus, recruited multiple stakeholder types) based on three factors: (1) variant relational roles—parent caring for a diagnosed child versus adult child caring for diagnosed parent; (2) different developmental phases in life (e.g., divergent intergenerational dynamics when caregiver is an adult child caring for an aging parent versus parents caring for an adolescent/young adult child; and (3) different blood cancers (e.g., an acute versus chronic disease type). With these influential variables in mind, we were able to capture and examine shared experiences as well as differences in needs related to communication challenges caregivers face across the disease trajectory, from diagnosis to treatment to treatment transitions as well as survivorship or end of life (Bagautdinova et al., 2022; Fisher et al., 2021; Kastrinos et al., 2022a; Kastrinos et al., 2022b; Mullis et al., 2023; Wollney et al., 2023). These findings helped us not only understand the unique needs of adult child blood cancer caregivers but also areas in which they need communication skill development to navigate communication challenges.

To further explore the communication needs of adult child caregivers specifically, we then conducted a survey study. We surveyed over 100 adult child caregivers to identify their communication skillset need in the three communication contexts we identified in our interview study: (1) communicating about online information in both family and clinical settings; (2) communicating with the parent's clinician in clinical, triadic encounters; and (3) facilitating open and supportive communication in the family, both with their diagnosed parent and family members in the broader system. We also explored links between how they communicate and psychosocial health outcomes to further demonstrate the need for a family-centered approach to blood cancer caregiving (Fisher et al., 2021; Wright et al., 2023; Vasquez et al., 2022). While our survey included validated scales, we used open-ended questions to expand on the communication challenges identified in the interview data, further enriching our initial narrative dataset (i.e., the interviews) for future intervention development (Fisher et al., 2021; Bagautdinova et al., 2022; Wright et al., 2023).

## Targeted Development: Overview of the Program

In addition to our multidisciplinary team, we developed the intervention with the input of an expert advisory board comprised of family caregivers, physicians, oncology social workers, psychologists, behavioral scientists, and instructional design experts who provided feedback across the entire development process. Our approach was also grounded in family systems, lifespan, communication, and education theories (Bylund et al., 2009; Fisher & Nussbaum, 2015; Hinyard & Kreuter, 2007; Koerner & Fitzpatrick, 2002; Mayer, 2014; Paige et al., 2018, 2019; Rolland, 2005). While we targeted it to midlife adult child family caregivers, we also considered their instructional needs. As adult learning theory recognizes that adults are independent learners as well as goal-oriented, we prioritized an asynchronous, interactive online learning approach. Not only was this supported by theory, but we also wanted to consider the feasibility of completing an intervention while navigating the unpredictable demands of being a cancer caregiver in midlife. Thus, an online approach ensured caregivers could complete it in the comfort of their own home, using different modalities (computer, phone, ipad), as well as stop and return to the program at any time.

We developed a 90-minute online, self-paced program that was divided into two parts (see Figure 4.1). Each part is focused on skill development in communication contexts central to caregiving. Part 1 helps caregivers build communication skills for navigating cancer information in online and clinical settings. Part 2 helps caregivers build skills critical to facilitating open and supportive communication in the family.

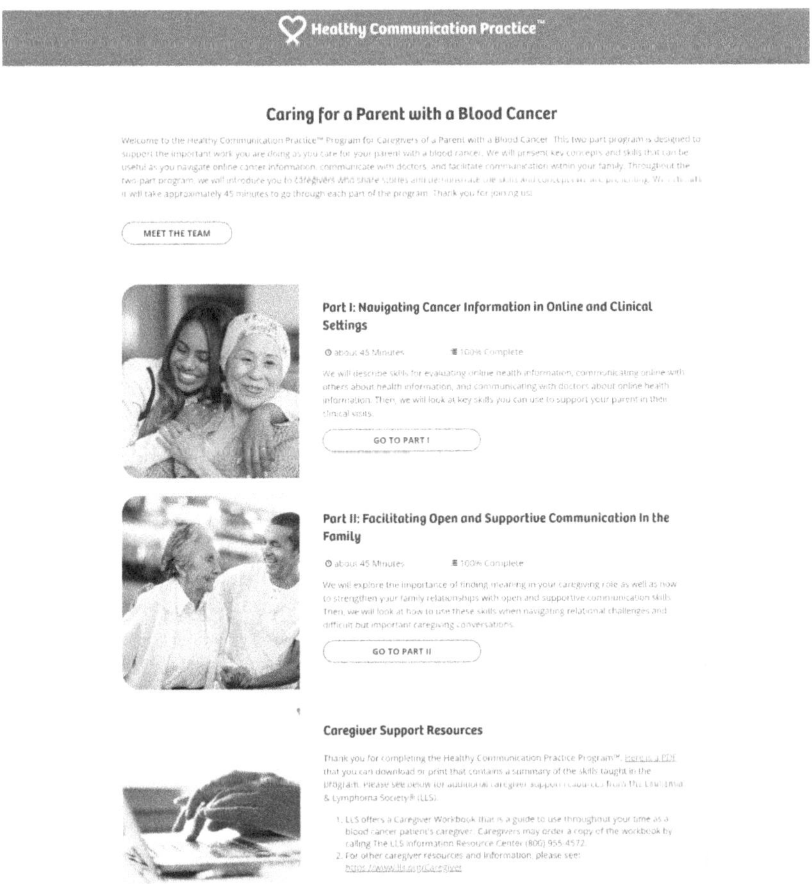


Figure 4.1: The *Healthy Communication Practice* intervention for blood cancer caregivers. Credit: Craig Fowler.

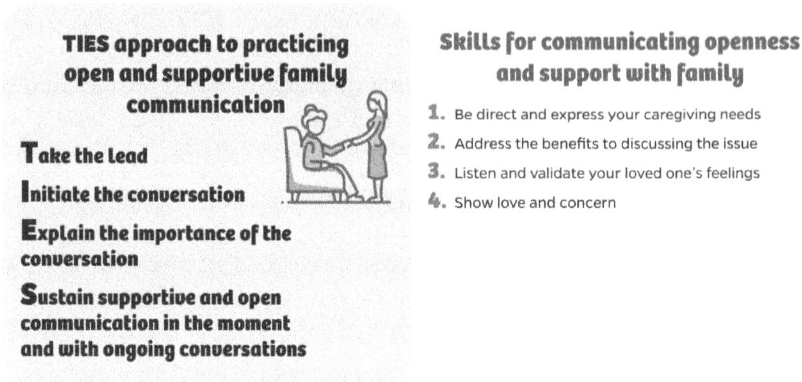


Figure 4.2: The TIES Model for teaching caregivers family communication skills.
Credit: Craig Fowler.

We also used a narrative-driven approach with a variety of instructional techniques to promote social learning and engagement. For instance, each subsection of Parts 1 and 2 begins with a video of an expert explaining concepts and skills related to the topic (e.g., talking openly about challenging topics). Each topic integrates a communication model to more easily teach the skills and promote learners' understanding of the concepts. For example, in Part 2 I teach the TIES model (Figure 4.2). I developed this model to illustrate the importance of family communication to strengthening family relationships—the ties that bind. Caregivers learn to *T*ake the lead in the family in facilitating openness and support by *I*nitiating the challenging care-related conversation, *E*xplain the importance of having the discussion, and then aim to *S*ustain the open and supportive communication in the moment and over time.

These concepts and skills are also modeled for caregivers using authentic caregiver narratives (i.e., behavioral modeling tools) that were drawn from our formative interview data. Different caregiver narratives are showcased in either audio form (e.g., caregivers sharing their story like challenges with being open) or video (e.g., caregivers interacting with clinicians and/or family members to illustrate the challenges and skills). Narratives represent diverse experiences to promote caregivers' ability to relate to the stories and promote their engagement. There are also two main caregivers whose stories we see across both Parts 1 and 2: Marco an African American, young adult, and only child of a diagnosed father who is single and Anne, a white, married, midlife, daughter (with children) who is caring for a diagnosed mother who has a living spouse and other adult children. Developed and implemented during the COVID-19 pandemic, our videos are also historically reflective of the shift we all experienced in both clinical and family interactions moving to online or telemedicine modalities. In each subsection, we also integrate different interactive activities caregivers complete to reflect on what they are learning and practice their communication skills. In turn, this can promote their intention and motivation to enact the skills in their lived experiences in both family and clinical settings.

## Pilot Testing the Intervention

We are currently conducting a single-arm trial of the intervention in which we are testing the impact of the intervention (post and three-months post) on caregivers' psychosocial outcomes (e.g., mental distress), communication skill development, and enactment of their personally set communication goals to enact the skills they learned to improve their family and clinical communication. We are also exploring differences based on their family communication environments (e.g., more open or less conforming communication patterns using FCP) to better understand their needs for future tailoring.

We also recently published a feasibility and acceptability test with 30 caregivers to obtain preliminary support that the *Healthy Communication Practice* intervention would work in action (Bylund et al., 2022). Caregivers found it acceptable and feasible, with participants perceiving it was easy to progress through the program without unexpected challenges. They liked the content and felt that it met their needs and described it as an "an eye-opener" and "an excellent learning experience." They also positively rated the caregiver narratives that we used as behavioral models to teach the communication skills, reporting that they could picture themselves in the stories, were mentally involved, were affected emotionally, and had vivid images of the caregivers (see Bylund et al., 2022). We also preliminarily looked at their pre-intervention mental distress scores and compared them with their post-intervention scores and saw improvements in their mental well-being, which were sustained three months after the intervention was completed. They also reported a willingness to change their communication with clinicians and family members and their intention to engage in communication with clinicians increased after the intervention.

## Future Adaptations of the Intervention

As we continue to test the *Healthy Communication Practice*, we are currently conducting formative research to adapt the program to other blood cancer caregiver types (e.g., spouses) and at specific phases of the lifespan (e.g., caregivers of diagnosed AYAs or AYA caregivers of diagnosed parents). Our long-term goal is to develop a larger *Healthy Communication Practice* program that serves as a core psychosocial map to all family caregivers that is personalized based on disease context (e.g., breast cancer versus dementia), relationship type (e.g., spouses versus mother-daughter), developmental phases (e.g., coping during young adulthood versus later life), and their family communication environments (e.g., low low openness versus high openness in families). In doing so, we can both move the needle on healthcare, making it more family-centered, while also providing a psychosocial map of coping with illness on a larger scale, thereby ensuring all family caregivers have an opportunity to develop communication skills critical to clinical and family communication.

## OVERVIEW OF TWO PART CHAPTERS

I now turn to the next two chapters of this part, written by my colleagues and Nussbaum family members. First is the chapter written by Kevin B. Wright, PhD (the "academic brother" as a fellow advisee of Nussbaum, whom I always admired and continue to look up to) and Mollie R. Canzona, PhD (my "academic daughter" who has impressed and inspired me since I had the privilege of being her advisor). They share their invaluable contributions to interpersonal health communication narrowing in on the importance of cultivating our willingness to communicate about health in clinical and family settings and the intersection of our openness with our ability to feel support (i.e., our social support communication skills). Wright shares his renowned work as one of the first scholars to examine family-focused computer-mediated communication and social support and shares a social action initiative we co-led in breast cancer risk communication for families in partnership with the NIH-funded Breast Cancer Environmental Research Program. Canzona shares her invaluable contributions in breaking down the barriers of silence in talking about sexual health (both at home and in clinical settings) in women's breast cancer survivorship care. She bridges the unique needs and perspectives of patients or survivors, their spouses, and clinicians across specialties to promote better care. She shares a social action initiative in this space implemented in conjunction with Wake Forest Comprehensive Cancer Center.

The second chapter is authored by Gemme Campbell-Salome, PhD, also a granddaughter of Nussbaum as my and Bylund's former joint post-doc and "academic daughter" whose work I've followed in great admiration since I knew her only in print during her graduate training. Now a boundary spanner at Geisinger (an integrated healthcare system in central Pennsylvania), Campbell-Salome's narrative-grounded work has greatly extended our understanding of the important role of family communication patterns and living with inherited disease risk and genomic conditions. She illustrates the powerful impact of narratives and communication patterns in families' health across generations, providing a social action example from her intervention work with families living with familial hypercholesterolemia (FH) and the use of innovative technology in genomic and precision medicine.

## REFERENCES


*American Cancer Society [ACS].* (2019). <https://www.cancer.org/research/cancer-facts-statistics/all-cancer-facts-figures/cancer-facts-figures-2019.html>

Bachner, Y. G., Karus, D. G., & Raveis, V. H. (2009). Examining the social context in the caregiving experience: Correlates of global self-esteem among adult daughter caregivers to an older parent with cancer. *Journal of Aging and Health*, *21*(7), 1016–1039. <https://doi.org/10.1177/0898264309344320>

Badr, H., Bakhshaie, J., & Chhabria, K. (2019). Dyadic interventions for cancer survivors and caregivers: State of the science and new directions. *Seminars in Oncology Nursing*, *35*(4), 337–341. <https://doi.org/10.1016/j.soncn.2019.06.004>

Bagautdinova, D., Bylund, C. L., Kastrinos, A., Hampton, C. N., Vasquez, T. S., Weiss, E. S., Sae-Hau, M., & Fisher, C. L. (2022). Adult sibling-related experiences while caring for a parent diagnosed with a blood cancer. *Families, Systems, & Health*, <https://doi.org/10.1037/fsh0000748>

Bandura, A. (1977). Self-efficacy: Toward a unifying theory of behavioral change. *Psychological Review*, *84*, 191–215. <https://doi.org/10.1037/0033-295X.84.2.191>

Beach, W., Buller, M., Dozier, D., Buller, D., & Gutzmer, K. (2013). The Conversations About Cancer (CAC) Project: Assessing feasibility and audience impacts from viewing the cancer play. *Health Communication*, *29*. <https://doi.org/10.1080/10410236.2013.767874>

Berterö, C., Eriksson, B.-E., & Ek, A.-C. (1997a). A substantive theory of quality of life of adults with chronic leukaemia. *International Journal of Nursing Studies*, *34*(1), 9–16. <https://doi.org/10.1016/S0020-7489(96)00025-9>

Berterö, C., Eriksson, B.-E., & Ek, A.-C. (1997b). Explaining different profiles in quality of life experiences in acute and chronic leukemia. *Cancer Nursing*, *20*(2), 100.

Bevan, J., Murphy, M., Lannutti, P., Slatcher, R., & Balzarini, R. (2022). A descriptive literature review of early research on COVID-19 and close relationships. *Communication Faculty Articles and Research*. <https://doi.org/10.1177/02654075221115387>

Bryant, A. L., Deal, A. M., Walton, A., Wood, W. A., Muss, H., & Mayer, D. K. (2015). Use of ED and hospital services for patients with acute leukemia after induction therapy: One year follow-up. *Leukemia Research*, *39*(4), 406–410. <https://doi.org/10.1016/j.leukres.2015.01.006>

Bylund, C. L., Fisher, C. L., Brashers, D., Edgerson, S., Glogowski, E. A., Boyar, S. R., Kemel, Y., Spencer, S., & Kissane, D. (2012). Sources of uncertainty about daughters' breast cancer risk that emerge during genetic counseling consultations. *Journal of Genetic Counseling*, *21*(2), 292–304. <https://doi.org/10.1007/s10897-011-9400-y>

Bylund, C. L., Gueguen, J. A., D'Agostino, T. A., Imes, R. S., & Sonet, E. (2009). Cancer patients' decisions about discussing Internet information with their doctors. *Psycho-Oncology*, *18*(11), 1139–1146. <https://doi.org/10.1002/pon.1511>

Bylund, C. L., Wollney, E. N., Campbell-Salome, G., Applebaum, A. J., Paige, S. R., DeGruccio, K., … & Fisher, C. L. (2022). Improving clinical and family communication for adult child caregivers of a parent with a blood cancer: Single-arm pre-post pilot intervention. *JMIR Cancer, 8*(3), e38722. <https://doi.org/doi:10.2196/38722/>.

Campbell-Salome, G., Fisher, C. L., Wright, K. B., Lincoln, G., Applebaum, A. J., Sae-Hau, M., Weiss, E. S., & Bylund, C. L. (2022). Impact of the family communication environment on burden and clinical communication in blood cancer caregiving. *Psycho-Oncology, 31*(7), 1212–1220. <https://doi.org/10.1002/pon.5910>

Cohen, M., & Pollack, S. (2005). Mothers with breast cancer and their adult daughters: The relationship between mothers' reaction to breast cancer and their daughters' emotional and neuroimmune status. *Psychosomatic Medicine, 67*(1), 64–71. <https://doi.org/10.1097/01.psy.0000151746.36540.6e>

Dean, M., & Fisher, C. L. (2019). Uncertainty and previvors' cancer risk management: Understanding the decision-making process. *Journal of Applied Communication Research, 47*(4), 460–483. <https://doi.org/10.1080/00909882.2019.1657236>

Dionne-Odom, J. N., Currie, E. R., Johnston, E. E., & Rosenberg, A. R. (2019). Supporting family caregivers of adult and pediatric persons with leukemia. *Seminars in Oncology Nursing, 35*(6), 150954. <https://doi.org/10.1016/j.soncn.2019.150954>

Fenton, A. T. H. R., Keating, N. L., Ornstein, K. A., Kent, E. E., Litzelman, K., Rowland, J. H., & Wright, A. A. (2022). Comparing adult-child and spousal caregiver burden and potential contributors. *Cancer, 128*(10), 2015–2024. <https://doi.org/10.1002/cncr.34164>

Fisher, C. L. (2010). Coping with breast cancer across adulthood: Emotional support communication in the mother–daughter bond. *Journal of Applied Communication Research, 38*(4), 386–411. <https://doi.org/10.1080/00909882.2010.513996>

Fisher, C. L. (2011). "Her pain was my pain": Mothers and daughters sharing the breast cancer journey. In M. Miller-Day (Ed.), *Family Communication, Connections, and Health Transitions: Going through This Together* (First printing edition, pp. 57–76). Peter Lang Inc., International Academic Publishers.

Fisher, C. L. (2014). *Coping Together, Side by Side: Enriching Mother-Daughter Communication Across the Breast Cancer Journey*. Hampton Press.

Fisher, C. L., Kastrinos, A., Piemonte, N., Canzona, M. R., Wolf, B., & Pipe, T. (2022a). Coping with breast cancer together: Challenging topics for mothers and their adolescent-young adult (AYA) daughters. *Journal of Psychosocial Oncology, 40*(6), 756–769. <https://doi.org/10.1080/07347332.2021.2005734>

Fisher, C. L., Kastrinos, A., Curley, A., Canzona, M. R., Piemonte, N., Wolf, B., & Pipe, T. (2022b). Helping diagnosed mothers and their adolescent-young adult daughters navigate challenging breast cancer conversations. *Cancer Care Research Online, 2*(3), e025. <https://doi.org/10.1097/CR9.0000000000000025>

Fisher, C. L., Maloney, E., Glogowski, E., Hurley, K., Edgerson, S., Lichtenthal, W. G., Kissane, D., & Bylund, C. (2014). Talking about familial breast cancer risk: Topics and strategies to enhance mother-daughter interactions. *Qualitative Health Research, 24*(4), 517–535. <https://doi.org/10.1177/1049732314524638>

Fisher, C. L., Miller-Day, M., & Nussbaum, J. F. (2012). Healing through healthy doses of positivity: Mothers' and daughters' positive communication when coping with breast cancer. In T. Socha & M. J. Pitts (Eds.), *Positive Communication in Health and Wellness* (New edition). Peter Lang Inc., International Academic Publishers.

Fisher, C. L., Mullis, M. D., Kastrinos, A., Wollney, E., Weiss, E. S., Sae-Hau, M., & Bylund, C. L. (2021). "Home wasn't really home anymore": Understanding caregivers' perspectives of the impact of blood cancer caregiving on the family system. *Supportive Care in Cancer*, *29*(6), 3069–3076. <https://doi.org/10.1007/s00520-020-05811-4>

Fisher, C. L., & Nussbaum, J. F. (2015). Maximizing wellness in successful aging and cancer coping: The importance of family communication from a socioemotional selectivity theoretical perspective. *Journal of Family Communication*, *15*, 3–19. <https://doi.org/10.1080/15267431.2014.946512>

Fisher, C. L., Roccotagliata, T., Rising, C. J., Kissane, D. W., Glogowski, E. A., & Bylund, C. L. (2017). "I Don't Want to Be an Ostrich": Managing Mothers' Uncertainty during BRCA1/2 Genetic Counseling. *Journal of Genetic Counseling*, *26*(3), 455–468. <https://doi.org/10.1007/s10897-016-9998-x>

Fisher, C. L., Wolf, B. M., Fowler, C., & Canzona, M. R. (2017). Experiences of "openness" between mothers and daughters during breast cancer: Implications for coping and healthy outcomes. *Psycho-Oncology*, *26*(11), 1872–1880. <https://doi.org/10.1002/pon.4253>

Fisher, C., Wright, K., Rising, C., Mullis, M., Afanaseva, D., Burke-Garcia, A., & Cai, X. (2019). Culturally appropriate breast cancer and environmental risk messages: Targeting racially and ethnically diverse mothers. *Journal of Cancer Education*, *36*. <https://doi.org/10.1007/s13187-019-01626-y>

Fisher, C. L., Wright, K. B., Hampton, C. N., Vasquez, T. S., Kastrinos, A., Applebaum, A. J., … & Bylund, C. L. (2021). Blood cancer caregiving during COVID-19: Understanding caregivers' needs. *Translational Behavioral Medicine*, *11*(5), 1187–1197.

Fletcher, B. S., Miaskowski, C., Given, B., & Schumacher, K. (2012). The cancer family caregiving experience: An updated and expanded conceptual model. *European Journal of Oncology Nursing: The Official Journal of European Oncology Nursing Society*, *16*(4), 387–398. <https://doi.org/10.1016/j.ejon.2011.09.001>

Galvin, K., & Young, M. (2010). Family systems theory. In Gaff, C. L., & Bylund, C. L. (Eds.), *Family communication and genetics: Theory and practice*, pp. 102–119. Oxford: Oxford University Press.

Green, M. C. (2006). Narratives and cancer communication. *Journal of Communication*, *56*(s1), S163–S183. <https://doi.org/10.1111/j.1460-2466.2006.00288.x>

Green, M. C., & Brock, T. C. (2000). The role of transportation in the persuasiveness of public narratives. *Journal of Personality and Social Psychology*, *79*, 701–721. <https://doi.org/10.1037/0022-3514.79.5.701>

Harter, L. M., Japp, P. M., & Beck, C. S. (Eds.). (2005). *Narratives, health, and healing: Communication theory, research, and practice* (pp. xvii, 516). Lawrence Erlbaum Associates Publishers.

Herr, P. M. (1995). Whither fact, artifact, and attitude: Reflections on the theory of reasoned action. *Journal of Consumer Psychology*, *4*(4), 371–380. <https://doi.org/10.1207/s15327663jcp0404_04>

Hinyard, L. J., & Kreuter, M. W. (2007). Using narrative communication as a tool for health behavior change: A conceptual, theoretical, and empirical overview. *Health Education & Behavior: The Official Publication of the Society for Public Health Education*, *34*(5), 777–792. <https://doi.org/10.1177/1090198106291963>

Howlander, N., Noone, A. M., Krapcho, M., Miller, D., Brest, A., Yu, M., Ruhl, J., Tatalovich, Z., Mariotto, A., Lewis, D. R., Chen, H. S., Feuer, E. J., & Kronin, K. A. (2019). *SEER Cancer Statistics Review, 1975–2016*. National Cancer Institute. <https://seer.cancer.gov/csr/1975_2016/index.html>

Hunt, G., Longacre, M., Kent, E., & Weber-Raley, L. (2016). *Cancer caregiving in the US: An intense, episodic, and challenging care experience* (p. 34). National Alliance for Caregiving.

<https://www.caregiving.org/wp-content/uploads/2020/05/CancerCaregivingReport_FINAL_June-17-2016.pdf>

Kastrinos, A. L., Bylund, C. L., Mullis, M. D., Wollney, E., Sae-Hau, M., Weiss, E., & Fisher, C. L. (2022a). Parents caring for children diagnosed with a blood cancer from infancy to emerging adulthood: A life span perspective. *Journal of Adolescent and Young Adult Oncology*, *11*(1), 61–67. <https://doi.org/10.1089/jayao.2021.0070>

Kastrinos, A. L., Fisher, C. L., Mullis, M. D., Wollney, E., Sae-Hau, M., Weiss, E. S., & Bylund, C. L. (2022b). A lifespan approach to understanding family caregiver experiences of a blood cancer diagnosis. *Palliative & Supportive Care*, *20*(1), 22–29. <https://doi.org/10.1017/S1478951521000389>

Koerner, A. F., & Fitzpatrick, M. A. (2002). Toward a Theory of Family Communication. *Communication Theory*, *12*(1), 70–91. <https://doi.org/10.1111/j.1468-2885.2002.tb00260.x>

Lambert, S. D., Harrison, J. D., Smith, E., Bonevski, B., Carey, M., Lawsin, C., Paul, C., & Girgis, A. (2012). The unmet needs of partners and caregivers of adults diagnosed with cancer: A systematic review. *BMJ Supportive & Palliative Care*, *2*(3), 224–230. <https://doi.org/10.1136/bmjspcare-2012-000226>

Magsamen-Conrad, K., Checton, M. G., Venetis, M. K., & Greene, K. (2015). Communication efficacy and couples' cancer management: Applying a dyadic appraisal model. *Communication Monographs*, *82*(2), 179–200. <https://doi.org/10.1080/03637751.2014.971415>

Matarazzo, J. D. (1980). Behavioral health and behavioral medicine: Frontiers for a new health psychology. *American Psychologist*, *35*, 807–817. <https://doi.org/10.1037/0003-066X.35.9.807>

Mayer, R. E. (Ed.). (2014). *The Cambridge Handbook of Multimedia Learning* (2nd ed.). Cambridge University Press. <https://doi.org/10.1017/CBO9781139547369>

McDaniel, S. H., Hepworth, J., & Doherty, W. J. (1992). *Medical family therapy: A biopsychosocial approach to families with health problems* (pp. xxi, 295). Basic Books.

Mcqueen, A., & Kreuter, M. (2010). Women's cognitive and affective reactions to breast cancer survivor stories: A structural equation analysis. *Patient Education and Counseling*, *81 Suppl*, S15–21. <https://doi.org/10.1016/j.pec.2010.08.015>

Mullis, M. D., Fisher, C. L., Kastrinos, A. L., Sae-Hau, M., Weiss, E. S., Rajotte, M., & Bylund, C. L. (2023). Survivorship transitions in blood cancer: Identifying experiences and supportive care needs for caregivers. *Journal of Cancer Survivorship*, 1–11.

Nussbaum, J. F. (1989). *Life-span Communication: Normative Processes*. L. Erlbaum Associates.

Nussbaum, J. F. (2014). The handbook of lifespan communication. *(No Title)*.

Paige, S. R., Stellefson, M., Krieger, J. L., Anderson-Lewis, C., Cheong, J., & Stopka, C. (2018). Proposing a Transactional Model of eHealth Literacy: Concept Analysis. *Journal of Medical Internet Research*, *20*(10), e10175. <https://doi.org/10.2196/10175>

Paige, S. R., Stellefson, M., Krieger, J. L., Miller, M. D., Cheong, J., & Anderson-Lewis, C. (2019). Transactional eHealth literacy: Developing and testing a multi-dimensional instrument. *Journal of Health Communication*, *24*(10), 737–748. <https://doi.org/10.1080/10810730.2019.1666940>

Pailler, M. E., Johnson, T. M., Kuszczak, S., Attwood, K. M., Zevon, M. A., Griffiths, E., Thompson, J., Wang, E. S., & Wetzler, M. (2016). Adjustment to acute leukemia: The impact of social support and marital satisfaction on distress and quality of life among newly diagnosed patients and their caregivers. *Journal of Clinical Psychology in Medical Settings*, *23*(3), 298–309. <https://doi.org/10.1007/s10880-016-9459-6>

Pecchioni, L. L., Wright, K. B., & Nussbaum, J. F. (2005). *Life-span communication*. Routledge Taylor & Francis Group. <https://doi.org/10.4324/9781410613233>

Rauscher, E., Hesse, C., & Campbell-Salome, G. (2020). Applying family communication patterns to patient-provider communication: Examining perceptions of patient involvement, satisfaction, and medical adherence. *Journal of Health Communication*, *25*, 1–10. <https://doi.org/10.1080/10810730.2020.1728596>

Reason, P. (1994). Three approaches to participative inquiry. *Handbook of qualitative research* (pp. 324–339). Sage Publications, Inc.

Regan, T. W., Lambert, S. D., Kelly, B., Falconier, M., Kissane, D., & Levesque, J. V. (2015). Couples coping with cancer: Exploration of theoretical frameworks from dyadic studies. *Psycho-Oncology*, *24*(12), 1605–1617. <https://doi.org/10.1002/pon.3854>

Rolland, J. S. (1994). *Families, illness, and disability: An integrative treatment model* (pp. xvi, 320). Basic Books.

Rolland, J. S. (2005). Cancer and the family: An integrative model. *Cancer*, *104*(11 Suppl), 2584–2595. <https://doi.org/10.1002/cncr.21489>

Rolland, J. S., & Walsh, F. (2006). Facilitating family resilience with childhood illness and disability. *Current Opinion in Pediatrics*, *18*(5), 527–538. <https://doi.org/10.1097/01.mop.0000245354.83454.68>

Rubin, H., & Rubin, I. (1986). *Community Organizing and Development*. <https://www.semanticscholar.org/paper/Community-Organizing-and-Development-Rubin-Rubin/25665078934002f8f8242fd159b07224a44c9d3a>

Samuelsson, M., Wennick, A., Jakobsson, J., & Bengtsson, M. (2021). Models of support to family members during the trajectory of cancer: A scoping review. *Journal of Clinical Nursing*, *30*(21–22), 3072–3098. <https://doi.org/10.1111/jocn.15832>

Schwartz, G. E., & Weiss, S. M. (1978). Yale conference on behavioral medicine: A proposed definition and statement of goals. *Journal of Behavioral Medicine*, *1*(1), 3–12. <https://doi.org/10.1007/BF00846582>

Spira, M., & Kenemore, E. (2000). Adolescent daughters of mothers with breast cancer: Impact and implications. *Clinical Social Work Journal*, *28*(2), 183–195. <https://doi.org/10.1023/A:1005106301713>

Stiffler, D., Barada, B., Hosei, B., & Haase, J. (2008). When mom has breast cancer: Adolescent daughters' experiences of being parented. *Oncology Nursing Forum*, *35*(6), 933–940. <https://doi.org/10.1188/08.ONF.933-940>

Sunwolf, Frey, L. R., & Keränen, L. Lynn M. Harter, Phyllis M. Japp, Christina S. Beck (2005). Rx story prescriptions: Healing effects of storytelling and storylistening in the practice of medicine. In *Narratives, health, and healing: Communication theory, research, and pratices* (pp. 237–257). Lawrence Erlbaum Associates Publishers. <https://www.academia.edu/15427515/Rx_Story_Prescriptions_The_Healing_Effects_of_Storytelling_and_Storylistening_in_the_Practice_of_Medicine_2005_>

Surbone A, Baider L, Weitzman TS, Brames MJ, Rittenberg CN, Johnson J (2010). Psychosocial care for patients and their families is integral to supportive care in cancer: MASCC position statement. *Support Care Cancer 18*, 255–263.

Teixeira, R., & Pereira, M. G. (2014). Family caregiver support to cancer patients: The relevance of adult children. In M. Paludi (Ed.), *The Praeger handbook on women's cancers: Personal and psychosocial insights* (pp. 305–333). Praeger.

Thompson, T., Ketcher, D., Gray, T. F., & Kent, E. E. (2021). The Dyadic Cancer Outcomes Framework: A general framework of the effects of cancer on patients and informal caregivers. *Social Science & Medicine, 287*, 114357.

Ussher, J. M., Perz, J., Hawkins, Y., & Brack, M. (2009). Evaluating the efficacy of psycho-social interventions for informal carers of cancer patients: A systematic review of the research literature. *Health Psychology Review*, *3*(1), 85–107. <https://doi.org/10.1080/17437190903033401>

Vasquez, T. S., Bylund, C. L., Fisher, C. L., & Paige, S. R. (2022). Validation of the transactional eHealth literacy instrument with cancer caregivers. *PEC Innovation*, *1*, 100075.

Wagner, D. (1991). Reviving the action research model: Combining case and cause with dislocated workers. *Social Work*, *36*(6), 477–482. <https://doi.org/10.1093/sw/36.6.477>

Wellisch, D. K., Ormseth, S. R., Hartoonian, N., & Owen, J. E. (2012). A retrospective study predicting psychological vulnerability in adult daughters of breast cancer patients. *Families, Systems, & Health*, *30*, 253–264. <https://doi.org/10.1037/a0029638>

Wollney, E. N., Bylund, C. L., Kastrinos, A. L., Campbell-Salome, G., Sae-Hau, M., Weiss, E. S., & Fisher, C. L. (2023). Understanding parents' uncertainty sources and management strategies while caring for a child diagnosed with a hematologic cancer. *PEC Innovation*, *3*, 100198.

Wright, K. B., Bylund, C. L., Vasquez, T. S., Mullis, M. D., Sae-Hau, M., Weiss, E. S., Bagautdinova, D., & Fisher, C. L. (2023). Adult-child caregivers' family communication experiences after an older parent's blood cancer diagnosis: a survey exploring their openness, avoidance, and social support. *Cancers*, *15*(12), 3177.

Yuen, E. Y. N., Dodson, S., Batterham, R. W., Knight, T., Chirgwin, J., & Livingston, P. M. (2016). Development of a conceptual model of cancer caregiver health literacy. *European Journal of Cancer Care*, *25*(2), 294–306. <https://doi.org/10.1111/ecc.12284>

Zimmermann, C., Yuen, D., Mischitelle, A., Minden, M. D., Brandwein, J. M., Schimmer, A., Gagliese, L., Lo, C., Rydall, A., & Rodin, G. (2013). Symptom burden and supportive care in patients with acute leukemia. *Leukemia Research*, *37*(7), 731–736. <https://doi.org/10.1016/j.leukres.2013.02.009>

CHAPTER FIVE

# Influence of Topic Avoidance, Willingness to Communicate about Health, and Social Support on Health Issues across the Life Span: Theoretical Underpinnings and Two Applied Studies

KEVIN B. WRIGHT AND MOLLIE R. CANZONA

Many health problems that individuals face across the lifespan present interpersonal communication challenges. For example, in close interpersonal networks such as families, it can be difficult for people to talk to their loved ones about topics such as death and dying, emotions they are experiencing due to an illness, or their family members may have insufficient information or understanding about the health issue a person is facing. Family members may wish to avoid talking about difficult topics, or patients may not be willing to discuss health problems or negative emotions with family members and close friends because they do not want to burden or alarm them. Researchers have found that weaker interpersonal ties, such as clergy, therapists, support group members, and online social network members are often able to help individuals who experience these types of issues when discussing health concerns with closer ties such as family members and close friends (Fingerman, 2009; Huxhold et al., 2020; Wright & Miller, 2010; Wright & Rains, 2013).

In recent years, health communication scholars have become interested in the ability of online social networks to help individuals facing health issues manage interpersonal communication issues such as topic avoidance and willingness to communicate about health (Sin et al., 2018; Wright et al., 2019). In addition, online social networks, such as online support communities, can be important sources of informational, emotional, and even tangible support (e.g., online communities that are associated with a certain city or region) (Rains & Wright, 2016). Online support has been linked to a variety of positive health outcomes, such as reduced stress, depression, increased quality of life, greater information about health issues, and lower incident rates of physical health problems in a variety of studies (Hong et al, 2012; Rains & Wright, 2016; Rains & Young, 2009).

Despite these positive aspects of online social networks when it comes to communicating about health, online networks can also lead to negative outcomes. These include the rapid spread of misinformation about health issues, encountering individuals in online communities who attempt to take advantage of people with health problems by suggesting ineffective remedies or treatments, or not being able to reach people online during times when support is needed (Harkin et al., 2020; Owen et al., 2017). In addition, people's perceptions of online social network members can be skewed by the characteristics of the online communication channels they use (Walther, 1996). For example, social media platforms that are text based or have reduced ability to transmit nonverbal information may limit a person's ability to decipher some messages or allow them to process social information about people they talk to online (Walther, 1996; Walther & Whitty, 2021).

While many individuals use online social networks for social support when communicating about difficult health-related topics, others prefer having such conversations in the face-to-face world, including supportive interactions with both strong and weak ties. In other cases, people may initiate difficult conversations about health and seek social support using a combination of online and face-to-face social networks (Reich et al., 2012). As we describe below, the decision to talk about sensitive health issues is complex and influenced by a number of interpersonal communication and relational factors (Hether et al., 2014).

As scholars have learned more about interpersonal communication processes in online social networks, a number of researchers have tried to gain a better understanding of the advantages of online social networks when developing health interventions (Maher et al., 2014; Wright et al., 2019). Social media health interventions can take advantage of online social network characteristics, such as working with trusted online community leaders or influencers to help disseminate health intervention messages to the larger online community. In addition, researchers can develop intervention messages that encourage people to talk to others in their interpersonal networks about specific health issues (both online and face-to-face), prevention behaviors they can take to avoid health problems, or information and other types of support that can help people manage health issues. Online social media networks allow researchers to create and spread health intervention messages that can provide more tailored information, reach large audiences more rapidly, and increase interactivity with others compared to traditional media interventions (see Günther et al., 2021; Maher et al., 2014).

This chapter examines three important interpersonal communication issues that are prevalent within a variety of health issues that individuals encounter across the lifespan, including coping with one's own health risks or issues as well as caring for a family member or loved one who is facing health problems. These include openness and avoidance of certain health-related topics or concerns, a person's willingness to communicate about health, and interpersonal benefits and challenges of supportive relationships (face-to-face and online). Toward that end, the chapter discusses the concepts of openness/avoidance, willingness to communicate about health (WTHC), interpersonal issues in social support from a lifespan perspective, and how this body of research was used to develop two different studies conducted by the authors. The chapter concludes by discussing how these concepts may help researchers develop similar types of health interventions in the future as well as the advantages and limitations of such approaches.

## INTERPERSONAL CHALLENGES ASSOCIATED WITH DISCUSSING HEALTH ISSUES: OPENNESS/AVOIDANCE

Topic avoidance (TA) occurs in close relationships when a person strategically decides not to disclose information (Afifi & Guerrero, 2000). Individuals are motivated to topic avoid for a variety of reasons, including self-, other-, and relationship-protection, conflict prevention, negative response avoidance, and to maintain "'normalcy' in close relationships" (Afifi & Guerrero, 2000; Caughlin & Afifi, 2004). Communicating about health issues can be difficult for relational partners, particularly in cases such as an illness diagnosis (or when a family member is diagnosed). Topic avoidance is important in terms of helping people cope with illness, manage distress, fulfill needs, and promote better health outcomes for themselves, the patient, and family members (Fisher, 2010; Wittenberg et al., 2017). Individuals may find it difficult to express the right words, fear saying the wrong thing, or family members and other close relational partners may not want to engage in conversations about difficult health-related topics. Family members do not always communicate openly about health and may avoid illness-related topics (Goldsmith et al., 2007; Wright & Frey, 2008).

Topic avoidance is seen frequently within family caregiver–patient relationships, and while sometimes beneficial, it has also been linked to negative mental health outcomes for patients and caregivers (Venetis et al., 2015). For example, Zhang and Siminoff (2003) found that among lung cancer patients, 65 % of family members reported reluctance to discuss particular topics. Moreover, not disclosing health concerns has been linked to increased depression, anxiety, and patient distress (Donovan-Kicken & Caughlin, 2010; Manne, 1999). In situations where patients do not have someone they can communicate their concerns about health issues, this can increase their risk for depression (Donovan-Kicken & Caughlin, 2010). In contrast, in relationships where partners communicate about health issues more openly, researchers have found that openness about discussing health issues is linked to physical and relational health outcomes (Fisher et al., 2017)

Avoidance and openness patterns tend to vary in terms of contextual factors like the specific relationship (e.g., spouses versus parent-child), type of illness, and cultural factors (Goldsmith & Miller, 2014). In the context of health interventions, resources for patients and their loved ones (particularly caregivers) should be tailored to a patient's specific needs as well as the caregiver's situation. One systematic review study found that caregiver interventions that teach communication skills may decrease caregiver burden and enhance quality of life (Waldron et al., 2013).

Relational partners may avoid health-related topics for a variety of reasons. In some cases, the decision to avoid discussing health-related topics might be motivated by the perception that one's health is a private issue (Fisher et al., 2017). For example, older generations in the United States were socialized to keep health issues private whereas younger generations experienced less privacy boundaries (Fisher et al., 2017). Avoiding discussions about health problems may help people maintain a sense of hope or normalcy (Goldsmith et al., 2007). Studies have found that patients and their close relational partners avoid excessive talk about cancer to maintain well-balanced lives, focus on enjoyable topics during what may be a limited remaining lifespan, or maintain a hopeful attitude (Fisher, 2010; Salander & Spetz, 2002). Patients report hesitancy when it comes to sharing distressing feelings (e.g., anger), believing such disclosures could exacerbate negative affect (Fisher et al, 2017). Additionally, midlife children of parents who have been diagnosed with a disease describe challenges with sharing information about the diagnosis, decisions, and mortality (Caughlin et al., 2011). They also avoid discussing their feeling of uncertainty about the future (e.g., their parent's prognosis) and are more open about non-emotional topics like treatment logistics (Caughlin et al.,

2011). Patterns of avoiding health-related discussions can differ depending upon the topic. For example, specific topics that are commonly avoided within cancer-related communication include death, emotions, fears, worries, sexuality, treatment, being a burden, future plans, and bodily change (Donovan-Kicken & Caughlin, 2010; Goldsmith et al., 2007).

Family social support is associated with health-related topic avoidance (Jeong et al., 2016). Various types of social support may be impeded if families avoid health-related topics (Boinon et al., 2014). Conversely, sharing health-related experiences can facilitate the receipt of support. When families engage in more health-related discussions, these interactions can be opportunities for social support exchanges (Salander & Spetz, 2002). For example, when patients and their family members or caregivers communicate openly about illness, they have opportunities to provide or exchange emotional support (Song et al., 2014). Additionally, perceived social support from family members can help facilitate the discussion of difficult topics (Jeong et al., 2016). For example, people feel more comfortable discussing difficult topics when they feel supported by family members. Social support has been linked with better health outcomes, including less burden and depressive symptoms for caregivers and less distress, side effects, and lower mortality rates for patients (Kronke et al., 2006).

## WILLINGNESS TO COMMUNICATE ABOUT HEALTH ISSUES

Similar to other contexts of communication (see MCroskey & Richmond, 1987), people vary in their willingness to communicate about a variety of topics in general, and there is evidence that individuals vary in their willingness to communicate about health issues (Canzona et al., 2019; Smith et al., 2004). In contrast to health-related topic avoidance, willingness to communicate about health is conceptualized as a general trait that influences communication patterns related to discussing health concerns (Wright & Frey, 2008; Wright et al., 2007;). In addition, willingness to communicate about health plays a key role in patient self-advocacy and patient empowerment, which has been linked to improved outcomes (Logan et al., 2016; Thomas et al., 2021; Thomas et al., 2023). Initiating conversations is a critical communication moment with its own motivations, features, and consequences (Smith et al., 2014). Decisions to initiate difficult conversations about health can influence subsequent interactions, help-seeking behaviors, and physical and psychological outcomes (Travers & Taylor, 2016; Wright & Frey, 2008).

There are many other situations where people may be more willing to communicate about their health with other people who share similar healthcare needs, such as in support groups (Smith et al., 2004; Wright & Rains, 2016). Online support communities often provide a space for people living with health problems to obtain experienced-based advice from other community members, information about disease trajectories, medications and other treatments, and reduced stigmatization of a person's health issue since others in the support group or community are dealing with similar health concerns (Wright & Miller, 2010). In addition, studies have found that people experience less stigmatization when communicating with weaker ties in contexts such as online support communities (Wright & Rains, 2013). Other studies have found that people are often more willing to communicate about health concerns with online weaker ties in online communities. Studies have found that it is less interpersonally risky to disclose sensitive information (especially to someone who has similar health problems) compared to closer interpersonal relationships where relational history, conflicts, and interpersonal boundary issues may make it more difficult to discuss health concerns (Wright & Miller, 2010).

## SOCIAL SUPPORT AND THE DYNAMIC NATURE OF RELATIONSHIPS ACROSS THE LIFESPAN

Decades of research studies have found that our social networks and interpersonal relationships have a substantial impact on our physical health and our psychological well-being (Berkman & Syme, 1979; Rains & Wright, 2016; Uchino et al., 2012). Studies have shown that people with low social support levels have a higher risk of mortality compared to people who have stronger and more satisfying support networks (Berkman & Syme, 1979; Uchino et al., 2012). In addition to being positively correlated with health, positive types of social network support can reinforce health behavior change, while negative types of social network influence can undermine health behavior change (Goldsmith, 2004). Research indicates that negative aspects of social networks and relationships can lead to negative health outcomes. For example, relational conflict, role obligations, and unwanted or insensitive advice from a friend can increase stress levels and lead to negative health outcomes (Goldsmith, 2004). Other problems related to social networks and social support can occur due to a variety of differing perceptions, cultural influences, and other environmental factors (Wright, 2016). Social network members may avoid communicating with a person or fail to provide satisfying support when it is needed most.

Researchers have found that this often happens when an individual is seeking support for a stigmatized health condition (Wright & Miller, 2010; Wright &

Rains, 2013). For example, cancer and other life-threatening disease sometimes frighten people into silence or avoidance. Moreover, inadequate support from friends may occur if they feel that you have brought on your own health problems through unhealthy lifestyle decisions, such as over-eating, smoking, or drinking alcohol (Goldsmith, 2004). Our social support networks are dynamic and often change dramatically throughout the life span, or due to positive and negative stressful life events, such as the birth of a child or a life-threatening illness diagnosis (Goldsmith, 2004). Health campaign researchers have become increasingly aware of the need to integrate social networks and interpersonal relationships into population-based healthcare interventions (Abroms & Maibach, 2008; Chee et al., 2016). These social relationships are often important in terms of helping target audience members change and maintain healthy behaviors, such as diet and exercise or screening for various health conditions.

With the rise of the Internet and the rise of social media platforms, numerous researchers have examined ways in which online communication may facilitate openness, willingness to communicate about health issues, and how online communities and relationships influence people's ability to mobilize social support (Rains et al., 2015, 2018; Rains & Wright, 2016). This body of research suggests that computer-mediated communication may make it easier to mitigate some of the relational challenges associated with seeking and providing support in face-to-face interaction (for a review, see Wright et al., 2011). One important factor motivating people to seek support online appears to be a preference for support from weak ties (Wright & Miller, 2010). Weak ties can be particularly valuable when strong ties such as family and friends are unable or unwilling to provide support, including due to health-related topic avoidance or unwillingness to communicate (Adelman et al., 1987; Wright & Bell, 2003; Wright & Miller, 2010). Relative to strong ties, weak ties can be more objective, provide novel information, and present less potential for role conflict (Wright & Miller, 2010).

Several studies have shown that individuals who prefer weak-tie support are more inclined to participate in computer-mediated support groups or experience greater benefits from their participation (Wright & Rains, 2013; Wright et al., 2012). Other research indicates that factors such as anonymity (Tanis, 2009), similarity (Wright, 2002), and accessibility (Walther & Boyd, 2002) are additional reasons that individuals may choose from computer-mediated resources for acquiring social support. Health-related online support groups/communities are frequently used by individuals with rare health conditions/issues, conditions/issues that are difficult for healthcare providers to explain in layperson terms, or if members of one's primary social network (i.e., friends and family members) have limited knowledge of their health condition (Tanis, 2008; Campbell-Grossman et al., 2009; Rains, 2018).

There is also evidence that online support is associated with beneficial health outcomes (De Jong et al., 2014; Hong et al., 2012; Rains & Young, 2009). Rains and Young (2009), for example, conducted a meta-analytic review of research on computer-mediated support group interventions and found that online support group participation resulted in increased social support, quality of life, and self-efficacy among members. However, many individuals may prefer to communicate about sensitive health issues with weak ties (or a combination of weak and strong ties) within their face-to-face social networks (Reich et al., 2012; Rozzell et al., 2014). In other cases, people may seek social support through a combination of online and face-to-face social networks depending upon a variety of factors, including trust, convenience, relational history, socialization, and cultural influences (Hether et al., 2014; Reich et al., 2012, Ye, 2006).

## APPLYING THE CONCEPTS OF HEALTH-RELATED TOPIC AVOIDANCE, WILLINGNESS TO COMMUNICATION ABOUT HEALTH, AND INTERPERSONAL ISSUES IN SOCIAL SUPPORT: TWO STUDIES

This section provides an overview of two studies conducted by the authors of this chapter that applied the concepts of health-related topic avoidance, willingness to communicate about health, and interpersonal issues related to social support. This is followed by a brief conclusion section that highlights the implications of both studies for future interpersonal health communication research from a life span perspective.

## SOCIAL MEDIA INTERVENTION TARGETING ENVIRONMENTAL BREAST CANCER RISK STUDY

Wright et al. (2019) developed a social media intervention targeting mother/daughter discussion about environmental breast cancer risk. The purpose of the study was to develop a partnership with bloggers who focus on motherhood/family issues to disseminate evidence-based information about environmental breast cancer risk to blog readers (mothers) as well as to encourage conversations about environmental breast cancer with daughters.

## Study Background

Social media intervention studies show that blogger-reader interactions can create a sense of immediacy about health topics that encourages readers' adoption of healthy behaviors (Bissonnette-Maheux et al., 2018). Moreover, the tailored context of the blog, in conjunction with readers' perceived source similarity (Lu, 2013), can influence women's adoption of recommended health behaviors (Bissonnette-Maheux et al., 2018). However, despite the potential for mommy bloggers to serve as trusted or relatable sources to disseminate breast cancer risk information to mothers, it is critical that bloggers disseminate accurate, scientifically informed content (Kulkami et al, 2018). Content should in part be *user-generated* with a target audience in mind, meaning that it should be produced in part with the bloggers' input (Korda & Itani, 2013). To achieve this, the researchers were interested in collaborative message development (between scientists and bloggers) to tailor messages to mothers and daughters in an effort to ensure that the women and their daughters received accurate information in a format they trust and relate to. The bloggers also encouraged readers to share this information with their daughters and provide emotional support in their conversations about environmental breast cancer risk.

The study was funded by an NIH grant through its Breast Cancer Environment Research Program (BCERP). The researchers posited that the intervention would influence women's exposure to, acceptance, and beliefs about environmental risks while promoting their intention to adopt risk-reducing behaviors. BCERP provides several educational materials online, including a toolkit for mothers with daughters. These mother-daughter–focused materials specifically address how mothers can reduce their own and their daughter's risk by adopting healthier lifestyle choices together (e.g., eliminating products with BPA and phthalates). Previous research suggested that when mothers advise daughters about how to reduce risk, daughters adhere to their mother's advice into adulthood (Sinicrope, 2009). Talking about breast cancer risk can be challenging. Younger daughters often avoid or withdraw from such conversations (Fisher, 2010), which can trigger a physiological stress response (Berlin et al., 2013).

## Participants and Recruitment

The researchers partnered with 75 mommy bloggers—mothers who write in "mommy blogs" about their maternal role. There are nearly 4 million female bloggers, and mothers increasingly turn to these blogs for health information (Sinicrope, 2009). Using BCERP scientific evidence, we developed an infographic that targets mothers and daughters on four lifestyle recommendations to reduce environmental risk of breast cancer. We asked a diverse group of bloggers to integrate the infographic and the BCERP toolkit hyperlink into a blog post.

The intervention group was comprised of 445 blog readers who followed one or more of the 75 bloggers the researchers partnered with in the intervention. The participating mommy bloggers were asked to recruit their readers and direct them to an online post-intervention survey link. A total of 353 blog readers made up the reader comparison group. To minimize contamination between the two groups, readers in the comparison group were recruited through a separate set of mommy bloggers who were affiliated with "The Motherhood" network, but who did not blog about breast cancer and were not involved in the intervention. The comparison group bloggers wrote about a wide range of issues, including parenting concerns and other health issues besides breast cancer. The intervention group completed an online post-intervention survey after the message exposure period. Blog readers recruited for the reader comparison group completed the same post-intervention online survey as the intervention group.

Our goal was to develop a message that was based on scientific evidence as well as informed by the community we sought to reach. First, to develop a scientifically informed message suitable for social media dissemination, the research team analyzed BCERP's online educational materials targeting mothers and daughters. Four (actionable steps) themes that would provide mothers with actionable steps they could take to reduce their own and their daughter's environmental risk for breast cancer development were identified. To facilitate social media dissemination, an infographic message with the four steps was created using language extracted from BCERP's materials to ensure that information was accurate and uneditable. Second, the authors sought to ensure that the message disseminated would also be community-informed (or user-generated) to better ensure women identified with the information. This aspect involved the bloggers adding their own content in addition to posting the infographic for their readers.

Participating bloggers were provided with a document that included the study protocol and instructions about when and how to integrate the image or intervention message into their blog post. Bloggers were asked to post these messages during the National Breast Cancer Awareness Month (October-November 2017) that included the infographic and narrative that encouraged mothers to talk with their daughters about environmental breast cancer risk. Bloggers were asked to include two sentences of text to identify the source of the information (BCERP). To ensure that information disseminated on the blog was in part user-generated, bloggers were asked to use their experience with their blog audience to integrate the infographic and required text in a manner that they felt would be appealing to them. Bloggers were not required but encouraged to promote their post via other social media channels. Finally, bloggers were asked to post a message with links to the surveys to remind readers to complete the online reader survey.

## Analysis of Online Engagement with Intervention Group Blog Messages

To assess the degree to which the intervention encouraged interaction about breast cancer risk messages among blog users, the researchers used an online tracking program (*Tracx*) to capture blog and related online social media content associated with the targeted online blog intervention. *Tracx* is a social media monitoring and analytics program that uses Boolean search querying to track posts, mentions, and conversations across different online channels (e.g., social media platforms, news outlets, blogs, and forums) through the program algorithms. Additionally, it populates the number of author's followers and total engagements per post. The sample was collected between October 1 and December 31, 2017, corresponding with the start of the intervention and two months following it.

## Study Findings

The intervention was successful in terms of diffusion (reaching more than 400 mothers) and impact. Compared to women (bloggers and readers) not exposed to the intervention group messages, women recalling the infographic/blog reported being significantly more satisfied with the information, significantly more likely to engage in risk-reducing behavior, and significantly more likely to share it with daughters than the comparison group. In terms of the online engagement analysis, the *Trax* analysis found that the original 75 seeded blog posts were shared by participants 2153 times across multiple social media platforms, and 524 users commented on the data (a content analysis of the comments was conducted in a subsequent study, see Wright et al., 2021). Moreover, the results indicated that blog readers who were exposed to (and specifically recalled) the seeded intervention message adapted from BCERP guidance had significantly higher breast cancer risk information exposure scores, higher breast cancer risk, and prevention information satisfaction and influence scores than those who did not see (or recall).

## Implications

The findings are consistent with previous theory and research on the influence of social networks and opinion leaders within them on health perceptions (see Chang et al., 2015). Online opinion leaders may be important sources of informational support for women facing health issues such as cancer. The findings of the

Wright et al. (2019) study suggest that these types of online opinion leaders may be key to enhancing health messages, tailoring health messages, as well as the delivery and impact of health risk information to audiences such as mothers. In addition, online opinion leaders may be influential despite typically being perceived as possessing relatively weaker social ties compared to friends or family members. Such sources of online social support may help obtain a variety of suggestions for how to talk to daughters and other family members about health risks by drawing upon the collective experiences of other blogger (or similar social media platforms) readers/participants. This type of informational support may be helpful in terms of helping people initiate sensitive (and often difficult) conversations between family members and other close ties about cancer risk or other health concerns. Future research should continue to test the efficacy of similar social media interventions that attempt to spur interpersonal conversations about health-related issues between family members and friends at different points in the life span. For example, scholars can tailor their interventions to at-risk groups who are at different points in their lifespan, such as attempts to increase interpersonal conversations about disease risk and prevention when people are younger, or interventions that focus on enhancing social support for caregivers for middle-aged or older individuals (when terminal illness is more likely to occur). Finally, future researchers should consider other factors that might influence topic avoidance, willingness to communicate about health, and supportive communication, including culture, relational history, and age or maturity, which make these types of conversations more challenging to navigate.

## UNDERSTANDING WHAT SHAPES BREAST CANCER SURVIVORS' WILLINGNESS TO COMMUNICATE WITH PROVIDERS ABOUT SEXUAL HEALTH STUDY

Canzona et al. (2019) examined breast cancer survivors (BCSs) willingness to communicate about sexual health (WTCSH). The purpose of this mixed-methods sequential explanatory study was (1) to understand what may impede survivors' ability to self-advocate and address sexual health-related quality of life concerns with healthcare providers, (2) to develop preliminary recommendations for clinical practice, and (3) to inform future development of communication resources to empower patients and providers to initiate and engage in these often-challenging conversations.

## Study Background

Sexual health (SH) can be defined as the physical, psychological, and social well-being experiences to sexual function (World Health Organization, 2020). SH concerns such as vaginal atrophy, difficulty with orgasm, body image and self-esteem concerns, and communication challenges with partners vary across adulthood and persist or worsen in survivorship for over 50 % of breast cancer survivors (Razaei et al., 2016; Tuinman et al., 2010). As women transition to survivorship, they begin to prioritize quality of life issues like SH but have few resources to have them manage conversations in the clinic (Ganz, 2000; Halley et al., 2014). One study found that up to 90 % of survivors said their oncologist seldom addresses SH (Halley et al., 2014). In another study, 40 % of BCSs indicated a desire to discuss SH with providers, but only 7 % of women reported they initiated those conversations (Hill et al., 2011).

Providers report hesitancy in initiating these conversations and suggest clinical barriers such as time constraints prevent them from treating SH issues (Canzona et al., 2018; Halley et al., 2014). This dynamic is complicated by the fact that BCSs see a range of providers. After primary treatment, women return to primary care but continue to see their cancer specialists for surveillance. Primary care providers and specialists like gynecology and oncology providers report conflicting perspectives about who is best suited to address SH concerns (Canzona et al., 2018). This is especially problematic because over time women can become resigned to SH distress, which is associated with disease interference, symptom severity, and poorer quality of life (Reese et al., 2010a, 2010b).

Self-advocacy is central component of patient empowerment, linked to a variety of health outcomes (Hagan et al., 2018; Wright et al., 2007). Healthcare-related self-advocacy involves (a) possessing medical knowledge to contribute to decision-making, (b) willingness to introduce topics and pursue clarification, and (3) willingness to challenge providers when treatments are inadequate or do not align with patient needs or values (Hagan et al., 2018). Thus, willingness to discuss this issue is probable factor contributing SH outcomes (Wright et al., 2007; Wright et al., 2008).

## Participants and Procedures

Recruitment materials were administered to cancer navigators and oncology social workers in hospitals and disseminated via support groups. BCSs who (1) completed primary cancer treatment (chemotherapy, radiation, or surgery) and (2) were at least 18 years old were eligible to patriciate. Representative samples from three stages of adulthood were pursued: young adults (under 40), middle adults (40–59), and older adults (60+) (Oktay & Walter, 1991). We collected and analyzed quantitative data to inform qualitative data collection and analysis (see also Canzona et al., 2019).

In the quantitative phase, 305 BCSs completed a 43-item survey to capture women's socio-demographics, medical information, SH outcomes, provider patterns, and willingness to communicate about sexual health. Sociodemographic/medical information included adulthood stage, marital status, race/ethnicity, education, employment, and income, as well as survivorship length, cancer stage, treatment type, and menopause/ovarian failure status (Smith et al., 2014). SH was measured using the 18-item Sexual Quality of Life—Female (SQOL-F) scale (Berger & Calabrese, 1975), with higher scores reflecting better SQOL. The SQOL-F demonstrated high reliability. According to the validation research, women without sexual dysfunction had mean scores of 80.1 (Berger & Calabrese, 1975). Provider patterns were assessed by asking women who they considered their primary general healthcare provider and which provider would they approach to discuss an SH concern. Wright et al.'s (2007) Willingness to Communicate about Health Scale (WTCH) scale was adapted to the Willingness to Communicate about Sexual Health (WTCSH) scale. Items included statements like "I'm comfortable talking about sexual health issues with healthcare providers in survivorship" on a 5-point Likert scale. Higher scores indicated more willingness to communicate. Principal component analysis extracted one factor for the WTCSH scale. The WTCSH demonstrated satisfactory reliability.

Quantitative findings suggested that (1) SH concerns were relevant for women across stages of adulthood and survivorship spectrums, (2) WTCSH was comparable across groups, (3) survivors interact with a range of provider types, and (4) women report confusion about whom to see for SH issues, and there is a reluctance to make appointments to discuss these concerns. Therefore, sampling for the qualitative phase sought representation from all developmental groups and survivorship lengths. Interview questions were designed to assess interaction with a range of providers and to explore what may contribute to confusion about provider selection and appointments.

During the qualitative phase, the Critical Incident Technique (CIT) was used to conduct interviews with 40 women from phase one (12 = young adulthood <40 years old; 16 = middle adulthood 41–59 years old; 12 = older adulthood 60+ years old). Before the interviews, women were instructed to write a reflection. The narrative prompt invited participants to write about a moment, conversation, or event she believed was a representative example of how her SH had changed after primary breast cancer treatment. Reflections were used to prime participants and interviewers. The interviewer first addressed the women's writing and subsequently elicited their SH concerns and their perceptions and experiences about SH communication in the clinic. Frequencies and hierarchical multiple regression were conducted to analyze the quantitative data. Regression analyses controlled for sociodemographic/medical data when testing the association between WTCSH on SQOL. The constant comparative method (Glaser & Strauss, 1967) was used to conduct thematic analyses of factors informing willingness to initiate SH conversations. Codes were attached to text demonstrating these factors. Related codes were clustered, and themes and their properties were developed and revised. Data associated with survivors from different stages of adulthood and survivorship lengths were compared to explore if and how themes and properties differed by place along the life span or time elapsed since primary treatment.

## Findings

No statistically significant differences in SQOL or WTCSH were found by age or survivorship length. However, there was a statistically significant positive relationship between WTCSH and SQOL. Additionally, we uncovered five themes that shaped women's WTCSH. Theme 1, comfort discussing SH, was influenced by the degree to which talking about SH was normalized in women's healthcare conversations: if discussing sex was taboo in their family or dominant culture; if women felt sharing SH concerns led to unfair, negative judgments; and if women were embarrassed by discussing body parts or physiological SH-related processes. Theme 2, perception of demographic similarity/discordance with provider, revealed that willingness to talk about SH was facilitated by feeling concordant with the provider in terms of age or gender. Theme 3, patient-centered communication behaviors, illustrated the ways in which perception of provider listening, provider prioritizing patients' concerns, and provider displaying nonverbals that convey discomfort shapes WTCSH. Theme 4, belief that SH is (un)treatable, revealed that when women think solutions to SH distress are unavailable and judge providers do not possess the knowledge needed to address SH issues, and they are less likely to be willing to bring up SH. Theme 5, inability to access timely or coordinated care, suggests that navigating poor communication/coordination among providers, confusion about which addresses SH, struggling with access issues, and feeling pressure to discuss other concerns due to time constraints shape women's communication choices.

## Implications

Our results connected lower WTCSH to lower SQOL, which contrasts research that found lower sexual satisfaction is related to a higher likelihood that patients will bring up SH with providers (Flynn et al., 2012). While both pathways are valid, it is important to consider how these dynamic intrapersonal-, interpersonal-, and organizational-level factors shape survivors' willingness to initiate these conversations—especially since previous work found that providers may assume if women have SH concerns, they will broach the topic themselves (Canzona et al., 2018). Results reveal three applied clinical recommendations to support women's WTCSH and SH healthcare: (1) assess the nature and impact of previous patient–provider messaging about QOL concerns, (2) recognize and honor patients' desire to be seen by and to relate to providers, and (3) explore patient perceptions about the feasibility of enhancing sexual health-related QOL.

Providers can explore if/how a history of patient–provider messaging can influence their patients' subsequent disclosures. When women reported their providers previously stated QOL concerns are important, and that the clinic was a "safe space" to discuss them participants said they were comfortable bringing up the topic. Participants who reported providers previously dismissed QOL concerns, or implied survivors should feel "lucky to be here" when they broached other topics like fatigue or headaches, suggested they were less likely to disclose SH concerns for fear providers would judge them. Communication behavior data with this level of specificity is needed to design effective communication training for providers (Canzona et al., 2016). Patient education resources and media campaigns that challenge erroneous notions of the appropriateness and importance of discussing SH may also facilitate disclosures.

Women reported a need for providers to see and relate to them as individuals. This was perceived to be more difficult when patients had appointments with providers who were dissimilar to them in terms of age or gender. Older BCSs encountered ageist stereotypes and younger women struggled to communicate with older providers perceived as "parental figures." Medical education can be designed to address stereotypes and make providers aware of intergenerational dynamics that may be impacting patient WTCSH. Providers can explore and validate patient concerns around discordant demographic dynamics and elicit their preferences for communicating with a clinician about SH. Further, patient education materials that represent women across adulthood and include examples of obstacles women face, connected to communication strategies for engaging with providers, may enhance their ability to self-advocate.

Our data suggest it would be beneficial to explore patient perceptions about the feasibility of treating SH distress. Women in this study suggested they "wouldn't bother" to broach the topic because it would be a "waste of time," because medical treatments for their SH do not exist, or that providers do not have the knowledge to help them. Specifically, women described an overarching belief that female sexuality was too complicated and that because (they believed) HRT was the only option, there was nothing that could be done to relieve SH distress. However, treatments such as counseling, HRT for patients in different preparation, and vaginal moisturizers/numbing creams are available, among other options, do exist (Reese et al., 2017). Furthermore, if concerns about provider training are informing women's WTCSH, providers can tell patients that even if they are not equipped to treat every QOL concern, they can connect survivors with suitable persons/resources. Women stated they felt like providers were sometimes "passing the buck" by offering "empty (non-specific) referrals" that were not coordinated. Organizing and following up on referrals specifically to discuss SH and including SH in survivorship care plans may increase the probability SH will be addressed.

## CONCLUSION

Both studies suggest several implications for the study of health-related topic avoidance, willingness to communicate about health, and supportive communication from a life span perspective as well as issues to consider for future research. For example, the findings from the Wright et al. (2019) intervention suggest the importance of providing target audience members with the option of discussing interpersonally sensitive health issues, such as breast cancer risk, with close ties (e.g., daughters and other family members) as well as online weaker ties (e.g., fellow blog readers or other weak ties across social media platforms). Generational differences in social media use as well as cultural factors may limit the degree to which people disclose sensitive health-related topics/information with weaker ties online. For example, studies drawing upon socioemotional selectivity theory (Löckenhoff & Carstensen, 2004) have found that people often prefer communicating with closer ties over weak ties when they have a limited time perspective (i.e., when facing a terminal illness like cancer). By comparison, individuals who have a more open-ended time perspective (i.e., not facing a terminal illness) tend to communicate more with weaker ties (Carstensen, 1992; Fisher & Nussbaum, 2015; Rui, 2022). In short, factors such as the type of illness and its stage of progression may influence who people are willing to talk to in terms of discussing sensitive health issues as well as the type of support they seek and receive (in both face-to-face and online social networks) (Chang et al., 2015a; Dudley & Multhaup, 2005; Huxhold et al, 2013; 2020). Such theoretical frameworks draw upon a lifespan perspective of relationships and communication and may be beneficial to future scholars interested in health-related topic avoidance, WTCH, and social support.

The Canzona et al. (2019) study underscores the difficulty that breast cancer survivors and individuals living with similar health issues often face when it comes to initiating conversations about stigmatized health issues. Sexual health (SH) issues are often considered to be a "taboo" topic among close relational partners, especially when dealing with stigmatized health issues such as cancer or other diseases that impact partners' physical and mental health. These conversations may become even more difficult when they occur between one relational partner who is the primary caregiver and the other who is the patient. Factors such as caregiver burden can exacerbate relational difficulties and impact interpersonal conversations about SH. Future studies should consider how weaker interpersonal ties (e.g., online support groups, etc.) may help people who are experiencing SH issues while simultaneously managing an illness like breast cancer. Studies that have examined online support as a form of weak-tie social network support (e.g., Wright & Miller, 2010; Wright & Rains, 2013) have found that people are often more willing to discuss sensitive health issues (such as SH) with weaker ties as these types of relationships tend to be of less interpersonally risk to self-disclose problems, ask questions, and obtain advice/support compared to closer ties. Moreover, online support groups can be important spaces for people to vent frustrations about relational partners in a low-risk environment as well as obtain multiple viewpoints on ways to talk to one's partner (Wright & Bell, 2003).

## REFERENCES

Abroms, L. C., & Maibach, E. W. (2008). The effectiveness of mass communication to change public health behavior. *Annual Review of Public Health*, *29*(1), 219–234. DOI: <https://doi.org/10.1146/annurev.publhealth.29.020907.090824>

Adelman, M. B., Parks, M. R., & Albrecht, T. L. (1987). Beyond close relationships: Support in weak ties. In T. L. Albrecht & M. B. Adelman (Eds.), *Communicating social support* (pp. 126–147). Newbury Park, CA: Sage.

Afifi, W. A., & Guerrero, G. L. (2000). Motivations underlying topic avoidance in close relationships. In S. Petronio (Ed.), *Balancing the secrets of private disclosures* (pp. 165–180). Mahwah, NJ: Erlbaum.

Berkman, L. F., & Syme, S. L. (1979). Social networks, host resistance, and mortality: A nine-year follow-up study of Alameda County residents. *American Journal of Epidemiology*, *109*(2), 186–204. DOI: <https://doi.org/10.1093/oxfordjournals.aje.a112674>

Berger, C. R., & Calabrese, R. J. (1974). Some explorations in initial interaction and beyond: Toward a developmental theory of interpersonal communication. *Human Communication Research*, *1*(2), 99–112. DOI: <https://doi.org/10.1111/j.1468-2958.1975.tb00258.x>

Berlin, K. L., Andreotti, C., Yull, F., Grau, A. M., & Compas, B. E. (2013). Mother-daughter communication about breast cancer risk: interpersonal and biological stress processes. *Journal of Behavioral Medicine*, *36*(3), 328–339. DOI: <https://doi.org/10.1007/s10865-012-9418-0>

Bissonnette-Maheux, V., Dumas, A. A., Provencher, V., Lapointe, A., Dugrenier, M., Straus, S., … & Desroches, S. (2018). Women's perceptions of usefulness and ease of use of four healthy eating blog characteristics: a qualitative study of 33 French-Canadian women. *Journal of the Academy of Nutrition and Dietetics*, *118*(7), 1220–1227. DOI: <https://doi.org/10.1016/j.jand.2017.08.012>

Boinon, D., Sultan, S., Charles, C., Stulz, A., Guillemeau, C., Delaloge, S., & Dauchy, S. (2014). Changes in psychological adjustment over the course of treatment for breast cancer: the predictive role of social sharing and social support. *Psycho-Oncology*, *23*(3), 291–298. DOI: <https://doi.org/10.1002/pon.3420>

Campbell-Grossman, C. K., Hudson, D. B., Keating-Lefler, R., & Heusinkvelt, S. (2009). New mothers network: The provision of social support to single, low-income, African American mothers via e-mail messages. *Journal of Family Nursing*, *15*(2), 220–236. DOI: <https://doi.org/10.1177/1074840708323048>

Canzona, M. R., Fisher, C. L., Wright, K. B., & Ledford, C. J. (2019). Talking about sexual health during survivorship: understanding what shapes breast cancer survivors' willingness to communicate with providers. *Journal of Cancer Survivorship*, *13*(6), 932–942. DOI: <https://doi.org/10.1007/s11764-019-00809-2>

Canzona, M. R., Garcia, D., Fisher, C. L., Raleigh, M., Kalish, V., & Ledford, C. J. (2016). Communication about sexual health with breast cancer survivors: Variation among patient and provider perspectives. *Patient Education and Counseling*, *99*(11), 1814–1820. DOI: <https://doi.org/10.1016/j.pec.2016.06.019>

Canzona, M. R., Ledford, C. J., Fisher, C. L., Garcia, D., Raleigh, M., & Kalish, V. B. (2018). Clinician barriers to initiating sexual health conversations with breast cancer survivors: The influence of assumptions and situational constraints. *Families, Systems, & Health*, *36*(1), 20. DOI: <https://doi.org/10.1037/fsh0000307>

Caughin, J. P., & Afifi, T. D. (2004). When is topic avoidance unsatisfying? Examining moderators of the association between avoidance and dissatisfaction. *Human Communication Research*, *30*, 479–513. DOI: <https://doi.org/10.1111/j.1468-2958.2004.tb00742.x>

Caughlin, J. P., Mikucki-Enyart, S. L., Middleton, A. V., Stone, A. M., & Brown, L. E. (2011). Being open without talking about it: A rhetorical/normative approach to understanding topic avoidance in families after a lung cancer diagnosis. *Communication Monographs*, *78*(4), 409–436. DOI: <https://doi.org/10.1080/03637751.2011.618141>

Chang, P. F., Choi, Y. H., Bazarova, N. N., & Löckenhoff, C. E. (2015a). Age differences in online social networking: Extending socioemotional selectivity theory to social network sites. *Journal of Broadcasting & Electronic Media*, *59*(2), 221–239. DOI: <https://doi.org/10.1080/08838151.2015.1029126>

Chang, Y. T., Yu, H., & Lu, H. P. (2015b). Persuasive messages, popularity cohesion, and message diffusion in social media marketing. *Journal of Business Research*, *68*(4), 777–782. DOI: <https://doi.org/10.1016/j.jbusres.2014.11.02>

Chee, W., Lee, Y., Im, E. O., Chee, E., Tsai, H. M., Nishigaki, M., … & Mao, J. J. (2017). A culturally tailored Internet cancer support group for Asian American breast cancer survivors: A randomized controlled pilot intervention study. *Journal of Telemedicine and Telecare*, *23*(6), 618–626. DOI: <https://doi.org/10.1177/1357633X16658369>

De Jong, C. C., Ros, W. J., & Schrijvers, G. (2014). The effects on health behavior and health outcomes of Internet-based asynchronous communication between health providers and patients with a chronic condition: a systematic review. *Journal of Medical Internet Research*, *16*(1), e3000. DOI: 10.2196/jmir.3000

Donovan-Kicken, E., & Caughlin, J. P. (2010). A multiple goals perspective on topic avoidance and relationship satisfaction in the context of breast cancer. *Communication Monographs*, *77*(2), 231–256. DOI: <https://doi.org/10.1080/03637751003758219>

Dudley, N. M., & Multhaup, K. S. (2005). When familiar social partners are selected in open-ended situations: Further tests of the socioemotional selectivity theory. *Experimental Aging Research*, *31*(3), 331–344. DOI: <https://doi.org/10.1080/03610730590948212>

Fingerman, K. L. (2009). Consequential strangers and peripheral ties: The importance of unimportant relationships. *Journal of Family Theory & Review*, *1*(2), 69–86. DOI: <https://doi.org/10.1111/j.1756-2589.2009.00010.x>

Fisher, C. L. (2010). Coping with breast cancer across adulthood: Emotional support communication in the mother–daughter bond. *Journal of Applied Communication Research*, *38*(4), 386–411. DOI: <https://doi.org/10.1080/00909882.2010.513996>

Fisher, C. L., & Nussbaum, J. F. (2015). Maximizing wellness in successful aging and cancer coping: The importance of family communication from a socioemotional selectivity theoretical perspective. *Journal of Family Communication*, *15*(1), 3–19. DOI: <https://doi.org/10.1080/15267431.2014.946512>

Fisher, C. L., Wolf, B. M., Fowler, C., & Canzona, M. R. (2017). Experiences of "openness" between mothers and daughters during breast cancer: implications for coping and healthy outcomes. *Psycho-Oncology*, *26*(11), 1872–1880. DOI: <https://doi.org/10.1002/pon.4253>

Flynn, K. E., Reese, J. B., Jeffery, D. D., Abernethy, A. P., Lin, L., Shelby, R. A., … & Weinfurt, K. P. (2012). Patient experiences with communication about sex during and after treatment for cancer. *Psycho-Oncology*, *21*(6), 594–601. DOI: <https://doi.org/10.1002/pon.1947>

Ganz, P. A. (2000). Quality of life across the continuum of breast cancer care. *The Breast Journal*, *6*(5), 324–330. DOI: <https://doi.org/10.1046/j.1524-4741.2000.20042.x>

Glaser, B. G., Strauss, A. L. (1967). *The discovery of grounded theory: strategies for qualitative research.* Chicago: Aldine Publications Company.

Goldsmith, D. J. (2004). *Communicating social support*. Cambridge University Press.

Goldsmith, D. J., & Miller, G. A. (2014). Conceptualizing how couples talk about cancer. *Health Communication*, *29*(1), 51–63. DOI: <https://doi.org/10.1080/10410236.2012.717215>

Goldsmith, D. J., Miller, L. E., & Caughlin, J. P. (2007). Openness and avoidance in couples communicating about cancer. *Annals of the International Communication Association*, *31*(1), 62–115. DOI: <https://doi.org/10.1080/23808985.2007.11679065>

Günther, L., Schleberger, S., & Pischke, C. R. (2021). Effectiveness of social media-based interventions for the Promotion of Physical Activity: Scoping Review. *International Journal of Environmental Research and Public Health*, *18*(24), 13018. DOI: <https://doi.org/10.3390/ijerph182413018>

Hagan, T. L., Cohen, S. M., Rosenzweig, M. Q., Zorn, K., Stone, C. A., & Donovan, H. S. (2018). The female self-advocacy in cancer survivorship scale: A validation study. *Journal of Advanced Nursing*, *74*(4), 976–987. DOI: <https://doi.org/10.1111/jan.13498>

Halley, M. C., May, S. G., Rendle, K. A., Frosch, D. L., & Kurian, A. W. (2014). Beyond barriers: Fundamental "disconnects" underlying the treatment of breast cancer patients' sexual health. *Culture, Health & Sexuality*, *16*(9), 1169–1180. DOI: <https://doi.org/10.1080/13691058.2014.939227>

Harkin, L. J., Beaver, K., Dey, P., & Choong, K. A. (2020). Secret groups and open forums: Defining online support communities from the perspective of people affected by cancer. *Digital Health*, *6*, DOI: 2055207619898993.

Hether, H. J., Murphy, S. T., & Valente, T. W. (2014). It's better to give than to receive: The role of social support, trust, and participation on health-related social networking sites. *Journal of Health Communication*, *19*(12), 1424–1439. DOI: <https://doi.org/10.1080/10810730.2014.894596>

Hong, Y., Pena-Purcell, N. C., & Ory, M. G. (2012). Outcomes of online support and resources for cancer survivors: A systematic literature review. *Patient Education and Counseling*, *86*(3), 288–296. DOI: <https://doi.org/10.1016/j.pec.2011.06.014>

Huxhold, O., Fiori, K. L., Webster, N. J., & Antonucci, T. C. (2020). The strength of weaker ties: An underexplored resource for maintaining emotional well-being in later life. *The Journals of Gerontology: Series B*, *75*(7), 1433–1442. DOI: doi:10.1093/geronb/gbaa019

Huxhold, O., Fiori, K. L., & Windsor, T. D. (2013). The dynamic interplay of social network characteristics, subjective well-being, and health: The costs and benefits of socio-emotional selectivity. *Psychology and Aging*, *28*(1), 3. DOI: <https://doi.org/10.1037/a0030170>

Jeong, A., Shin, D. W., Kim, S. Y., Yang, H. K., & Park, J. H. (2016). Avoidance of cancer communication, perceived social support, and anxiety and depression among patients with cancer. *Psycho-Oncology*, *25*(11), 1301–1307. DOI: <https://doi.org/10.1002/pon.4060>

Korda, H., & Itani, Z. (2013). Harnessing social media for health promotion and behavior change. *Health Promotion Practice*, *14*(1), 15–23. DOI: <https://doi.org/10.1177/1524839911405850>

Kroenke, C. H., Kubzansky, L. D., Schernhammer, E. S., Holmes, M. D., & Kawachi, I. (2006). Social networks, social support, and survival after breast cancer diagnosis. *Journal of Clinical Oncology*, *24*(7), 1105–1111. DOI: 10.1200/JCO.2005.04.2846

Kulkarni, S., Lewis, K., Arp Adams, S., Brandt, H. M., Lead, J. R., Ureda, J. R., … & Friedman, D. B. (2018). A comprehensive analysis of how environmental risks of breast cancer are portrayed on the internet. *American Journal of Health Education*, *49*(4), 222–233. DOI: <https://doi.org/10.1080/19325037.2018.1473182>

Löckenhoff, C. E., & Carstensen, L. L. (2004). Socioemotional selectivity theory, aging, and health: The increasingly delicate balance between regulating emotions and making tough choices. *Journal of Personality*, *72*(6), 1395–1424. DOI: <https://doi.org/10.1111/j.1467-6494.2004.00301.x>

Logan, S., Steel, Z., & Hunt, C. (2016). Intercultural willingness to communicate within health services: Investigating anxiety, uncertainty, ethnocentrism and help seeking behaviour. *International Journal of Intercultural Relations*, *54*, 77–86. DOI: <https://doi.org/10.1016/j.ijintrel.2016.07.007>

Maher, C. A., Lewis, L. K., Ferrar, K., Marshall, S., De Bourdeaudhuij, I., & Vandelanotte, C. (2014). Are health behavior change interventions that use online social networks effective? A systematic review. *Journal of Medical Internet Research*, *16*(2), e2952. DOI: 10.2196/jmir.2952

Manne, S. L. (1999). Intrusive thoughts and psychological distress among cancer patients: the role of spouse avoidance and criticism. *Journal of Consulting and Clinical Psychology*, *67*(4), 539. DOI: <https://doi.org/10.1037/0022-006X.67.4.539>

McCroskey, J. C., & Richmond, V. P. (1987). Willingness to communicate. In J.C. McCroskey, & J.A. Daly (Eds.), Personality and interpersonal communication (pp. 129–156). Newbury Park, CA: Sage.

Oktay, J. S., & Walter C. A. (1991). *Breast cancer in the life course: Women's experiences.* New York: Springer.

Tim Owen, Wayne Noble, &Faye Christabel Speed. (2017). New Perspectives on Cybercrime (1st ed. 2017 edition.). Springer International Publishing. https://doi.org/10.1007/978-3-319-53856-3

Owen, T., Noble, W., & Speed, F. C. (2017). The challenges posed by scammers to online support groups: The "deserving" and the "undeserving" victims of scams. In *New perspectives on cybercrime* (pp. 213–240). Cham: Palgrave Macmillan.

Rains, S. A. (2018). *Coping with illness digitally*. MIT Press.

Rains, S. A., Peterson, E. B., & Wright, K. B. (2015). Communicating social support in computer-mediated contexts: A meta-analytic review of content analyses examining support messages shared online among individuals coping with illness. *Communication Monographs*, *82*(4), 403–430. DOI: <https://doi.org/10.1080/03637751.2015.1019530>

Rains, S. A., & Wright, K. B. (2016). Social support and computer-mediated communication: A state-of-the-art review and agenda for future research. *Annals of the International Communication Association*, *40*(1), 175–211. DOI: <https://doi.org/10.1080/23808985.2015.11735260>

Rains, S. A., & Young, V. (2009). A meta-analysis of research on formal computer-mediated support groups: Examining group characteristics and health outcomes. *Human Communication Research*, *35*(3), 309–336. DOI: <https://doi.org/10.1111/j.1468-2958.2009.01353.x>

Reese, J. B., Bober, S. L., & Daly, M. B. (2017). Talking about women's sexual health after cancer: Why is it so hard to move the needle?. *Cancer*, *123*(24), 4757–4763. DOI: <https://doi.org/10.1002/cncr.31084>

Reese, J. B., Keefe, F. J., Somers, T. J., & Abernethy, A. P. (2010). Coping with sexual concerns after cancer: The use of flexible coping. *Supportive Care in Cancer*, *18*(7), 785–800. DOI: <https://doi.org/10.1007/s00520-010-0819-8>

Reese, J. B., Shelby, R. A., Keefe, F. J., Porter, L. S., & Abernethy, A. P. (2010a). Sexual concerns in cancer patients: A comparison of GI and breast cancer patients. *Supportive Care in Cancer*, *18*(9), 1179–1189. DOI: <https://doi.org/10.1007/s00520-009-0738-8>.

Reich, S. M., Subrahmanyam, K., & Espinoza, G. (2012). Friending, IMing, and hanging out face-to-face: Overlap in adolescents' online and offline social networks. *Developmental Psychology*, *48*(2), 356. DOI: <https://doi.org/10.1037/a0026980>

Rezaei, M., Elyasi, F., Janbabai, G., Moosazadeh, M., & Hamzehgardeshi, Z. (2016). Factors influencing body image in women with breast cancer: A comprehensive literature review. *Iranian Red Crescent Medical Journal*, *18*(10). DOI: 10.5812/ircmj.39465

Rozzell, B., Piercy, C. W., Carr, C. T., King, S., Lane, B. L., Tornes, M., … & Wright, K. B. (2014). Notification pending: Online social support from close and nonclose relational ties via Facebook. *Computers in Human Behavior*, *38*, 272–280. DOI: <https://doi.org/10.1016/j.chb.2014.06.006>

Rui, J. R. (2022). Health information sharing via social ntwork sites (SNSs): Integrating social support and socioemotional selectivity theory. *Health Communication*, 1–11. DOI: <https://doi.org/10.1080/10410236.2022.2074779>

Salander, P., & Spetz, A. (2002). How do patients and spouses deal with the serious facts of malignant glioma? *Palliative Medicine*, *16*(4), 305–313. DOI: <https://doi.org/10.1191/0269216302pm569oa>

Sin, J., Henderson, C., Spain, D., Cornelius, V., Chen, T., & Gillard, S. (2018). eHealth interventions for family carers of people with long term illness: A promising approach? *Clinical Psychology Review*, *60*, 109–125. DOI: <https://doi.org/10.1016/j.cpr.2018.01.008>

Sinicrope, P. S., Patten, C. A., Clark, L. P., Brockman, T. A., Frost, M. H., Petersen, L. R., … & Cerhan, J. R. (2009). Adult daughters' reports of breast cancer risk reduction and early detection advice received from their mothers: An exploratory study. *Psycho-Oncology: Journal of the Psychological, Social and Behavioral Dimensions of Cancer*, *18*(2), 169–178. DOI: <https://doi.org/10.1002/pon.1393>

Smith, R. A., Hernandez, R., & Catona, D. (2014). Investigating initial disclosures and reactions to unexpected, positive HPV diagnosis. *Western Journal of Communication*, *78*(4), 426–440. DOI: <https://doi.org/10.1080/10570314.2013.786120>

Song, L., Northouse, L. L., Zhang, L., Braun, T. M., Cimprich, B., Ronis, D. L., & Mood, D. W. (2012). Study of dyadic communication in couples managing prostate cancer: A longitudinal perspective. *Psycho-Oncology*, *21*(1), 72–81. DOI: <https://doi.org/10.1002/pon.1861>

Tanis, M. (2009). What makes the Internet a place to seek social support. In E. A. Konijin, S. Utz, M. Tanis & S. B. Barnes (Eds.), *Mediated interpersonal communication* (pp. 290–308). New York, NY: Routledge.

Thomas, T. H., Donovan, H. S., Rosenzweig, M. Q., Bender, C. M., & Schenker, Y. (2021). A conceptual framework of self-advocacy in women with cancer. *ANS. Advances in Nursing Science*, *44*(1), E1. DOI: 10.1097/ANS.0000000000000342

Thomas, T. H., Bender, C., Rosenzweig, M., Taylor, S., Sereika, S. M., Babichenko, D., … & Schenker, Y. (2023). Testing the effects of the Strong Together self-advocacy serious game among women with advanced cancer: Protocol for the STRONG randomized clinical trial. *Contemporary Clinical Trials*, *124*, 107003. DOI: <https://doi.org/10.1016/j.cct.2022.107003>

Travers, A., & Taylor, V. (2016). What are the barriers to initiating end-of-life conversations with patients in the last year of life? *International journal of palliative nursing*, *22*(9), 454–462. DOI: <https://doi.org/10.12968/ijpn.2016.22.9.454>

Tuinman, M. A., Hoekstra, H. J., Vidrine, D. J., Gritz, E. R., Sleijfer, D. T., Fleer, J., & Hoekstra-Weebers, J. E. (2010). Sexual function, depressive symptoms and marital status in nonseminoma testicular cancer patients: A longitudinal study. *Psycho-Oncology: Journal of the Psychological, Social and Behavioral Dimensions of Cancer*, *19*(3), 238–247. DOI: <https://doi.org/10.1002/pon.1560>

Uchino, B. N. (2009). Understanding the links between social support and physical health: Alifespan perspective with emphasis on the separability of perceived and received support. *Perspectives in Psychological Science*, *4*, 236–255. DOI: <https://doi.org/10.1111/j.1745-6924.2009.01122.x>

Uchino, B. N., Bowen, K., Carlisle, M., & Birmingham, W. (2012). Psychological pathways linking social support to health outcomes: A visit with the "ghosts" of research past, present, and future. *Social Science & Medicine*, *74*(7), 949–957. DOI: <https://doi.org/10.1016/j.socscimed.2011.11.023>

Venetis, M. K., Greene, K., Checton, M. G., & Magsamen-Conrad, K. (2015). Decision making in cancer-related topic avoidance. *Journal of Health Communication*, *20*(3), 306–313. DOI: <https://doi.org/10.1080/10810730.2014.965364>

Waldron, E. A., Janke, E. A., Bechtel, C. F., Ramirez, M., & Cohen, A. (2013). A systematic review of psychosocial interventions to improve cancer caregiver quality of life. *Psycho-Oncology*, *22*(6), 1200–1207. DOI: <https://doi.org/10.1002/pon.3118>

Walther, J. B. (1996). Computer-mediated communication: Impersonal, interpersonal, and hyperpersonal interaction. *Communication Research*, *23*(1), 3–43. DOI: <https://doi.org/10.1177/009365096023001001>

Walther, J. B., & Boyd, S. (2002). Attraction to computer-mediated social support. In C. A. Lin & D. Atkin (Eds.), *Communication technology and society: Audience adoption and uses* (pp. 153–188). Cresskill, NJ: Hampton Press.

Walther, J. B., & Whitty, M. T. (2021). Language, psychology, and new new media: The hyperpersonal model of mediated communication at twenty-five years. *Journal of Language and Social Psychology, 40*(1), 120–135. DOI: <https://doi.org/10.1177/0261927X20967703>

Wittenberg, E., Buller, H., Ferrell, B., Koczywas, M., & Borneman, T. (2017, December). Understanding family caregiver communication to provide family-centered cancer care. In *Seminars in oncology nursing* (Vol. 33, No. 5, pp. 507–516). WB Saunders.

Wright, K. (2002). Social support within an on-line cancer community: An assessment of emotional support, perceptions of advantages and disadvantages, and motives for using the community from a communication perspective. *Journal of Applied Communication Research, 30*(3), 195–209. DOI: <https://doi.org/10.1080/00909880216586>

Wright, K. (2016). Social networks, interpersonal social support, and health outcomes: A health communication perspective. *Frontiers in Communication, 1*, 10. DOI: <https://doi.org/10.3389/fcomm.2016.00010>

Wright, K. B., & Bell, S. B. (2003). Health-related support groups on the Internet: Linking empirical findings to social support and computer-mediated communication theory. *Journal of Health Psychology, 8*(1), 39–54. DOI: <https://doi.org/10.1177/1359105303008001429>

Wright, K. B., Cai, X., Fisher, C., Rising, C. J., Burke-Garcia, A., & Afanaseva, D. (2021). A content analysis of social support messages about environmental breast cancer risk within blogs for mothers. *Health Communication, 36*(13), 1796–1804. DOI: <https://doi.org/10.1080/10410236.2020.1800241>

Wright, K. B., Fisher, C. L., Rising, C. J., Afanaseva, D., Burke-Garcia, A., & Cai, X. (2019). Partnering with mommy bloggers to disseminate breast cancer risk information: A social media intervention. *Journal of Medical Internet Research, 21*(3), e12441. DOI:10.2196/12441

Wright, K. B., & Frey, L. R. (2008). Communication and care in an acute cancer center: The effects of patients' willingness to communicate about health, health-care environment perceptions, and health status on information seeking, participation in care practices, and satisfaction. *Health Communication, 23*(4), 369–379. DOI: <https://doi.org/10.1080/10410230802229886>

Wright, K. B., Johnson, A. J., Averbeck, J., & Bernard, D. (2011). Computer-mediated social support groups: Promises and pitfalls for individuals coping with health concerns. In T. L. Thompson, R. Parrott & J. F. Nussbaum (Eds.) *Handbook of health communication* (pp. 349–362). Thousand Oaks, CA: Sage.

Wright, K. B., & Miller, C. H. (2010). A measure of weak-tie/strong-tie support network preference. *Communication Monographs, 77*(4), 500–517. DOI: <https://doi.org/10.1080/03637751.2010.502538>

Wright, K. B., & Rains, S. A. (2013). Weak-tie support network preference, health-related stigma, and health outcomes in computer-mediated support groups. *Journal of Applied Communication Research, 41*(3), 309–324. DOI: <https://doi.org/10.1080/00909882.2013.792435>

Wright, K. B., Frey, L., & Sopory, P. (2007). Willingness to communicate about health as an underlying trait of patient self-advocacy: The development of the willingness to communicate about health (WTCH) measure. *Communication Studies, 58*(1), 35–51. DOI: <https://doi.org/10.1080/10510970601168673>

Ye, J. (2006). Traditional and online support networks in the cross-cultural adaptation of Chinese international students in the United States. *Journal of Computer-Mediated Communication*, *11*(3), 863–876. DOI: <https://doi.org/10.1111/j.1083-6101.2006.00039.x>

Zhang, A. Y., & Siminoff, L. A. (2003). Silence and cancer: Why do families and patients fail to communicate?. *Health Communication*, *15*(4), 415–429. DOI: <https://doi.org/10.1207/S15327027HC1504_03>

CHAPTER SIX

# Family Health Legacies: Inherited Familial Health Risks and Patterns of Communication

GEMME CAMPBELL-SALOME

Families as social constructions create expectations and rules for how to behave within and outside of the family system (Baxter, 2011; Braithwaite, Foster, & Bergen, 2017; Klein & White, 2002). As such, the socially constructed and shared worldviews of families can (un)consciously pattern attitudes, behaviors, and ideals for communication across generations (Bylund, 2010). Families also communicate and model health attitudes, behaviors, and expectations (Baiocchi-Wagner & Talley, 2013; Dorrance Hall et al., 2021), which can influence how its members make health decisions (Campbell-Salome & Barbour, 2022; Fisher, 2011; Rauscher, Young, Durham, & Barbour, 2017). Further, family members are often expected to provide support and caregiving, especially in contexts of managing long-term health risks (Campbell-Salome & Rauscher, 2020; Fisher et al., 2021). One key area illuminating the intersection of family and health across the lifespan is genomic medicine, as families with hereditary conditions inherit both familial rules for interaction and a complex family health history and heightened future risk for disease.

To have a hereditary condition is to face lifelong uncertainty for individual health risks and manage the familial health legacy (Campbell-Salome & Barbour, 2022). Individuals with autosomal dominant conditions, such as Hereditary Breast and Ovarian Cancer syndrome (HBOC), Lynch syndrome, and Familial Hypercholesterolemia (FH), have a 50 % chance of passing on the pathogenic variant (also known as a mutation) and inherited risk to their offspring (CDC, March

6, 2014). Hereditary risk status also carries serious implications for other close relatives (Sobel & Cowan, 2003). Family communication about these conditions, the related family health history, and adaptive sensemaking can alert relatives to their genetic risks and motivate their adherence to recommended medical management (e.g., genetic testing, advanced screenings, surveillance, and prophylactic surgeries). Thus, family communication can provide potentially lifesaving information and support decision-making to reduce health risks.

Families with a hereditary condition make sense of their illness experiences and future risks through storytelling, in which they interactionally structure past health experiences and perceptions of risk (Campbell-Salome & Rauscher, 2020). Often these stories become family narratives, passed down through generations teaching relatives how to assess and manage their risk and what the condition means for their family (Trees, Kellas, & Roche, 2010; Werner-Lin & Gardner, 2009). For instance, Paige and Nancy (sisters) described how past health events in the family related to the hereditary cancer condition shaped their perceptions of risk and gave them a sense of knowing that they would get cancer:

> *Paige: I knew I was always going to get cancer. I just had that feeling, and I ended up getting breast cancer. It was just caught very early during a mammogram, and actually, it was stage zero. I elected to have double mastectomy, which is probably the best decision I could have made. Because last year my daughter, who was 29, she had just given birth to her third son, my third grandchild. A few weeks later she was diagnosed with stage four sarcoma. That was very unexpected, very surprising, and it happened very quickly. She passed away 10 weeks later. That's when we found out we had the genetic mutation, and my immediate family got tested. I'm positive, my brother's positive, my nephew is positive, and my grandson is also positive.*

> *Nancy: Just to pick up on some of the things that Paige said. She said that we have a lot of history on both sides of the family. I always felt the same way she did. I haven't had any cancer, but I always feel like, and I still feel like it's probably inevitable that I might get some sort of cancer at some point in my life.*

Paige and Nancy discuss how they expected to get cancer growing up before they even knew they had a hereditary predisposition for cancer. Paige reflects on how she lost her daughter to a cancer related to the condition, how it reinforced her health decision to get a double mastectomy, and considered future health risks for her family members. Notably, Nancy who does not have a genetic variant for the condition still feels she is at risk for cancer and describes difficulty coping with these feelings of heightened risk. Often, families with these conditions have long, painful family histories of loss that make the risk more tangible, and sharing stories about this health history can aid in coping (Campbell-Salome & Rauscher, 2020). Additionally, these stories can also help relatives consider their own risk and how they fit into the family health narrative, which can be updated with each generation's new health experiences. Thus, these families grapple with legacies of hereditary disease while also passing down legacies for how to communicate and make sense of these health risks.

In this chapter we will discuss the lifespan lens in the context of familial inheritance of health conditions, patterns for communicating about health, and health narratives. I will use the context of genomic and precision medicine to illustrate these points as it has been a ripe area to explore the persistent influence of family on health communication and apply a lifespan lens. Finally, this chapter will examine the social action related to the research presented that can support coping and healthy decision-making for families with genetic conditions.

## COMMUNICATION IN GENOMIC AND PRECISION MEDICINE: THE CENTRALITY OF FAMILY COMMUNICATION

Family communication about hereditary disease is pivotal in alerting relatives to their own risks, which can strengthen or challenge how these families interact about health issues. Family members may feel betrayed if a relative's genetic test results are not shared with them or feel burdened by this information, creating additional dialectical tensions for how these families communicate (Baxter, 2011). Managing personal health information for these families is not just personal, it is inherently familial. While all families grapple with tensions related to connection-autonomy and openness-privacy, families with hereditary diseases also face potentially serious health implications for how they manage such tensions (Campbell-Salome & Barbour, 2022). To illustrate, Pam and Abigail (sisters) described how a family member not sharing news of a pathogenic *BRCA1* variant result with their immediate family contributed to the death of their mother:

> *Abigail: About two weeks before my mom dies, [our aunt] called, just to say goodbye to my mother. She goes, "Well, you know [your mother's nephew] was BRCA1 positive, and that's why he died of pancreatic cancer, and two of his three girls also tested positive a number of years back and had all the preventive surgery." They knew my mother had had cancer twice...No one in their family ever called my mother and said, "Hey this is a possibility." If she had been tested the first time she had cancer, 12 years before she died, things might have happened differently and if I hadn't been lucky enough to be tested before I developed cancer, I could be dead...I still harbor anger that they didn't reach out to my mother. I remember that a lot.*

> *Pam: I believe that somehow the import of it kind of escaped me. I think I was just in too much shock from other stuff at that time for it.*

As the sisters told their family's story of HBOC, they described this lack of sharing as intentionally "withholding information" and "lousy" and explained how they severed contact with that family after this revelation. This example further illustrates how potentially mis-managing risk information and dialectical tensions for these families can alter family relationships and networks. Further, it demonstrates the potential long-lasting impacts of family communication decisions and how families can view these decisions as life or death.

Clinical variables of hereditary diseases such as HBOC, Lynch syndrome, and FH can shape the psychosocial demands individuals and families face in managing hereditary risks across the lifespan (Rolland & Williams, 2006). Specifically, how families make sense of hereditary risk is based on four clinical variables including the likelihood of developing the hereditary condition (penetrance), timing of onset in an individual's lifecycle, the existence of effective treatment or preventive medicine, and clinical severity. These variables and their impacts have been well documented in previous research on how individuals with hereditary risks grapple with medical uncertainty (Campbell-Salome & Barbour, 2022; Dean & Fisher, 2019), disclose personal health information about genetic risk to family members (Dean & Rauscher, 2018; Rauscher, Hesse, Miller, Ford, & Youngs, 2015), and exchange support (Koehly et al., 2009; Koehly et al., 2008; Koehly et al., 2003). These variables contribute to rules for familial interaction such as when to discuss the hereditary condition, who should be informed of genetic information, and expectations for how individuals should manage their health for the family.

## PATTERNS OF FAMILY COMMUNICATION: THE PERSISTENT INFLUENCE ON HEALTH

Family creates a shared social reality through communication. Family communication is governed by the family's communication patterns, which are the taken-for-granted ways we expect our relatives to interact and behave (Koerner, & Fitzpatrick, 2002). Patterns of family communication, such as how open the family is about topics (conversation orientation) and how their power structure functions (conformity orientation), create a shared social reality for families that informs and governs actions (Koerner, & Fitzpatrick, 2002). These patterns represent a relatively stable and predictable schema that helps individuals understand and communicate with the world. Moreover, these patterns for interaction can be passed down through generations of family (Rauscher, Schrodt, Campbell-Salome, & Freytag, 2020). All families inherit rules for interaction, which can shape how families talk about health and establish expectations for how families with hereditary risks should communicate about the condition.

The family communication patterns follow family over the lifespan and have been found to influence individual's health communication and behaviors. For example, how openly a family communicates can impact how likely members are to discuss complex or emotional health topics, the rules regarding the depth of these conversations, and the frequency of the conversations (Hays, Maliski, & Warner, 2017). Additionally, conversation orientation is positively related to talking about diet and exercise and shaping young adults' health attitudes and behaviors (Baiocchi-Wagner & Talley, 2013) as well as indirectly socializing children's health lifestyle choices (Baxter, Bylund, Imes, & Scheive, 2005). These effects on early life and development can also impact adult child–parent relationships and health (Goldsmith, Wittenberg, Platt, Iannarino, & Reno, 2016; Wittenberg-Lyles, Goldsmith, Demiris, Oliver, & Stone, 2012). For instance, conversation orientation was found to indirectly reduce caregiver burden for adult children caring for a parent with a blood cancer. Additionally, conversation orientation also indirectly improved caregivers' report of their own skills clinically communicating with their parent's healthcare providers (Campbell-Salome et al., 2022). This degree of openness can also impact if individuals can gather family health history information or disclose genetic cancer risks (Campbell Salome, Rauscher, & Freytag, 2019; Koerner, LeRoy, Veach, 2010; Rauscher et al., 2015). Conversation orientation has been found to have an inverse relationship with conformity orientation.

In health contexts, conformity orientation has had a complex relationship with family health outcomes. Families high on this orientation (i.e., reinforcing hierarchy, obedience to parents and elders, and putting family before individuals) tend to stress homogeneity of beliefs and attitudes, avoid conflict, and have a strong sense of duty to family (Koerner & Fitzpatrick, 2006). These characteristics may impede open conversations about health, reinforce problematic health attitudes and beliefs of previous generations, and create conflicts for individual medical decision-making. For instance, conformity orientation has been associated with negative attitudes and intentions toward child vaccination (Hesse & Rauscher, 2016) and reduced likelihood of young adults disclosing health issues to parents (Hays et al., 2017). However, some scholars argue that previous research and measures of conformity have be biased toward seeing this dimension as a negative family characteristic (Hesse, Rauscher, Goodman, & Couvrette, 2017; Kranstuber Horstman et al., 2018). Recent research using updated measures have actually found that conformity orientation can promote family unity and the family hierarchy can pass down important lessons that may improve health outcomes. For example, a new measure of conformity demonstrated a positive association with patients' perceptions of their involvement in medical encounters, satisfaction with clinicians, and intentions toward medical adherence (Rauscher, Hesse, & Campbell-Salome, 2020). There has also been recent research finding these positive connections between conformity orientation and genetic risk. For instance, a recent study found that conversation orientation and conformity orientation (parental control, in particular) promoted systematic processing of persuasive family health history messages, leading to more positive attitudes and intentions to seek this information from family (Hovick, Thomas, Watts, & Tan, 2021). In the context of hereditary disease, families with these conditions may prioritize health communication behaviors and medical decisions that fulfill familial obligations and the family's definition of the "right way" to manage risks (Campbell-Salome & Barbour, 2022). More work is needed in this area to explicate the ways in which family communication patterns shape rules and decisions for those with hereditary disease risks.

Dimensions of family communication patterns are inherited and relatively stable across lifespans, making them a force for shaping interactions and decisions including health behaviors. One way that these family communication patterns can present themselves is in family narratives, wherein families craft myths, a sense of identity, and use stories to teach lessons across generations. We will next discuss how family health narratives can further socialize relatives, and pass down information and lessons to guide individuals.

## FAMILY HEALTH NARRATIVES: AN INHERENT LIFESPAN PERSPECTIVE

Storytelling is an easy and natural form of communication for human beings, which can help families make sense of who they are and the world around them. Storytelling is a key mechanism for sharing coherent information across branches and generations of the family, engaging in communal sensemaking about hardship and risk, and shaping how individual members define their identities and roles (Koenig Kellas, 2005; Koenig Kellas & Trees, 2006). While stories can be told individually, people usually collaborate to jointly tell stories and lace individual stories together into larger narratives that make sense of relationships and experiences. For instance, families may have narratives of courtship (the story of how your parents met) and stories of genesis (the story of how you were born) (Langellier & Peterson, 2017). Families with hereditary disease may also have narratives of diagnostic odysseys (how we learned we have this hereditary disease). Additionally, Langellier and Peterson (2017) posit that "not only do families tell stories, but making stories is one way of doing family" (p.210). Narratives are a powerful tool to communicate and socialize family members toward certain values, attitudes, and behaviors, which can impact health.

Creating narratives in families with hereditary conditions can help relatives make sense of and cope with challenging, yet meaningful, health experiences (Koenig Kellas & Kranstuber Horstman, 2014). These family narratives can be especially important as individuals often pull from family health histories and describe health conditions as stories during health consultations when providing information to clinicians (Trees, Koenig Kellas, & Roche, 2010). These stories contain family health details and risk perceptions related to penetrance (e.g., who in the family may have the condition, how likely someone with a pathogenic variant will get cancer) (D'Agincourt-Canning, 2001; Kenen, Ardern-Jones, & Eeles, 2003), danger zones for the onset of disease (Werner-Lin, 2007; Werner-Lin & Gardner, 2009), if and how to reduce disease risks and the family's judgments of medical recommendations (Lloyd et al., 2000), and memories of how severely family members were affected (Campbell-Salome & Rauscher, 2020). Family health narratives related to hereditary disease knit together individual stories and health experiences that can span generations, change or be updated with each new diagnosis or procedure, and shape each generations' health attitudes and behaviors (Campbell-Salome & Rauscher, 2020).

Families with hereditary conditions can use these narratives to contextualize their experience in relation to previous generations, which can affirm their identity and motivate proactive decision-making. For instance, Agnes described to her cousin how she uses her mother's example as a model for how to manage her health:

> *[I] tackle [the cancer risks] aggressively, and know it's always just the way to be a fighter like my mom. That's what she would always advocate for me, taking care of myself, and being more involved with the family, and just reaching out more about what I was going through and what I was doing.*

Agnes earlier explained how her mother passed away due to cancer, but how her mother motivated her when she was living and now after she's passed to be an advocate for her own health and her family. This family narrative encourages fighting against cancer and aggressively reducing risks, as well as idolizes family members who engage in this fight. However, these family narratives can also use guilt to motivate medical decision-making that can complicate coping. For example, Helen and Hannah (sisters) describe how the loss of their mother and what she may have wanted motivated their genetic testing, but that trauma also makes it hard to adhere long-term to more medical recommendations:

> *Helen: Basically, the reason I [got genetic testing] is because when we had found out [about HBOC when] my mom was still alive but she was getting near the end, so I did it because I wanted to give my mom peace of mind that we tested because I wanted her to have that peace of mind and know that we got it taken care of and that we would be on top of it.*

> *Hannah: I really didn't want to do it at first, I had a really hard time going to do it because I didn't really [know if] that would really change my mind or not, I was just so sad about my mom. And, then I just decided that I should after my mom passed, I went and then I tested positive.*

> *Helen: I go every six months and I go get a breast MRI and then I alternate, so every six months I get a pelvic and vaginal ultrasound and then either a breast MRI and then it switches off between the breast MRI and a breast mammogram…So, we're just doing that preventative measures and stuff like that. There's a lot more than I need to be doing as far as food and taking care of my body in a healthier manner. I take those precautions right now.*

> *Hannah: I haven't done anything in about a year now because I sometimes shut down and I just don't really like to deal with it sometimes because a lot of times I've had false results and then it's just been really stressful and we're already dealing with a lot of trauma in our lives. Sometimes I don't care, I'd rather just not deal with it and I know that's not the best way but sometimes I just shut down so I haven't been in probably a year and I'm supposed to be doing every six months. I've been pretty good with it but I'm not consistent and I have recently in the last year or so, for some reason, it's just been the least of my priorities even though it shouldn't be.*

Helen and Hannah's account illustrates how family narratives of loss can motivate health decisions, but also impede them or complicate psychosocial well-being. These narratives cast family members as characters such as martyrs and survivors, which can provide examples for behavior for other generations to emulate. However, these narratives can also be a mechanism for sharing family traumas, loss, and crises and preparing other relatives for their potential roles.

Family health narratives about genetic conditions carry elements of the clinical variables detailed above (Rolland, 2005), demonstrate shared sensemaking about health between and among generations, and the type of health legacies that are passed down in these families. Indeed, the clinical variables of their genetic condition can help in identifying defining moments in a family health narrative and shifts in relationships or behaviors. For instance, Campbell-Salome and Barbour (2022) found that individuals with hereditary cancer conditions prioritized family goals and shifted their approach to testing and care from individual goals to familial goals around salient time points. The time points driving those shifts were after a family crisis, trauma, or loss (e.g., parent died, children watched their parent suffer in treatment), when making family planning decisions, and when considering how to manage health threats for young or fully grown children (Campbell-Salome et al., 2022). These events in a relative's lifespan and potential threats to the next generation were described as altering health decisions and becoming part of the narrative they would pass down to teach future generations of the family how to manage health.

## SOCIAL ACTION: PUTTING RESEARCH INTO PRACTICE

A key component of my own research in the areas described above is to develop and test health communication interventions to support families with hereditary diseases. My research explores the experiences and needs of individuals and families with hereditary conditions to implement interventions that can improve coping and resilience, support uncertainty and information management about complex medical information, and promote healthy decision-making to reduce disease risks. Given my research focus and the potential impact of this work for families with hereditary diseases, I work in a learning healthcare system. Learning healthcare systems are designed to generate and apply the best scientific evidence to support patients, providers, and the system overall. Geisinger, an integrated healthcare system in central Pennsylvania, is a learning healthcare system engaging in cutting-edge research in patient-centered precision health and genomic medicine (Davis, Williams, & Stametz, 2021; Williams et al., 2018). In my role, I primarily conduct research related to the MyCode® Community Health Initiative, which is a population screening program that returns clinically actionable genetic results (Carey et al., 2016; Schwartz et al., 2018). In this context, patients and families may be learning about their genetic risk for the first time and have unique needs to aid in family communication and sensemaking (McCormick et al., 2022).

Many health communication scientists work in university systems, situated in departments or colleges with other experts in their field. In my current role, I am the only health communication scientist at my institution. This pushes me to conduct collaborative and interdisciplinary research with experts in implementation science, public health, and genomic medicine to reach my research goals. Additionally, as I am situated in a learning healthcare system, I also collaborate with clinicians and healthcare stakeholders, who both participate in and contribute to the research as well as implement the evidence into care. This allows me and other health communication scientists in similar positions to span boundaries outside of communication science into other fields as well as span from academic research to clinical integration (Hoffmann-Longtin et al., 2020). Spanning these boundaries can facilitate the further reach and impact of health communication research and better recognition of the field and its contributions outside of academia. Thus, I want to stress the importance of and opportunities for health communication scientists to also step into the spaces of medical academia, learning healthcare systems, and other nontraditional research paths to ensure our field's work reaches the people that can most benefit.

## RESEARCH APPLICATIONS IN GENOMIC MEDICINE

In my work I aim to apply communication science and previous research in health communication to projects that can improve well-being and health. One of the projects that integrates health communication seamlessly is the development of chatbots, or digital conversation agents, to deliver information and support at different points in a patient's journey after receiving a genetic result from MyCode (Schmidlen, Schwartz, DiLoreto, Kirchner, & Sturm, 2019; Snir et al., 2021). In collaboration with genetic counselors and engineers, we developed chatbots to facilitate family communication about genetic results, provide information to at-risk relatives to motivate their screening, and reengage patients who do not immediately act on their results (Schmidlen et al., 2022; Schmidlen et al., 2019). With these collaborators, we are currently developing a chatbot to help patients prepare for a genetic counseling appointment and provide information on patient sensemaking about their results to tailor the genetic counseling appointment. We are currently engaging in user-testing of our "Pre-Visit Chatbot" to ensure it fits with patients' needs and desires for this type of tool so we can further iterate on it before pilot testing (Kuniavsky, 2003). This chatbot applies health communication research on family storytelling to identify the sensemaking frames patients and their families utilize (Campbell-Salome & Rauscher, 2020) and their willingness to communicate and disclose results to their families (Greene et al., 2012; Wright, Frey, & Sopory, 2007). We also partnered with genetic counselors in our system to design components of the chatbot that prepare the patient for what to expect for their appointment and common questions healthcare stakeholders encounter. While this communication tool is still in development and refinement, it demonstrates the potential benefit of applying health communication science in collaboration with other fields to create an intervention that may improve patient–clinician communication outcomes.

Another example of recent research applying health communication science to genomic medicine comes from my work on the Identification Methods, Patient Activation, and Cascade Testing for Familial Hypercholesterolemia (IMPACT-FH) R01 from the National Heart, Lung, and Blood Institute. The overall goal of this grant is to improve FH identification through innovative methods like automated approaches to EHR data and developing communication strategies to facilitate family communication about FH and follow-up screening for at-risk relatives (Campbell-Salome et al., 2021). Based on feedback from individuals and families with FH, we optimized communication strategies including a letter, chatbots, and a direct contact program (i.e., a program in which a genetic counselor can directly contact at-risk relatives with the permission of the patient to share their genetic result information) using the Extended Parallel Process Model (EPPM) (Witte & Allen, 2000). Participants gave feedback on how to design and optimize the communication strategies as well as how to message the information about FH to their relatives to overcome ambivalence and motivate screening (Campbell-Salome et al., 2022). Using their feedback and the EPPM, our team re-designed messages within each of the communication strategies and tested them in a pragmatic trial. Currently, we are assessing the outcomes of the trial and analyzing interviews from clinicians, patients, and relatives who used these strategies to assess their experiences. Findings from this study will shape how we communicate with patients and at-risk relatives for FH in the future and may also be applied to other hereditary conditions to motivate screening and adherence to medical recommendations.

## CONCLUSION

All families inherit patterns for interaction and narratives that shape individual and familial identities. Families with unique health experiences like having a hereditary condition also inherit complex health legacies that can shape and be shaped by family communication patterns and health narratives. Studying how these families communicate has been a rich area of study for applying health and family communication theories as well as a lifespan lens to explore how these family health legacies impact generations. However, these types of health legacies may also exist for other family health contexts such as addiction, mental health, and chronic diseases. Future research should continue to examine familial inheritance of both health conditions and how the ways family communication shapes health behaviors. Further, for this research to potentially have more impact in supporting these families, researchers working in the intersections of health and family or interpersonal communication may need to step into new roles. Collaborating with complementary sciences and clinical stakeholders in organizations that allow us to translate research into practice can enhance our impact and the benefits from our work.

## REFERENCES

Baiocchi-Wagner, E. A., & Talley, A. E. (2013). The role of family communication in individual health attitudes and behaviors concerning diet and physical activity. *Health Commun, 28*(2), 193–205.

Baxter, L. A. (2011). *Voicing relationships: A dialogic perspective.* Sage Publications.

Baxter, L. A., Bylund, C. L., Imes, R. S., & Scheive, D. M. (2005). Family communication environments and rule-based social control of adolescents' healthy lifestyle choices. *The Journal of Family Communication, 5*(3), 209–227.

Braithwaite, D. O., Foster, E., & Bergen, K. M. (2017). Social construction theory: Communication co-creating families. *Engaging theories in family communication* (pp. 267–278). Routledge.

Bylund, C. L. (2010). Improving clinical communication and promoting health through concordance-based patient education. *Communication Education, 59*(3), 294–311.

Campbell-Salome, G., & Barbour, J. B. (2022). Managing Uncertainty for and With Family: Communication Strategies and Motivations in Familial Uncertainty Management for Hereditary Cancer. *Qual Health Res*, 10497323221090191.

Campbell-Salome, G., Fisher, C. L., Wright, K. B., Lincoln, G., Applebaum, A. J., Sae-Hau, M., . . . Bylund, C. L. (2022). Impact of the family communication environment on burden and clinical communication in blood cancer caregiving. *Psychooncology, 31*(7). doi:10.1002/pon.5910

Campbell-Salome, G., Jones, L. K., Masnick, M. F., Walton, N. A., Ahmed, C. D., Buchanan, A. H., . . . Sturm, A. C. (2021). Developing and optimizing innovative tools to address familial hypercholesterolemia underdiagnosis: Identification methods, patient activation, and cascade testing for familial hypercholesterolemia. *Circ Genom Precis Med, 14*(1), e003120. doi:10.1161/circgen.120.003120

Campbell-Salome, G., Rauscher, E. A., & Freytag, J. (2019). Patterns of communicating about family health history: Exploring differences in family types, age, and sex. *Health Educ Behav, 46*(5), 809–817. doi:10.1177/1090198119853002

Campbell-Salome, G., Walters, N. L., Ladd, I. G., Sheldon, A., Ahmed, C. D., Brangan, A., . . . Sturm, A. C. (2022). Motivating cascade testing for familial hypercholesterolemia: applying the extended parallel process model for clinician communication. *Transl Behav Med.* doi:10.1093/tbm/ibac018

Campbell-Salome, G., & Rauscher, E. A. (2020). Family storytelling about hereditary cancer: Framing shared understandings of risk. *Journal of Genetic Counseling, 29*(6), 936–948.

Carey, D. J., Fetterolf, S. N., Davis, F. D., Faucett, W. A., Kirchner, H. L., Mirshahi, U., . . . Ledbetter, D. H. (2016). The Geisinger MyCode community health initiative: an electronic health record-linked biobank for precision medicine research. *Genet Med, 18*(9), 906–913. doi:10.1038/gim.2015.187

CDC. (March 6, 2014). Tier 1 Genomics Applications and their Importance to Public Health. Retrieved from <https://www.cdc.gov/genomics/implementation/toolkit/tier1.htm>

D'Agincourt-Canning, L. (2001). Experiences of genetic risk: disclosure and the gendering of responsibility. *Bioethics, 15*(3), 231–247.

Davis, F. D., Williams, M. S., & Stametz, R. A. (2021). Geisinger's effort to realize its potential as a learning health system: A progress report. *Learning Health Systems, 5*(2), e10221.

Dean, M., & Fisher, C. L. (2019). Uncertainty and previvors' cancer risk management: understanding the decision-making process. *Journal of Applied Communication Research, 47*(4), 460–483.

Dean, M., & Rauscher, E. A. (2018). Men's and women's approaches to disclosure about BRCA-related cancer risks and family planning decision-making. *Qual Health Res, 28*(14), 2155–2168. doi:10.1177/1049732318788377

Dorrance Hall, E., Ma, M., Azimova, D., Campbell, N., Ellithorpe, M., Plasencia, J., . . . Hennessy, M. (2021). The mediating role of family and cultural food beliefs on the relationship between family communication patterns and diet and health issues across racial/ethnic groups. *Health Commun, 36*(5), 593–605. doi:10.1080/10410236.2020.1733213

Fisher, C. (2011). "Her pain was my pain": Mothers and daughters sharing the breast cancer journey. *Family communication, connections, and health transitions*, 56–76.

Fisher, C. L., Wright, K. B., Hampton, C. N., Vasquez, T. S., Kastrinos, A., Applebaum, A. J., . . . Bylund, C. L. (2021). Blood cancer caregiving during COVID-19: understanding caregivers' needs. *Transl Behav Med, 11*(5), 1187–1197. doi:10.1093/tbm/ibab021

Goldsmith, J., Wittenberg, E., Platt, C. S., Iannarino, N. T., & Reno, J. (2016). Family caregiver communication in oncology: advancing a typology. *Psycho-Oncology, 25*(4), 463–470.

Greene, K., Magsamen-Conrad, K., Venetis, M. K., Checton, M. G., Bagdasarov, Z., & Banerjee, S. C. (2012). Assessing health diagnosis disclosure decisions in relationships: Testing the disclosure decision-making model. *Health Commun, 27*(4), 356–368.

Hays, A., Maliski, R., & Warner, B. (2017). Analyzing the effects of family communication patterns on the decision to disclose a health issue to a parent: The benefits of conversation and dangers of conformity. *Health Commun, 32*(7), 837–844.

Hesse, C., & Rauscher, E. A. (2016). The relationship between family communication patterns and child vaccination intentions. *Communication Research Reports, 33*(1), 61–67.

Hesse, C., Rauscher, E. A., Goodman, R. B., & Couvrette, M. A. (2017). Reconceptualizing the role of conformity behaviors in family communication patterns theory. *Journal of Family Communication, 17*(4), 319–337.

Hoffmann-Longtin, K., Kerr, A. M., Shaunfield, S., Koenig, C. J., Bylund, C. L., & Clayton, M. F. (2020). Fostering interdisciplinary boundary spanning in health communication: A call for a paradigm shift. *Health Commun*, 1–9. doi:10.1080/10410236.2020.1857517

Horstman, H. K., Schrodt, P., Warner, B., Koerner, A., Maliski, R., Hays, A., & Colaner, C. W. (2018). Expanding the conceptual and empirical boundaries of family communication patterns: The development and validation of an expanded conformity orientation scale. *Communication Monographs, 85*(2), 157–180.

Hovick, S. R., Thomas, S. N., Watts, J., & Tan, N. Q. (2021). The influence of family communication patterns on the processing of messages to increase family health history seeking intentions. *Health Commun, 36*(4), 424–432.

Kenen, R., Ardern-Jones, A., & Eeles, R. (2003). Family stories and the use of heuristics: women from suspected hereditary breast and ovarian cancer (HBOC) families. *Sociology of health & illness, 25*(7), 838–865.

Klein, D., & White, J. (2002). Family theories: An introduction (pp. 32–55): Thousand Oaks, CA: Sage Publications.

Koehly, L. M., Peters, J. A., Kenen, R., Hoskins, L. M., Ersig, A. L., Kuhn, N. R., . . . Greene, M. H. (2009). Characteristics of health information gatherers, disseminators, and blockers within families at risk of hereditary cancer: Implications for family health communication interventions. *American Journal of Public Health, 99*(12), 2203–2209.

Koehly, L. M., Peters, J. A., Kuhn, N., Hoskins, L., Letocha, A., Kenen, R., . . . Greene, M. H. (2008). Sisters in hereditary breast and ovarian cancer families: communal coping, social integration, and psychological well-being. *Psycho-Oncology, 17*(8), 812–821.

Koehly, L. M., Peterson, S. K., Watts, B. G., Kempf, K. K., Vernon, S. W., & Gritz, E. R. (2003). A social network analysis of communication about hereditary nonpolyposis colorectal cancer genetic testing and family functioning. *Cancer Epidemiology Biomarkers & Prevention, 12*(4), 304–313.

Koenig Kellas, J., & Kranstuber Horstman, H. (2014). Communicated narrative sense-making: Understanding family narratives, storytelling, and the construction of meaning through a communicative lens. *The Sage handbook of family communication* (pp. 76–90). SAGE Publications Inc.

Koenig Kellas, J. K. (2005). Family ties: Communicating identity through jointly told family stories. *Communication Monographs, 72*(4), 365–389.

Koenig Kellas, J., & Trees, A. R. (2006). Finding meaning in difficult family experiences: Sense-making and interaction processes during joint family storytelling. *The Journal of Family Communication, 6*(1), 49–76.

Koerner, A. F., & Fitzpatrick, M.A. (2002). Toward a theory of family communication. *Communication Theory, 12*(1), 70–91.

Koerner, A. F., & Fitzpatrick, M. A. (2006). Family communication patterns theory: A social cognitive approach. *Engaging theories in family communication: Multiple perspectives*, 50–65.

Koerner, A. F., LeRoy, B., Veach, P. . (2010). Family communication patterns: Theory and practice. In C. L. G. a. C. L. Bylund (Ed.), *Family communication about genetics: Theory and practice* (pp. 184–198): Oxford University Press.

Kuniavsky, M. (2003). *Observing the user experience: a practitioner's guide to user research*: Elsevier.

Langellier, K. M., & Peterson, E. E. (2017). Narrative performance theory: Making stories, doing family *Engaging Theories in Family Communication* (pp. 210–220): Routledge.

Lloyd, S., Watson, M., Oaker, G., Sacks, N., Querci della Rovere, U., & Gui, G. (2000). Understanding the experience of prophylactic bilateral mastectomy: A qualitative study of ten women. *Psycho-Oncology: Journal of the Psychological, Social and Behavioral Dimensions of Cancer, 9*(6), 473–485.

McCormick, C. Z., Yu, K. D., Johns, A., Campbell-Salome, G., Hallquist, M. L., Sturm, A. C., & Buchanan, A. H. (2022). Investigating Psychological Impact after Receiving Genetic Risk Results—A Survey of Participants in a Population Genomic Screening Program. *J Pers Med, 12*(12), 1943.

Rauscher, E. A., Hesse, C., & Campbell-Salome, G. (2020). Applying family communication patterns to patient-provider communication: Examining perceptions of patient involvement, satisfaction, and medical aAdherence. *J Health Commun, 25*(2), 180–189. doi:10.1080/10810730.2020.1728596

Rauscher, E. A., Hesse, C., Miller, S., Ford, W., & Youngs, E. L. (2015). Privacy and family communication about genetic cancer risk: Investigating factors promoting women's disclosure decisions. *Journal of Family Communication, 15*(4), 368–386.

Rauscher, E. A., Schrodt, P., Campbell-Salome, G., & Freytag, J. . (2020). The intergenerational transmission of family communication patterns: (In)Consistencies in conversation and conformity orientations across two generations of family. *Journal of Family Communication, 20*(2), 97–113.

Rauscher, E. A., Young, S. L., Durham, W. T., & Barbour, J. B. (2017). "I'd know that my child was out there": Egg donation, the institutionalized "ideal" family, and health care decision making. *Health Commun, 32*(5), 550–559.

Rolland, J. S. (2005). Cancer and the family: An integrative model. *Cancer, 104*(11 Suppl), 2584–2595. doi:10.1002/cncr.21489

Rolland, J. S., & Williams, J. K. (2006). Toward a Psychosocial Model. *Individuals, families, and the new era of genetics: Biopsychosocial perspectives*, 36.

Schmidlen, T., Jones, C. L., Campbell-Salome, G., McCormick, C. Z., Vanenkevort, E., & Sturm, A. C. (2022). Use of a chatbot to increase uptake of cascade genetic testing. *J Genet Couns, 31*(5), 1219–1230. doi:10.1002/jgc4.1592

Schmidlen, T., Schwartz, M., DiLoreto, K., Kirchner, H. L., & Sturm, A. C. (2019). Patient assessment of chatbots for the scalable delivery of genetic counseling. *J Genet Couns, 28*(6), 1166–1177. doi:10.1002/jgc4.1169

Schwartz, M. L. B., McCormick, C. Z., Lazzeri, A. L., Lindbuchler, D. M., Hallquist, M. L. G., Manickam, K., . . . Murray, M. F. (2018). A model for genome-first care: Returning secondary genomic findings to participants and their healthcare providers in a large research cohort. *Am J Hum Genet, 103*(3), 328–337. doi:10.1016/j.ajhg.2018.07.009

Snir, M., Nazareth, S., Simmons, E., Hayward, L., Ashcraft, K., Bristow, S. L., . . . Aradhya, S. (2021). Democratizing genomics: Leveraging software to make genetics an integral part of routine care. *Am J Med Genet C Semin Med Genet, 187*(1), 14–27. doi:10.1002/ajmg.c.31866

Sobel, S., & Cowan, C. B. (2003). Ambiguous loss and disenfranchised grief: the impact of DNA predictive testing on the family as a system. *Fam Process, 42*(1), 47–57.

Trees, A. R., Koenig Kellas, J., & Roche, M. I. (2010). Family narratives. In C. L. G. C. L. Bylund (Ed.), *Family communication about genetics: Theory and practice* (pp. 68–86). New York, NY: Oxford University Press.

Werner-Lin, A. (2007). Danger zones: Risk perceptions of young women from families with hereditary breast and ovarian cancer. *Fam Process, 46*(3), 335–349.

Werner-Lin, A., & Gardner, D. S. (2009). Family illness narratives of inherited cancer risk: continuity and transformation. *Families, Systems, & Health, 27*(3), 201.

Williams, M. S., Buchanan, A. H., Davis, F. D., Faucett, W. A., Hallquist, M. L., Leader, J. B., . . . Murray, M. F. (2018). Patient-centered precision health in a learning health care system: Geisinger's genomic medicine experience. *Health Affairs, 37*(5), 757–764.

Witte, K., & Allen, M. (2000). A meta-analysis of fear appeals: implications for effective public health campaigns. *Health Educ Behav, 27*(5), 591–615. doi:10.1177/109019810002700506

Wittenberg-Lyles, E., Goldsmith, J., Demiris, G., Oliver, D. P., & Stone, J. (2012). The impact of family communication patterns on hospice family caregivers: A new typology. *Journal of hospice and palliative nursing: JHPN: the official journal of the Hospice and Palliative Nurses Association, 14*(1), 25.

Wright, K. B., Frey, L., & Sopory, P. (2007). Willingness to communicate about health as an underlying trait of patient self-advocacy: The development of the willingness to communicate about health (WTCH) measure. *Communication Studies, 58*(1), 35–51.

PART THREE

# Social Environments Conducive to Successful Aging

CHAPTER SEVEN

# Word by Word, Not Brick by Brick: Building Spaces for Successful Aging through Social Interaction and Communication

CRAIG FOWLER

From working with Jon (Nussbaum), I learned that communication was an essential means by which older adults could maintain identity, facilitate social connection, and raise awareness of needs (Nussbaum et al., 2000). In immediate, pragmatic ways such as this, I discovered, communication was necessary if a person wished to age successfully, and I made sure to say as much in the courses I taught in communication and aging as a newly hired assistant professor!

Almost a decade after graduating as one of Jon's graduate students (during which time the research projects I took on mostly addressed some element of intergenerational family communication), a chance conversation with Howie Giles renewed my interest in the role communication played in successful aging. Through a series of projects carried out with Howie and Jessica Gasiorek (who was one of Howie's graduate students when this work began), I began to study and write about the ways in which people communicatively construct social environments within which they can age more successfully.

The phrasing of that previous sentence has become so familiar to me that it just rolls off my tongue, but it's the sort of sentence that can make other people's eyes glaze over. After all, isn't aging successfully primarily a matter of "genetics or good luck" (Carstensen, 2009, p. 7)? And don't tangible, *physical* environments have a far greater importance impact on whether a person ages well than these nebulous, vaguely hippy-ish sounding "social environments"? Howie, Jessica, and

I try to avoid implying that communication is the panacea to all challenges associated with aging. Nonetheless, we *do* argue that whether we age successfully or not is affected by how we *communicate* about age. We view this as something to be grateful for: we have no control over our genetics, limited control over our physical environments, and are subject to the whims of fate and luck. Every one of us, however, is able to exert control over our communication!

Before going further, it's useful to consider what it actually *means* to "age successfully." Aging is, of course, a biological process that involves significant physical and cognitive changes (Crosnoe & Elder, 2002), and some schools of thought recommend using objective standards to gauge whether a person is aging successfully. There are advantages to this. It is relatively straightforward, for instance, to determine whether a given individual can walk a certain distance or grip an object with a certain degree of strength, to gauge whether that person's memory is reasonably sound, or to assess whether they can complete a certain number of activities of daily living unaided. Some research, however, indicates that (depending on the criteria employed) the proportion of people who meet objective standards for successful aging is relatively low (Depp & Jeste, 2006). Moreover, people who do not meet objective criteria for successful aging may nonetheless perceive themselves to be aging perfectly well, thank you very much (e.g., Pruchno et al., 2010)!

Because of this, many scholars think it is important to let people decide for themselves whether they are aging successfully. To a large degree, Howie, Jessica, and I share this view, and much of our work therefore privileges people's subjective assessments of how successfully they are aging. However, while this ameliorates some of the problems that result from relying on a set of fixed criteria to gauge successful aging, it introduces others! Most notably, previous research has shown that people have *wildly* different ideas about what it means to age well. Even when only a small number of lay people are asked to define what it means to *them* to age well, a range of suggestions emerges. According to one small-scale survey ($n = 53$), people aged 60 or older defined successful aging as involving activity/exercise, good physical health, social relationships, and psychological/cognitive health (Ferri et al., 2009). In a separate interview-based study ($n = 22$) with persons aged 64–96, however, a different set of priorities was voiced: Older adults believed themselves to be aging successfully to the extent that they felt a sense of self-acceptance and perceived themselves to be growing or engaging with life (Reichstadt et al., 2010). Obviously, as the number of participants involved in a study increases, there is greater potential for disparate perspectives to emerge regarding what it means to age successfully. Perhaps nowhere is this better illustrated than in a five-wave longitudinal study conducted between 1996 and 2006. During this period, Tate et al. (2013) studied 1,745 men ($M_{age} = 78$ years at baseline) who provided almost 6,000 responses to the question "What is your definition of successful aging?" Such was the breadth of open-ended responses that 21 main themes and 86 subthemes were required to capture them!

In light of such research, Howie, Jessica, and I conceptualized successful aging in our own work as a phenomenon that—while it may have biomedical components—must also be understood as psychosocial in nature (see Bowling, 2006). This approach acknowledges that there are multiple routes people can take to arrive at a "successful" old age (Hsu & Jones, 2012), that there is considerable heterogeneity with respect to what "successful aging" looks and sounds like (Gasiorek et al., 2015), and that how well we age is, in part, a product of the social and psychological experiences we encounter during our lives. Central to the work we've been doing is the belief not only that these experiences are constituted through communication and interaction but also that it is through communication and interaction that we constitute our understanding of *aging* itself.

In this chapter, I begin by outlining the *Communicative Ecology Model of Successful Aging* (CEMSA) developed by myself, Jessica and Howie, paying particular attention to the model's roots in social constructivism, which is something that has not always been made as explicit as it could have been. After sketching this outline, I discuss the ways in which the model has been developed and extended, summarizing findings from this program of research along the way. Finally, I try to convey that although our model seeks to explain why and how communication is vital for successful aging, it is a model that has implications for people of all ages—not just people who already consider themselves to be old!

## THE CONSTRUCTION OF AGING SPACES, AND THE DEVELOPMENT OF THE CEMSA

### Aging and Social Constructivism

The CEMSA was born out of applied scholarship that sought to offer prescriptions for how to communicate in ways that bolstered one's chances of aging well (see Giles et al., 2013). Nonetheless, to understand some of the assumptions that guided the development of the CEMSA, it is helpful to review some slightly more abstract and philosophical ideas regarding communication and ontology (i.e., the nature of being and reality; Frey et al., 1999).

Anderson and Baym (2004) suggest that communication scholars differ in terms of how they understand the nature of reality. For scholars who adopt what they refer to as a *communicative* stance, communication is not merely referential but is "ontologically constitutive" (p. 601). That is, people are conceived as "linguistic beings" who exist "within and through dialogue and interaction," and for whom language is the basis of experience, perception, cognition, and action.

A second group of communication scholars adhere to a *discursive* view, according to which the existence of any "stable, underlying foundation" is dubious. For such scholars, reality is something that is unmoored, and subject to "ever-shifting processes of representation" (p. 602) through language and communication. Adopting either of these positions carries significant implications, for in both views, "ontology is shifted…from the material and the biological to the domain of language and action" (Anderson and Baym, 2004, p. 602). As a consequence, "the real must be reconceptualized not as preexistent, but as socially constructed, not as universally singular, but as contingent upon communicative contexts and therefore local and unavoidably multiple" (p. 602).

I began undergraduate study of communication in 1995, which has given me plenty of exposure to conversations where terms such as *social constructivism* and *symbolic interactionism* have been bandied about. Mindful of the adage that it is better to be thought a fool than to open your mouth and prove it, I've typically participated in these conversations more as a listener than a speaker. Presented with a written account of the socially constructed nature of reality, I tend to think *ahhh, that makes sense! Of course! How could it be otherwise?* Yet when required to explain what social constructivism is (and isn't) in my own words, I flounder. This is, in part, why I have quoted quite extensively from Anderson and Baym in the previous paragraph rather than risk butchering their very helpful explanations.

One area of confusion concerning social constructivism pertains to "just exactly what is being socially constructed" (Keaton and Bodie, 2011, p. 192). Depending on how these ideas are introduced, there is a risk that communication can be seen as practically alchemic in nature, calling into existence "the physical composition of an object (i.e., its material arrangement)" (p. 192). This is not the case, of course! Instead, what is meant when we talk of a socially constructed reality is simply that communication creates an object's "social composition." That is, "communication changes how objects are perceived and the range of potential meanings they can embody" (p. 192).

The "object" of interest to me is *aging*. Obviously, the way in which we communicate does not change the physical materiality of aging. Telling an ageist joke does not decrease the amount of collagen in our skin, increase the thickness of hair that for some of us sprouts unbidden from our ears, or prompt the emergence of liver spots. However, telling an ageist joke *does*, perhaps, modify the social definition of aging. It changes how we view aging and older people, and it changes what aging *means* to us. Through processes of social interaction, then, we engage in the process of actively creating, maintaining, and transforming our psychological selves and social worlds (Lindlof, 2008). Whereas *physical* aging spaces may be constructed brick-by-brick, the *social* aging spaces within which we age are constructed word-by-word and conversation-by-conversation. Indeed, what it means to get older or to be a certain age is symbolically constructed through communication: In Carstensen's words, "Life stages are social constructions, not absolute realities" (2009, p. 7).

As Taylor (1994) illustrates, any attempt to grasp what it means to be old or grow older can only be made by grappling with cultural vocabularies that "segment, theorize, and moralize the aging process" (p. 199). These vocabularies shift over time and place, and what it means to be "old," to be a particular age, or to be aging successfully is something that must be continually negotiated and renegotiated as discourses shift "in relation to worldly forces of economics, politics, technology, and history" (Taylor, 1994, p. 190). Such discursive shifts can be profound. Taylor notes, for instance, that societal discourse about older adults in the colonial period led to older persons being "venerated…as repositories of wisdom and morality" (p. 197). Following the Industrial Revolution, however, these discourses redefined what it meant to be old in far more negative terms, culminating (during the 1970s) in the symbolic construction of aging as an "illness" and as a "social problem" (p. 198). Given that the meaning of age is inherently unstable, it is little wonder that some people find the aging process to be fraught with uncertainty. After all, in the absence of fixed waypoints and pre-defined meanings, it is a journey that must be improvised; we must feel our way as we go.

## Postulates of the CEMSA

Uncertainty about aging can center on all manner of issues, from the deeply existential to the pragmatic. As an example of the former, Taylor (1994) writes that aging and agedness may prompt individuals to question, *Who* <u>*am*</u> *I now that I am not what I was? What will I be after this?* (p. 186). As individuals adapt to changes in health and work status, uncertainties about one's purpose, meaning, value, and legacy become particularly salient (e.g., Nuttman-Shwartz, 2004). At a more practical level, as people age they may grapple with unknowns about matters such as whether they will have enough money, whether they will be lonely (Neikrug, 2003), and whether they will need long-term care (Kemper et al., 2005).

When we developed the CEMSA, our conceptualization of uncertainty was informed by the theory of motivated information management (TMIM: Afifi & Weiner, 2004). That is, we emphasized the importance of *uncertainty discrepancy* rather than the mere existence of uncertainty itself. In the context of aging, an uncertainty discrepancy occurs when a gap exists between (a) what a person *knows* about getting older and (b) what they would *like to know* about getting older. Part of what makes the TMIM distinctive is that it does not treat uncertainty as inherently problematic or undesirable; rather, the theory allows for the possibility that people may feel more *uncertain* than they want to be, more *certain* that they want to be, or to be fortunate enough to experience just the *right* amount of uncertainty or certainty. The measurement choices we made in our original studies, however, nonetheless betrayed an implicit assumption that uncertainty about aging is likely to be experienced as problematic or undesirable[1].

Uncertainty discrepancy was positioned in the CEMSA as a factor that might instantiate seven kinds of age-related communication behavior. More specifically, we anticipated that uncertainty about aging would influence the degree to which individuals (a) invoked age to account for their behavior or circumstances; (b) expressed optimism about aging; (c) colluded in age-related teasing and stereotyping; (d) responded to being the recipient of ageist remarks or teasing; (e) resisted (or felt psychological reactance in response to) advertising messages predicated on the notion that being old is problematic; (f) discussed their future care needs with family and other loved ones; and (g) were able to use and appreciate new technologies (e.g., Skype; social media; the internet) that might facilitate communication with friends and family.

We also anticipated that experiencing age-related uncertainty discrepancy—in conjunction with engaging in these seven forms of age-related communication—would influence the degree to which the thought of growing older elicited positive (e.g., interest or optimism) and/or negative (e.g., anxiety or distress) affective reactions. Together, uncertainty discrepancy, communication about aging, and affect were expected to predict the extent to which individuals experienced *aging efficacy*. We defined aging efficacy as the felt ability to cope with changes experienced as a result of getting older and positioned it as the direct antecedent of successful aging itself (gauged by people's subjective judgments that they were aging well). There's a lot going on here, and if it's helpful to see these relationships depicted visually, take a look at Figure 7.1.

1 Operationally, we adapted scales used in TMIM studies, gauging the level of uncertainty discrepancy by asking people to respond to scale items such as "I am less certain than I would like to be about what my future holds," and "I know less than I would like to about what my life will be like as I get older."

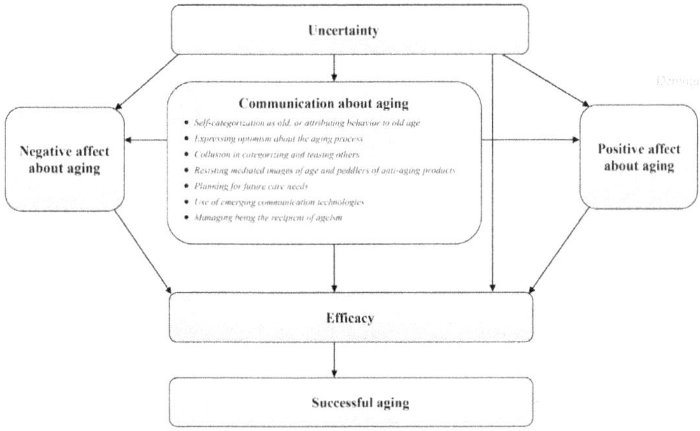


Figure 7.1: The original communicative ecology model of successful aging (from Fowler et al., 2015)

## Initial Results

The first test of the model was carried out with a sample of middle-aged and older New Zealanders. Some components of the model worked largely as expected. In particular, we found support for the hypothesized relationships between uncertainty, affect, efficacy, and successful aging. Moreover, the CEMSA explained a large proportion of the variance in participants' judgments that they were aging well, by virtue of a very strong relationship between self-reported aging efficacy and successful aging. We found more equivocal support for the role of communication in the model, however. Expressing optimism about aging was the communicative domain that yielded the most consistent results, being associated in the expected manner with uncertainty, affect, and efficacy. We also found that using new communication technology was associated with affect and efficacy, that invoking age to explain behavior (or as we also refer to it, self-categorization as old) was associated as expected with uncertainty, and that discussing future care needs was associated with affect.

In sum, the initial results were encouraging but not as consistent as we would have hoped. We interpreted them as suggesting that the overarching CEMSA framework was pretty sound, but that there was still work to be done with respect to pinning down theoretically salient communication variables and figuring out how to measure them.

## Profiles

Arguably, a better sense of the communication ecology individuals create and inhabit might be obtained by assessing people's patterns of communication about aging *across* domains, rather than by examining isolated dimensions of age-related talk. By way of analogy, examining the impact of an individual domain of talk might be akin to examining a length of a 2×4, whereas examining a *profile* is more like examining a structure assembled from multiple 2×4s. In this pursuit, CEMSA researchers have employed latent class analysis (LCA; sometimes also called latent profile analysis, or LPA). This analytic approach has not only helped identify more holistic patterns of age-related communication but has also allowed us to examine whether engaging in a particular pattern of age-related communication predicts people's affect or efficacy related to aging.

I'll touch on recent profile-based CEMSA research shortly. For now, though, I'd like to highlight findings emerging from the first three LCAs conducted on CEMSA data. Two of these analyses were reported by Gasiorek et al. (2015), who ran a pair of LCAs; one on data from the original New Zealand sample, and a second on a new dataset comprising adults aged 40+ living in the United States. The third analysis (see Gasiorek & Fowler, 2016) was conducted on data collected from *younger* adults (aged 18–39) living in the United States.

Three very similar profiles of communication about age and aging emerged in each of the samples. *Disengaged* agers reported low levels of talk about age and aging across all seven domains. *Engaged* agers tended not to self-categorize as old or tease others about their age, but reported expressing quite high levels of optimism, resistance of anti-aging media messages, and discussion of future care needs. Finally, *bantering* agers self-reported high levels of both positive and negative age-focused talk—i.e., self-categorization, optimism, and teasing, but only moderate levels of discussion of future care needs.

In the two middle-aged and older-adult samples, *engaged agers* reported somewhat lower levels of negative affect and higher levels of positive affect, efficacy, and self-reported successful aging. However, people in *all* profiles seemed to be experiencing aging quite positively. Curiously, the advantages bestowed by being an engaged ager (with respect to attitudes and emotions concerning aging) and the disadvantages deriving from being a *disengaged* ager were more pronounced in the young-adult sample (Gasiorek & Fowler, 2016). It may be tempting to shrug off the importance of this by questioning whether it even matters what young people think and feel about aging. To do so would be a mistake, however, for—at the risk of stating the obvious—the beliefs and mindsets people adopt about aging early in life are the precursors to the beliefs and mindsets about aging that they hold as older adults. Consequently, the views of aging people when they are young can have associations with long-term health outcomes that only appear later in life (Levy, 2009).

## EVOLUTION OF THE CEMSA

Since the first CEMSA-based papers were published in 2015, researchers have poked and prodded at the model Jessica, Howie, and I proposed. Indeed, we have done a fair amount of this poking ourselves! In this section, I describe how elements of the CEMSA have evolved. First, I highlight how we have grappled with the way uncertainty is incorporated into the CEMSA. Second, I describe how CEMSA researchers have begun to consider alternative conceptualizations of successful aging. Third, I discuss research seeking to broaden the scope of what constitutes age-related talk. Fourth, I review a concept Gasiorek et al. (2016) introduced in a revised formulation of the CEMSA; namely, *environmental chatter* (see Figure 7.2).

### The Role of Uncertainty

In one way or another, uncertainty has been at the heart of the CEMSA since the model was merely a gleam in Howie's eye. We remain committed to the belief that uncertainty should be a central component of a model seeking to examine how communication facilitates successful aging. After all, some scholars have gone so far as to argue that the aging process is "permeated" (Pecchioni et al., 2004, p. 179) by "radical uncertainty" (Coupland, 2004, p. 83). And not only is this uncertainty something that individuals must "battle against" (Nussbaum & Coupland, 2004, p. xii) but also among the weapons with which Coupland (2004) believes this battle should be fought are "language and discourse" (p. 83). With that said, it is worth reiterating that we shy away from suggesting in the CEMSA that these "weapons" should be employed to *reduce* uncertainty (as might be inferred by those familiar with classic communication theories concerning uncertainty such as uncertainty reduction theory; Berger, 1987). Rather, we argue that uncertainty may stimulate a wide range of communicative behaviors via which individuals—more or less successfully—negotiate ambiguities that accompany aging.

#### Theorizing Uncertainty in the CEMSA

As noted earlier, our thinking regarding uncertainty in the CEMSA has always owed a debt to Afifi and Weiner's (2004) TMIM. In part, we drew on the TMIM because it offers a very flexible, pragmatic view of uncertainty, holding that

(a) uncertainty is not always experienced as aversive, and (b) it is people's appraisals of their level of uncertainty rather than the mere *presence* of uncertainty that evokes emotional reactions from individuals. It seemed to us that these characteristics lent themselves particularly well to the context of aging. Nonetheless, findings from our early studies forced us to consider whether we ought to rely solely on a conceptualization of uncertainty grounded in the TMIM. We discovered, for instance, that whereas in early TMIM studies relatively few people (well under 10 % according to Afifi, 2010) appeared to desire more uncertainty (or less certainty) than they experienced, over *half* of participants in our first CEMSA study (Fowler et al., 2015) were in this position.

What this suggested to us was that the majority of respondents in our initial tests of the CEMSA "were *not* experiencing 'radical uncertainty' about aging" (Gasiorek et al., 2019, p. 232). In fact, rather than wrestling with what they *didn't* know about aging, our participants were, we began to suspect, "daunted by what they believe they already know" about aging, namely that it would be a predominantly undesirable experience (Gasiorek et al., 2019, p. 232). This suspicion prompted us to consider how else we might think about the role of uncertainty within the CEMSA.

The more we pondered, the more we realized that how people perceived and appraised the certainties and vagaries associated with the aging process was particularly well captured by *problematic integration theory* (PIT; Babrow, 1992, 2001). According to PIT, individuals assess a given situation (or an event; an outcome, and so on) with respect to both (i) the likelihood or probability that it will occur, and (ii) the desirability of its occurrence. For instance, people may assess both the probability that they will live far away from family when they are older and the degree to which this prospect troubles or delights them. Together, these assessments are then held to shape how people approach, encounter, and communicate about the situation (or event; outcome, etc.).

We found PIT appealing not only because it seemed to more accurately capture how people think about the aging process but also because it positions communicative behavior as a resource: Communication is treated as something people can use to work through and manage episodes when something is deemed desirable but improbable or undesirable but probable (i.e., when their combined assessments of desirability and likelihood result in the *problematic integration* from which the theory gets its name). Yet another advantage of PIT is that Babrow (1992) considers communicative behavior itself to shape whether ambiguous situations are seen to be problematic or unconcerning, avoidable or inevitable, threatening or challenging, and so on. In short, communication is positioned as "the vehicle for…transformations" (p. 99) with respect to how we view (un)ambiguous or (un) certain situations. This framing is particularly appropriate for how we view the role of communication with respect to facilitating successful aging.

### Operationalizing Uncertainty in the CEMSA

To incorporate insights from PIT into the CEMSA, we developed a measure of the *perceived probability of negative experiences* (PPNE) associated with aging (Gasiorek et al., 2019). We envisioned this PIT-based operationalization of uncertainty supplementing rather than replacing the TMIM-based operationalization because the two theories treat uncertainty in different but complementary ways: Whereas *uncertainty discrepancy* measures generalized "unwanted uncertainty or certainty about aging" (Gasiorek et al., 2019, p. 243), PPNE assesses the degree to which people believe it is likely (or not) that they will experience specific problematic age-related phenomena such as loneliness, ill-health, and financial difficulties.

From two studies, Gasiorek et al. (2019) determined that—relative to UD—PPNE more consistently predicted CEMSA variables. PPNE predicted positive affect about aging, negative affect about aging, efficacy about aging, and (indirectly) successful aging, *regardless* of whether individuals were classified as bantering, engaged, or disengaged agers. Uncertainty discrepancy predicted positive and negative affect about aging for people in some profiles of aging, albeit not as strongly as did PPNE. Likewise, there were fewer associations between UD and efficacy, and the magnitude of this association was smaller than the comparable association between PPNE and efficacy.

Ultimately, Gasiorek et al. (2019) concluded that "people's emotional responses to the prospect of getting older...are better explained by their expectations for their future than their appraisals of gaps in uncertainty" (p. 244). However, they also acknowledged that both UD and PPNE contributed independently to the prediction of attitudes toward aging. As such they recommended that, where possible, CEMSA studies include both operationalizations of uncertainty.

## Expansion to Include Objective Indicators of Successful Aging

I noted over the first two or three pages of this chapter that research grounded in the CEMSA has usually operationalized "successful aging" by asking participants to provide a subjective judgment of their state of affairs (Fowler et al., 2015). This assessment has typically been the "end point" of CEMSA-studies; the "ultimate" dependent variable that all antecedents are working to predict. And the model has often, in this sense, done its job very well! In our first test of the CEMSA, for example, the model accounted for 78 % of the variance in successful aging (Fowler et al., 2015).

Beginning with a 2018 paper by Gasiorek and Barile, however, CEMSA researchers began to explore alternative endpoints of the model, typically by examining whether membership in a given communicative profile of aging (e.g., engaged, bantering, disengaged) predicted health-related outcomes. Several of the selected endpoints in Gasiorek and Barile's study were natural extensions of existing CEMSA research, for they comprised quite subjective judgments regarding life satisfaction and perceived stress levels. Additionally, however, Gasiorek and Barile employed the 4-item Health-related quality of life (HRQoL-4) index to obtain more objective estimates from participants of the number of days (during the preceding thirty days) on which they experienced poor mental and physical health, or on which their mental or physical health kept them from engaging in their usual activities.

Subsequently, in collaboration with Jessica and Howie, Quinten Bernhold extended the range of potential outcomes affected by age-related communication to include healthy eating (Bernhold & Giles, 2020), mental health and depression (Bernhold & Gasiorek, 2020; Bernhold et al., 2020), and alcohol use (Bernhold & Gasiorek, 2020; Bernhold et al., 2020). Although these behaviors may appear to be somewhat removed from the simple, subjective assessment of successful aging used in the first few tests of the CEMSA, they reflect how lay adults themselves define what constitutes or indicates successful aging (e.g., Ferri et al., 2009; Reichstadt et al., 2010; Tate et al., 2013).

In general, being an "engaged ager" seems to be positively associated with health and well-being. For instance, communicating like an engaged ager has been found to predict higher levels of life satisfaction (relative to disengaged agers; Gasiorek & Barile, 2018). Further, being an engaged ager predicted more consumption of healthy food (specifically, fruit) and less consumption of unhealthy beverages (specifically, soft drinks; Bernhold & Giles, 2020). And, in studies that have examined how membership in a given communication profile might affect health outcomes indirectly via efficacy, people who are engaged agers report fewer symptoms of depression and alcohol use disorder (relative to disengaged agers; Bernhold & Gasiorek, 2020), as well as lower levels of loneliness (Bernhold et al., 2020)[2].

Although I have tried to cover what I consider to be the key findings of this research program here, this is not intended to be an exhaustive review of CEMSA studies that have employed LCA. In particular, for reasons of space I have not

2 There are also indications that *bantering* agers may fare more poorly than engaged agers with respect to levels of stress (Gasiorek & Barile, 2018), depressive symptomology (Bernhold & Gasiorek, 2020), and that bantering agers may consume less fruit and vegetables (Bernhold & Giles, 2020).

discussed findings relating to comparisons between disengaged and bantering agers (see Gasiorek & Barile, 2018). Nor have I touched on outcomes associated with a fourth communicative profile of aging identified by Bernhold et al. (2020); namely, the *gloomy* ager[3]. Nonetheless, the findings summarized in this section do, I think, support the argument that engaging in certain systematic patterns of age-related communication can have important consequences for a variety of indicators of (or proxies for) successful aging.

## Expansion to Include Additional Domains of (Not Necessarily) Age-Related Talk

The CEMSA originally identified seven foci of age-related talk (usually referred to as *domains*; for a refresher on these, see Figure 7.1). Recently, however, Gettings and Kuang (2022) made a case for incorporating two additional domains of age-related talk[4]. The first of these is *talk about retirement*, which was operationalized by Gettings and Kuang via items such as *I talk with others about what retirement will look like* and *I talk to family or friends about how I will financially support myself as I age*.

I find the argument for including this domain of talk in the CEMSA compelling. After all, retirement is a stage of life that involves considerable uncertainty! Retirees (or retirees-to-be) may be unsure of *when* they should retire, *where* they should live when they retire, *what* they will do when they retire, *how* they will manage financially during retirement, and so on. Indeed, when we first articulated the CEMSA, we referenced uncertainty about retirement as a particularly important area of ambiguity, noting Carstensen's (2009) observation that "[n]obody told us what to do with a retirement that could…last forty years" (p. 4). This is an aspect of age-related talk that I wish we'd included in the CEMSA from the outset; it sits very naturally alongside the domain of age-related talk that focuses on preparation for future care needs.

The second "new" domain of talk Gettings and Kuang propose concerns *career meaning*. At a conceptual level, this domain captures the degree to which individuals talk about the significance they attach to their career and work. At an operational level, *career meaning* is assessed via items such as, *When talking about*

3 People fitting this communication profile are characterized by "high levels of self-categorization [as old], low levels of expressed optimism and teasing, moderate-to-low levels of talk about future care, and low levels of engagement with technology" (Bernhold et al., 2020, p. 119).

4 A few days before this chapter was due to be sent to the publisher, Bernhold et al. (2023) published an article identifying another potentially important domain of communication that could be incorporated into the CEMSA; namely, communicating about religion.

*my career, I often comment on how meaningful it was*, and *I talk about how the work I did served a greater purpose*.

While I'm enthusiastic about including *talk about retirement* in the CEMSA, I'm conflicted about the domain of *career meaning*, largely because I think the domains of talk should be *explicitly* related to age and aging[5]. Nonetheless, I'm mindful that as we developed the CEMSA, we were very much inspired by Ouwehand et al.'s (2007) argument that aging well requires a person to "create environments, which make success possible while effectively dealing with losses due to aging" (p. 874). And, to the extent that internalized and self-directed ageism leads individuals to feel diminished by age (or that one's time of being procreative, productive, and creative may be drawing to a close; Erikson, 1997), talking about the meaningfulness of one's labors (past, present, or even future) may be an important way of "dealing with losses." As such, perhaps it is unfair to insist that any new domain explicitly address aging. Moreover, such insistence could be seen as hypocritical. After all, while most of the CEMSA's original domains of talk referenced age or aging in an explicit way, at least one domain—*using technology to foster communication*—did not. And, although using communication technology may take on particular significance in the context of aging (especially if geographic separation from intimates or physical infirmity renders face-to-face interaction difficult), none of the items used to measure this domain make any reference to age (Fowler et al., 2015; Gasiorek & Fowler, 2019).

On the matter of adding further domains of talk to the CEMSA, my feeling is that this should be done with care. I don't think Jessica, Howie, or I believed we'd offered an exhaustive account of the various forms of talk that might construct social environments conducive to successful aging. At the same time, there is a risk of opening the doors too wide, for many forms of communication potentially help individuals create social environments conducive to aging successfully! Should we include in the CEMSA, for instance, measures to assess domains of communicative behavior such as support-seeking? Or how clearly or completely is a person able to articulate symptoms during conversations with health professionals? Or how often (and with what level of success) an individual initiates conversation with potential friends? Obviously, being able to solicit needed support, convey where precisely one's body hurts and the nature of that pain, and to form new connections are likely to help a person age more successfully. Nonetheless, to incorporate such broad, non-age-specific domains of talk risks erasing what makes the CEMSA distinctive, which is its focus on age-related talk. By including

5 This was certainly the case for most of the CEMSA's original domains of talk: expressing optimism about aging, teasing people about their age or stereotyping them on the basis of age, attributing one's behaviour to old age, preparing for future care needs, and managing ageism.

"anything and everything," in the CEMSA, there is a danger that it is left with nothing unique to say.

At a purely pragmatic level, including additional domains of talk (whether they are explicitly age-related or not!) also has implications for researchers who take a profile-based approach to examining the CEMSA. The typology of *engaged*, *bantering*, and *disengaged* profiles has been detected and replicated in numerous samples (Bernhold, 2021; Bernhold & Giles, 2020; Gasiorek & Barile, 2018; Gasiorek & Fowler, 2016; Gasiorek et al., 2015). This is encouraging and suggests that (as Jessica once put it to me) this general distinction of different kinds of agers is a "real thing"!

This consistency, however, has likely been facilitated by the fact that researchers conducting LCAs have typically been working with the same set of 21 items (i.e., those used in Fowler et al., 2015). If studies using LCA begin to also include the 16 items used to capture *talk about retirement* and *career meaning*—as well as items intended to measure any further domains that are proposed—the configuration of profiles could shift substantially. This is not in itself a reason to shy away from including new domains of talk in CEMSA studies—but researchers who take seriously the value of parsimony should weigh whether what is gained justifies both the increased complexity and reduced comparability with existing CEMSA research.

## Expansion to Include Environmental Chatter

In the original version of the CEMSA, we focused almost exclusively on the possibility that a person's *own* age-related communication might influence their attitudes and emotions concerning aging, thereby influencing the degree to which they age successfully. This ascribes a great deal of agency to individuals and reflects that the CEMSA builds on ideas first expressed in a book written with the express purpose of empowering people to age better (Giles et al., 2013). However, we paid much less attention to the possibility that the degree to which aging elicits an emotional response and is seen as controllable is also shaped by the communication an individual *experiences from others,* and by the messages about aging they absorb from their environment. As we observed in an earlier chapter (Gasiorek et al., 2016), "Individuals are rarely in complete control of their social and communicative environments; they are also subject to what others say and do" (p. 39).

Jessica, Howie, and I have since argued that we encounter a sort of low-grade (or at times, quite loud!) background noise. This noise often, we think, comprises messages about aging that are often relatively negative. Regardless of whether a person attends deeply to such messages (or even notices them) at the time, the accumulated and ongoing "hum" about aging that people encounter in the form of "environmental chatter" may have important consequences for how they come to think and feel about the aging process. When we began to consider the broad forms that environmental chatter might take, four variants stood out. In the following discussion, I examine each of these forms of chatter in turn[6].

## Explicit Messages about Aging

Explicit messages about aging involve conversations and comments that openly reference some element of the aging process. Although these messages might occur in the context of interactions with age-peers (e.g., a teen might observe to a friend that "old people are so gross!"), we have mostly focused on explicit messages about aging communicated by older adults themselves. Thus far, the majority of studies that have invoked the concept of environmental chatter have addressed explicit messages about aging.

The term *environmental chatter* is intended to reflect that we encounter a huge number of messages about aging over the course of our lives, often in ways that are experienced or processed as being in the background. As Knapp et al. (1981) point out, most of the messages we encounter about *anything* "have a relatively short life; they are processed, responded to, and forgotten" (p. 27). However, some messages stay with us, influencing our lives in profound ways. Such messages are *memorable messages*, which are an important kind of explicit message about aging.

A neat—albeit fictional—example of a memorable message about aging can be found in the 2019 movie *Jumanji: The next level*. In this film, "Grandpa Eddie" (played by Danny DeVito) repeatedly tells his grandson (Spencer; played by Alex Wolff) that "Getting older sucks. Don't let anybody tell you any different." You get the impression that poor Spencer has grown up hearing repeatedly that old age is something to be feared or resented.

The *memorable messages* framework was first applied to the study of explicit messages people receive about aging long before the CEMSA was developed, when Holladay (2002) asked people aged 18–77 to describe the substance, wording, and source of a memorable message they had encountered about aging. She found, perhaps predictably, that the majority of such messages seem to be passed down from people who are considerably older than recipients (the mean age difference

6 I do not, however, address recent efforts to identify environmental chatter profiles (see Bernhold & Giles, 2020). Nor do I try to cover studies that have examined environmental chatter from a specific source, such as one's romantic partner's communication about aging (Bernhold & Gasiorek, 2020).

between sender and receiver was approximately 35 years), and that the majority (more than three-quarters) of message senders were family members of recipients.

So far, then, Grandpa Eddie seems to be a typical *source* of a memorable message about aging! The *content* of Grandpa Eddie's memorable message about aging (which is prompted by the pain and temporary loss of independence caused by a recent hip surgery) is also a fairly good representation of real-life messages, for Holladay (2002) found that the messages her participants recalled about aging often addressed negative aspects of aging, such as the probability or experience of "physical decline" or "cognitive decline," and the likelihood of facing "social network losses." Interestingly, however, Holladay learned that other memorable message themes were more positive, emphasizing the "benefits of aging," the need to "enjoy life," and the beliefs that aging is both a "natural process" and a "state of mind." By the end of *Jumanji: The next level*, Grandpa Eddie's explicit—and likely memorable—messaging about aging starts to reflect these more favorable beliefs as he states: "Getting old is a gift; I forget that sometimes."

For me, there are two important "takeaways" from Holladay's study. First, a majority of messages included a positive element. Indeed, almost half the messages were *exclusively* positive in valence! Second, more than 70 % of respondents believed the message they recalled had impacted them in some way; for example, by making them view aging differently, or by making them decide to live life more fully. In other words, environmental chatter (which in this instance constituted a single, isolated message) had a significant impact on how recipients viewed, felt about, and in some cases approached the aging process! The importance of Holladay's findings regarding the importance of explicit memorable messages about aging were recently underscored by Bernhold and Giles (2019). These researchers learned that memorable messages about aging indirectly enhanced perceptions of successful aging by increasing participants' beliefs that they could exert control over the aging process, and cope with or adapt to challenges associated with it (i.e., by increasing aging efficacy).

Working outside the memorable messages framework, other researchers have also shed light on the potential of encountering explicit messages about aging. From a survey of young adults, for instance, Gasiorek and Fowler (2022) found that the frequency with which young adults perceived their mothers and fathers to complain about aging predicted (respectively) more negative affect about aging and reduced efficacy about aging. And, in a vignette-based study, Fowler and Bernhold (2023) varied the explanations provided by an older person to a younger adult for an age-typed behavior. Specifically, they tested the effects of invoking a positively valenced reference to age, a negatively valenced reference to age, or an age-neutral reason. For instance, an older adult who was unable to perform a physical task could reference being sore from exercise (which was important at their age!), having been affected by the wear-and-tear that inevitably accompanies aging, or simply having a bad back that runs in the family (and perhaps needing a more supportive mattress). Young adults who read the positive age-based explanations perceived the aging process to have been portrayed more favorably. Consequently, the prospect of their own aging elicited more positive emotions, which in turn predicted not only feeling better able to manage their *own* aging but also having more positive expectations regarding the aging process writ large.

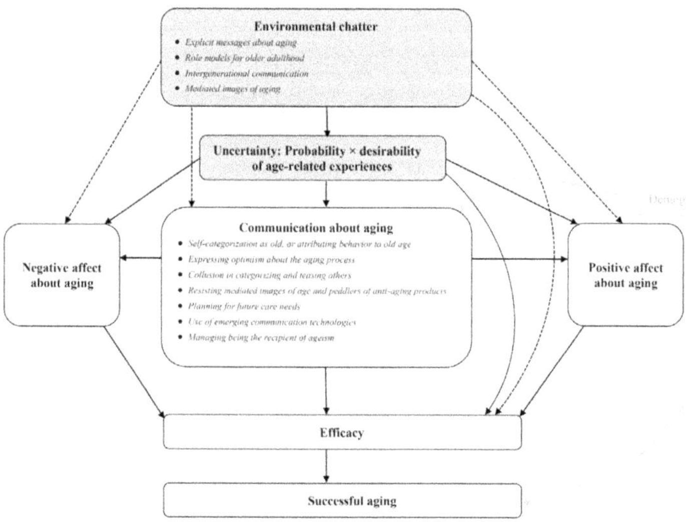


Figure 7.2: The revised communicative ecology model of successful aging (from Gasiorek et al., 2016)

## Role Models

Even when they do not provide explicit messages about aging, older adults (through what they say and how they behave) provide powerful demonstrations of what it means to age well—or in some cases, to age poorly. Let's go back to Grandpa Eddie for a moment: Perhaps Spencer never hears his grandfather overtly remark on how much "being old sucks." Instead, perhaps Grandpa Eddie merely—without referencing age—conveys that he is in a constant state of misery, despite the fact that all around the house are old family photos featuring a youthful and grinning Eddie. These observations can serve as implicit messages, and Spencer may infer for himself that old age is the source of his grandfather's unhappiness. Lest I appear to be making too much of what Spencer is learning from Grandpa Eddie, it is worth noting that close kin provides particularly accessible models of aging: When we picture our own futures, we often "extrapolate from our limited family experiences" (Carstensen, 2009, p. 14) and whether we come away with positive ideas about what aging entails will depend much on whether, as Carstensen puts it, "Aunt Betty baked cookies or had dementia" (p. 14).

The older adults who serve as our role models for aging probably do so unconsciously for the most part. We might infer from Aunt Betty's baking bonanzas that older adults are hospitable, active, and know their way around a stand mixer. Nonetheless, it seems unlikely that Aunt Betty whips up a batch of cookies with the express purpose of cultivating in her younger relatives a particular understanding of the aging process! My parents are both in their 70s, and although I doubt that they intentionally set out to model what it is to age successfully, they do so anyway by volunteering, nurturing, taking classes in Te reo Māori, exercising, socializing, and philosophizing. Since retiring (and relocating from England to New Zealand after reaching pensionable age), both my parents have found new ways to have meaning-filled lives—and witnessing this makes me feel more optimistic about what my *own* life will be like when I am older.

Non-familial older adults who are members of our wider social networks can also act as positive or negative aging role models. At the risk of being too "on the nose," despite having officially retired, Howie continues to edit journals, publish articles faster than I can read them, and train members of his local police force. He is the very embodiment of Hummert et al.'s (1994) stereotype of the "golden-ager" and an example of somebody demonstrating how to do old age "well." Intriguingly, older people we've never met—and even those who don't really exist—can also serve as role models for how to age well: Schiappa et al.'s (2005) parasocial contact hypothesis speaks to the fact that mass-mediated contact with members of a group—whether real or fictional—can shape the attitudes we hold regarding that group as a whole. Whether we look to David Attenborough, Albus Dumbledore, Morgan Freeman, or Betty White, potential aging role models abound in popular media (Gasiorek et al., 2016).

Gasiorek et al. (2016) argued that having role models who demonstrate positive aspects of growing older should enhance the positive affect and efficacy a person feels with respect to aging while diminishing negative affect. Having role models whose behavior signals that aging is unpleasant or undesirable should have the opposite effect. Although it is only in its nascent stages, research so far seems to support this thinking. Gasiorek and Fowler (2020) discovered, for instance, that young adults' reports of having positive role models about aging positively predicted the degree to which they felt efficacious about aging.

### Media Messages

A third—and particularly pervasive—form of environmental chatter about aging comprises messages communicated by the mass media, which tends to underrepresent older adults (Gerbner et al., 1980; Harwood & Anderson, 2002, Roy & Harwood, 1997; Robinson & Skill, 1995; Vasil & Wass, 1993), and depict them in unflattering, stereotypical ways (Robinson et al., 2004). In so doing, mass media may affect the judgments people make regarding the vitality and longevity of older adults (Gerbner et al., 2002), the traits ascribed to older adults (Robinson & Anderson, 2006), and the belief that looking or feeling old should at all costs be avoided (Coupland, 2007; Mehlman et al., 2004).

Only one study has so far examined potential links between mass media–centered forms of chatter and constructs included in the CEMSA. In this study, Bernhold (2021) asked participants aged 55 or older to rate how positively or negatively they believed ten kinds of media portrayed aging. Almost half of the respondents perceived all ten media variants to depict aging negatively. The responses of slightly fewer than a third of participants were consistently around the scale midpoint, indicating that they viewed the media as depicting neither a negative nor positive view of aging. Just over one-fifth of participants believed that aging was portrayed at least somewhat positively in each of the types of media.

Interestingly, Bernhold's (2021) findings did not support the expectation that people who encountered more negative media messages about aging would have more negative attitudes about aging (i.e., lower levels of positive affect and efficacy about aging, and higher levels of negative affect about aging). Instead, relative to people who felt media portrayals of aging were mostly positive, those who thought portrayals were neutral or negative had higher levels of aging efficacy and, consequently, reported aging *more* successfully. One explanation for these counter-intuitive findings is that although people may frequently encounter negative depictions of aging in the media, they also recognize that these portrayals are inaccurate or commercially motivated. As such, they may not be inclined to draw on such portrayals when reflecting on their own feelings about aging (Bernhold, 2021). In accounting for why—seemingly paradoxically—participants who felt mass media depicted aging favorably were actually those with the lowest levels of aging efficacy (and consequently, of successful aging), Bernhold suggested that seeing older characters portrayed in a highly positive way, viewers may feel that their own lives "pale by comparison, thereby reducing their aging efficacy and successful aging" (p. 25).

### Accommodative and Nonaccommodative Communication

The final form of environmental chatter Gasiorek et al. (2016) identified comprises accommodative and nonaccommodative communication. According to communication accommodation theory (Giles, 2016), accommodative interactions tend to be prosocial in nature, featuring positive and/or appropriately adapted messages. Interactions that are nonaccommodative, however, involve negative and/or inappropriately adjusted communication (Giles & Gasiorek, 2011).

To illustrate how (non)accommodative communication might shape attitudes to aging, consider a scenario in which an older adult encounters an accommodative younger adult who listens carefully to what the older person has to say, conveys respect (and perhaps admiration), and communicates in a way that is supportive or encouraging (Williams et al., 1997). Arguably, such interactions support the older adult's positive sense of identity: the younger person's behavior implicitly (or even explicitly) expresses that older adults are worthy of attention and engagement—and old age is something to be valued and appreciated. As such, a younger person who engages in accommodative communication with an older adult might enhance the older interactant's positive affect and efficacy about aging while damping their negative affect about aging. Nonaccommodative interactions, in which young adults patronize, demean, or ignore older adults may have the opposite effect (Gasiorek & Fowler, 2020).

Results from two recent studies seem to support this reasoning. In a study of middle-aged and older adults, Gasiorek & Fowler (2020) found that receiving accommodative communication had a direct positive effect on efficacy about aging whereas receiving nonaccommodative communication had a direct negative effect on aging efficacy. Similarly, in a study of *younger* adults (aged 18–28), Gasiorek (2022) found that having received nonaccommodation from older people predicted greater anxiety about aging, lower efficacy about aging, and more negative views of older adults.

## CONCLUSION

The degree to which people are considered to be aging successfully is often thought to be a matter of "genetics or good luck" (Carstensen, 2009, p. 7). And, while this may be true to some extent, it is not the *whole* truth: People's sense of whether or not they are aging well also hinges on their ability to communicatively construct social environments that facilitate well-being as they move through the life course. In this final section, I have tried to capture our developing thoughts regarding how people shape their trajectories of aging via communication, and how the "aging spaces" we inhabit may be shaped—for better or worse—by the communication of others.

Although this goal ostensibly separates what we refer to as a person's own "age-related talk" from the "environmental chatter" that they encounter, this division is somewhat artificial: In the context of social interaction, the two inevitably mingle together. Fowler and Bernhold (2023) noted, for instance:

> When an older person offers an age-based attribution or account, it constitutes an example of their own age-related communication. At the same time, however, such a remark may constitute environmental chatter to the person to whom it is directed (or indeed, anyone who overhears it). (p. 5)

There are also suggestions from research that encountering certain kinds of chatter in their environment may actually modify an individual's *own* age-related communication. Gasiorek and Fowler (2020), for example, discovered that more exposure to (negative) explicit messages about aging predicted more self-reported self-categorization as old and teasing about their age. Consequently, there is a danger that negative messages about aging become self-perpetuating: One person complains about the struggles of growing old to another person, who experiences that complaint as chatter...but then becomes more apt to make their own complaints about growing old to someone else, who experiences that complaint as chatter, ad infinitum.

Of course, such a "doom-spiral" is far from inevitable. For one thing, the relationship between encountering explicit negative messages about aging and self-categorizing as old is simply not that strong (Gasiorek & Fowler, 2020)! As such, all I'm describing is a troublesome *potential* circularity. Second, and perhaps more importantly, the existence of a possible negative spiral also hints at the possible existence of a comparable *positive* spiral. The communication predicament model of aging (Ryan et al., 1986), for example, articulates a process by which negative stereotypes of aging elicit certain communication behaviors that elicit stereotype-conforming behavior that appears to legitimate and reinforce negative stereotypes and start the "vicious cycle" anew. However, the communication *enhancement* model (Ryan et al., 1995) identifies sites of potential disruption in this process that not only break the negative cycle but also hint that a positive, *virtuous* cycle is possible: In their model, a younger person's recognition of an older individual's unique characteristics may prompt the younger person to engage in personalized, non-stereotype-dependent communication with the older adult that creates opportunities for the older person to disconfirm negative stereotypes. In turn, this facilitates the younger person's continued and deeper recognition of the older person's unique characteristics, thereby perpetuating more individualized communication. Following similar logic, perhaps experiencing *positive* explicit messages about aging in the form of chatter, could lead an individual to express greater optimism about aging in their own age-related talk to others. For those hearing such expressions of optimism, of course, such messages serve as chatter, which perhaps dispose them, in turn, to express their own optimistic thoughts about aging to others…and so on (again—but this time, more cheerfully)!

When Randy Pausch delivered his "Last Lecture" before dying of pancreatic cancer, he observed, "We cannot change the cards we are dealt, just how we play the hand" (p. 17). By this, he meant that although he could not control whether or not he developed cancer, he *could* exert some level of control over how he responded to (and lived with) his diagnosis. Similarly, there are many factors affecting how we age that are beyond our ability to control: We have no say, for example, in whether our genetic makeup predisposes us to certain illness or protects us against them; in whether quality medical care is available to and affordable for us; in whether the timing of our retirement means we cash out any investments during the height of an economic boom or during the depth of an unanticipated recession. Even so, we can, through our communicative behavior, exert or reclaim a degree of agency over how we encounter the aging process. If nothing else from this chapter sticks with you, I hope that you will remember this: With our words we shape not only our *own* aging environments but also those occupied by people dear to us. How we talk about aging *matters.*

## REFERENCES


Afifi, W. A. (2010). Uncertainty and information management in interpersonal contexts. In S. W Smith & S. R. Wilson (Eds.), *New directions in interpersonal communication research* (pp. 94–114). Sage.

Afifi, W. A., & Weiner, J. L. (2004). Toward a theory of motivated information management. *Communication Theory, 14*(2), 167–190. <https://doi.org/10.1111/j.1468-2885.2004.tb00310.x>

Anderson, J. A., & Baym, G. (2004). Philosophies and philosophic issues in communication, 1995–2004. *Journal of Communication, 54*(4), 589–615. <https://doi.org/10.1111/j.1460-2466.2004.tb02647.x>

Babrow, A. S. (1992). Communication and problematic integration: Understanding diverging probability and value, ambiguity, ambivalence, and impossibility. *Communication Theory, 2*(2), 95–130. <https://doi.org/10.1111/j.1468-2885.1992.tb00031.x>

Babrow, A. S. (2001). Uncertainty, value, communication, and problematic integration. *Journal of Communication, 51*(3), 553–573. <https://doi.org/10.1111/j.1460-2466.2001.tb02896.x>

Berger, C. R. (1987). Communicating under uncertainty. In M. E. Roloff and G. R. Miller (Eds.), *Interpersonal processes: New directions in communication research* (pp. 39–62). Sage.

Bernhold, Q. S. (2021). The role of media in predicting older adults' own age-related communication and successful aging. *Mass Communication and Society, 24*(1), 1–30. <https://doi.org/10.1080/15205436.2020.1743862>

Bernhold, Q. S., Blue, J., Devereux, S., Bertram, V., & Janus, K. (2023). Expanding the boundary conditions of the Communicative Ecology Model of Successful Aging to include communication about religion. *Communication Research*. <https://doi.org/10.1177/00936502231165844>

Bernhold, Q. S., & Gasiorek, J. (2020). Older adults' perceptions of their own and their romantic partners' age-related communication and their associations with aging well, depressive symptoms, and alcohol use disorder symptoms. *Journal of Social and Personal Relationships, 37*(4), 1172–1192. <https://doi.org/10.1177/0265407519890413>

Bernhold, Q. S., Gasiorek, J., & Giles, H. (2020). Communicative predictors of older adults' successful aging, mental health, and alcohol use. *International Journal of Aging and Human Development, 90*(2), 107–134. <https://doi.org/10.1177/0091415018784715>

Bernhold, Q. S., & Giles, H. (2019). Older adults' recalled memorable messages about aging and their associations with successful aging. *Human Communication Research, 45*(4), 474–507. <https://doi.org/10.1093/hcr/hqz011>

Bernhold, Q. S., & Giles, H. (2020). Older adults' age-related communication and routine dietary habits. *Health Communication, 35*(12), 1556–1564. <https://doi.org/10.1080/10410236.2019.1652391>

Bowling, A. (2006). Lay perceptions of successful aging: findings from a national survey of middle aged and older adults in Britain. *European Journal of Ageing, 3*(3), 123–136. <https://doi.org/10.1007/s10433-006-0032-2>

Carstensen, L. L. (2009). *A long bright future: An action plan for a lifetime of happiness, health, and financial security*. Random House.

Coupland, N. (2004). Age in social and sociolinguistic theory. In J. F. Nussbaum & J. Coupland (Eds.), *Handbook of communication and aging research* (2nd ed.), (pp. 69–90). Lawrence Erlbaum Associates.

Coupland, J. (2007). Gendered discourse on the "problem" of ageing: Consumerized solutions. *Discourse and Communication, 1*(1), 37–61. <https://doi.org/10.1177/1750481307071984>

Crosnoe, R., & Elder Jr,, G. H. (2002). Successful adaptation in the later years: A life course approach to aging. *Social Psychology Quarterly, 65*(4), 309–328. <https://doi.org/10.2307/3090105>

Depp, C. A., & Jeste, D. V. (2006). Definitions and predictors of successful aging: A comprehensive review of larger quantitative studies. *American Journal of Geriatric Psychiatry, 14*(1), 6–20. <https://doi.org/10.1097/01.JGP.0000192501.03069.bc>

Erikson, E. H. (1997). *Life cycle completed*. Norton.

Ferri, C., James, I., & Pruchno, R. (2009). Successful aging: Definitions and subjective assessment according to older adults. *Clinical Gerontologist, 32*(4), 379–388. <https://doi.org/10.1080/07317110802677302>

Fowler, C. A., & Bernhold, Q. S. (2023). Implications of older adults' attributions for young adults' attitudes to aging: A vignette study. *Journal of Language and Social Psychology, 42*(1), 31–59. <https://doi.org/10.1177/0261927X221105096>

Fowler, C. A., Gasiorek, J., & Giles, H. (2015). The role of communication in aging well: Introducing the Communicative ecology model of successful aging. *Communication Monographs, 82*(4), 431–457. <https://doi.org/10.1080/03637751.2015.1024701>

Frey, L., Botan, C., & Kreps, G. (1999). *Investigating communication: An introduction to research methods* (2nd ed.). Allyn & Bacon.

Gasiorek, J. (2022). Present-future self-continuity and intergenerational communication as predictors of young adults' evaluations of older adults and attitudes toward aging. *Journal of Language and Social Psychology, 41*(4), 476–489. <https://doi.org/10.1177/0261927X211068539>

Gasiorek, J., & Barile, J. P. (2018). Associations between profiles of communication about aging and quality of life for middle-aged and older American adults. *International Journal of Aging and Human Development, 87*(2), 141–155. <https://doi.org/10.1177/0091415017724546>

Gasiorek, J., & Fowler, C. A. (2016). Profiling younger adults' communication about aging. *Communication Studies, 67*(2), 163–182. <https://doi.org/10.1080/10510974.2015.1121159>

Gasiorek, J., & Fowler, C. A. (2020). Effects of "environmental chatter" about age and aging on middle-aged and older adults' communication and perceptions of aging efficacy. *Western Journal of Communication, 84*(1), 98–122. <https://doi.org/10.1080/10570314.2019.1637930>

Gasiorek, J., & Fowler, C. A. (2022). Associations between parents' negative talk about aging and young adults' negative affect and efficacy related to aging. *Journal of Family Communication, 22*(4), 374–386. <https://doi.org/10.1080/15267431.2022.2108428>

Gasiorek, J., Fowler, C. A., & Giles, H. (2015). What does successful aging sound like? Profiling communication about aging. *Human Communication Research. 41*(4), 577–602. <https://doi.org/10.1111/hcre.12060>

Gasiorek, J., Fowler, C. A., & Giles, H. (2016). Communication and successful aging. In J. F. Nussbaum (Ed.), *Communication across the lifespan* (pp. 35–50). Peter Lang.

Gasiorek, J., Fowler, C. A., & Giles, H. (2019). Communication and successful aging: Testing alternative conceptualizations of uncertainty. *Communication Monographs, 86*(2), 229–250. <https://doi.org/10.1080/03637751.2018.1538561>

Gerbner, G., Gross, L., Morgan, M., Signorelli, N., & Shanahan, J. (2002). Growing up with television: Cultivation processes. In J. Bryant & D. Zillmann (Eds.), *Media effects: Advances in theory and research* (2nd ed.), (pp. 43–67). Lawrence Erlbaum.

Gerbner, G., Gross, L., Signorelli, N., & Morgan, M. (1980). Aging with television: Images on television drama and conceptions of social reality. *Journal of Communication, 30*(1), 37–47. <https://doi.org/10.1111/j.1460-2466.1980.tb01766.x>

Gettings, P. E., & Kuang, K. (2022). Extending the communicative ecology model of successful aging using talk about careers and retirement. *Communication Monographs, 89*(4), 493–514. <https://doi.org/10.1080/03637751.2021.2025410>

Giles, H. (Ed.) (2016). *Communication accommodation theory: Negotiating personal and social identities across contexts.* Cambridge University Press.

Giles, H., Davis, S., Gasiorek, J., & Giles, J. (2013). *Successful aging: A communication guide to empowerment.* Editorial Aresta.

Giles, H., & Gasiorek, J. (2011). Intergenerational communication practices. In K. W. Schaie & S. Willis (Eds.), *Handbook of the psychology of aging* (7th ed.), (pp. 231–245). Elsevier. <https://doi.org/10.1016/B978-0-12-380882-0.00015-2>

Harwood, J., & Anderson, K. (2002). The presence and portrayal of social groups on prime-time television. *Communication Reports, 15*(2), 81–97. <https://doi.org/10.1080/08934210209367756>

Holladay, S. J. (2002). "Have fun while you can," "You're only as old as you feel," and "Don't ever get old!": An examination of memorable messages about aging. *Journal of Communication, 52*(4), 681–697. <https://doi.org/10.1111/j.1460-2466.2002.tb02568.x>

Hsu, H.-C., & Jones, B. L. (2012). Multiple trajectories of successful aging of older and younger cohorts. *The Gerontologist, 52*(6), 843–856. <https://doi.org/10.1093/geront/gns005>

Hummert, M. L., Garstka, T. A., Shaner, J. L., & Strahm, S. (1994). Stereotypes of the elderly held by young, middle-aged, and elderly adults. *Journal of Gerontology, 49*(5), 240–249. <https://doi.org/10.1093/geronj/49.5.P240>

Keaton, S. A., & Bodie, G. D. (2011). Explaining social constructivism. *Communication Teacher, 25*(4), 192–196. https://doi.org/10.1080/17404622.2011.601725

Kemper P, Komisar, H. L., Alecxih, L. (2005). Long-Term Care over an Uncertain Future: What Can Current Retirees Expect? *INQUIRY: The Journal of Health Care Organization, Provision, and Financing, 42*(4),335-350. https://doi.org/10.5034/inquiryjrnl_42.4.335

Knapp, M. L., Stohl, C., & Reardon, K. K. (1981). "Memorable" messages. *Journal of Communication, 31*(4), 27–41. <https://doi.org/10.1111/j.1460-2466.1981.tb00448.x>

Levy, B. R. (2009). Stereotype embodiment: A psychosocial approach to aging. *Current Directions in Psychological Science, 18*(6), 332–336. <https://doi.org/10.1111/j.1467-8721.2009.01662.x>

Lindlof, T. R. (2008). Constructivism. In W. Donsbach (Ed.), *The International Encyclopedia of Communication* (1st ed.). John Wiley & Sons. <https://doi.org/10.1002/9781405186407.wbiecc129>

Mehlman, M. J., Binstock, R. H., Juengst, E. T., Ponsaran, R. S., & Whitehouse, P. J. (2004). Anti-aging medicine: Can consumers be better protected? *The Gerontologist, 44*(3), 304–310. <https://doi.org/10.1093/geront/44.3.304>

Neikrug, S. M. (2003). Worrying about a frightening old age. *Aging and Mental Health, 7*(5), 326–333. <https://doi.org/10.1080/1360786031000150702>

Nussbaum, J. F., & Coupland, J. (Eds.). (2004). *Handbook of communication and aging research* (2nd ed.). Lawrence Erlbaum.

Nussbaum, J. F., Pecchioni, L. L., Robinson, J. D., & Thompson T. L. (2000). *Communication and aging* (2nd ed.). Lawrence Erlbaum.

Nuttman-Shwartz, O. (2004). Like a high wave: Adjustment to retirement. *The Gerontologist, 44*(2), 229–236. <https://doi.org/10.1093/geront/44.2.229>

Ouwehand, C., de Ridder, D. T. D., & Bensing, J. M. (2007). A review of successful aging models: Proposing proactive coping as an important additional strategy. *Clinical Psychology Review, 27*(8), 873–884. <https://doi.org/10.1016/j.cpr.2006.11.003>

Pausch, R. (2008). *The last lecture.* Hyperion.

Pecchioni, L. L., Ota, H., & Sparks, L. (2004). Cultural issues in communication and aging. In J. F. Nussbaum & J. Coupland (Eds.), *Handbook of communication and aging research* (2nd ed.), (pp. 167–207). Lawrence Erlbaum.

Pruchno, R. A., Wilson-Genderson, M., Rose, M., & Cartwright, F. (2010). Successful aging: Early influences and contemporary characteristics. *The Gerontologist, 50*(6), 821– 833. <https://doi.org/10.1093/geront/gnq041>

Reichstadt J., Sengupta, G., Depp, C. A., Palinkas, L. A., & Jeste, D. V. (2010). Older adults' perspectives on successful aging: Qualitative interviews. *American Journal of Geriatric Psychiatry, 18*(7), 567–575. <https://doi.org/10.1097/JGP.0b013e3181e040bb>

Robinson, T., & Anderson, C. (2006). Older characters in children's animated television programs: A content analysis of their portrayal. *Journal of Broadcasting and Electronic Media, 50*(2), 287–304. <https://doi.org/10.1207/s15506878jobem5002_7>

Robinson, J. D., & Skill, T. (1995). The invisible generation: Portrayals of the elderly on prime-time television. *Communication Reports, 8*(2), 111–119. <https://doi.org/10.1080/08934219509367617>

Robinson, J. D., Skill, T., & Turner, J. T. (2004). Media usage patterns and portrayals of seniors. In J. Coupland & J. F. Nussbaum (Eds.), *Handbook of communication and aging research* (pp. 423– 446). Lawrence Erlbaum.

Roy, A., & Harwood, J. (1997). Underrepresented, positively portrayed: Older adults in television commercials. *Journal of Applied Communication Research, 25*(1), 39–56. <https://doi.org/10.1080/00909889709365464>

Ryan, E. B., Giles, H., Bartolucci, G., & Henwood, K. (1986). Psycholinguistic and social psychological components of communication by and with the elderly. *Language & Communication, 6*(1–2), 1–24. <https://doi.org/10.1016/0271-5309(86)90002-9>

Ryan, E. B., Meredith, S. D., Maclean, M. J., & Orange, J. B. (1995). Changing the way we talk with elders: Promoting health using the communication enhancement model. *International Journal of Aging and Human Development, 41*(2), 89–107. <https://doi.org/10.2190/FP05-FM8V-0Y9F-53FX>

Schiappa, E., Gregg, P. B., & Hewes, D. E. (2005). The parasocial contact hypothesis. *Communication Monographs, 72*(1), 92–115. <https://doi.org/10.1080/0363775052000342544>

Tate, R. B., Swift, A. U., & Bayomi, D. J. (2013). Older men's lay definitions of successful aging over time: The Manitoba follow-up study. *International Journal of Aging and Human Development, 76*(4), 297–322. <https://doi.org/10.2190/AG.76.4.b>

Taylor, B. C. (1994). Frailty, language, and elderly identity: Interpretive and critical perspectives on the aging subject. In M. L. Hummert, J. M. Wiemann, and J. F. Nussbaum (Eds.), *Interpersonal communication in older adulthood: Interdisciplinary theory and research* (pp. 185–208). Sage. <https://dx.doi.org/10.4135/9781483326832.n9>

Vasil, L., & Wass, H. (1993). Portrayal of the elderly in the media: A literature review and implications for educational gerontologists. *Educational Gerontology, 19*(1), 71–85. <https://doi.org/10.1080/0360127930190107>

Williams, A., Ota, H., Giles, H., Pierson, H. D., Gallois, C., Ng, S., Lim, T-S., Ryan, E. B., Somera, L., Maher, J., Cai, D., & Harwood, J. (1997). Young people's beliefs about intergenerational communication: An initial cross-cultural comparison. *Communication Research, 24*(4), 370–393. <https://doi.org/10.1177/009365097024004003>

CHAPTER EIGHT

# Comparing Baby Boomer Women's and Men's Sensemaking about the Transition to Retirement

PATRICIA E. GETTINGS

Baby boomer women in the United States blazed new trails in the workplace and are continuing to do so as they transition to retirement. In contrast to the work and educational experiences of previous generations, many boomer women entered the paid workforce, developed careers outside the home, and/or earned college degrees (Bialik & Fry, 2019), while simultaneously engaging in unpaid work (e.g., raising children). Scholars have (re)developed career theories to account for the complex career experiences of women, which have been characterized as discontinuous, non-linear, and relational (e.g., Pringle & McCulloch Dixon, 2003; Mainiero & Sullivan, 2005). However, much of the retirement literature is still framed using a male-as-breadwinner norm and, hence, tends to overlook how the gendered nature of the life course shapes retirement (for exceptions see Duberley et al., 2014; Loretto & Vickerstaff, 2013). A life course perspective focuses on how structural, social, and cultural factors influence the way lives unfold and how earlier life events enable and constrain future possibilities (Elder et al., 2003). The study described in this chapter responds to calls for deeper exploration of the gendered nature of career pathways into retirement (Duberley & Carmichael, 2016; Sawyer & James, 2018) by considering how recently retired boomer women in the United States make sense of their transitions to retirement, and comparing the emergent framework to a comparable sample of men. Such an examination is an important step in understanding the role that communication about work and retirement plays in (un)successful aging (Gettings & Kuang, 2022).

A successful transition to retirement involves adjusting to more than simply a change in employment status. When viewed as a communicative process (Gettings & Anderson, 2018), retiring involves negotiations around instrumental issues like finances or where to live in retirement; identity issues like reframing who one is as a result of a shift in work arrangements; or relational issues such as how to renegotiate daily routines with a spouse or partner (e.g., Loe & Johnston, 2016). It is during these times of transition and equivocality when one's identities, routines, and relationships are challenged that sensemaking becomes most necessary and apparent (Weick, 1995). Sensemaking is particularly important because of its association with health and well-being (e.g., Koenig Kellas, 2017). The goal of this study is to analyze the discourses and practices of a particular group of retirees (U.S. baby boomer women in the first three years of their transition from professional employment to retirement) to examine how they "thread their way through the complexities of everyday social life" (Weick, 1992, p. 172). This group warrants focus because their disengagement from the paid labor force may be distinct from women in other kinds of work (e.g., non-professional work, Birkett, 2013) as they likely have the financial resources to make a range of choices about retirement timing, forms, and activities. These women are entering retirement under circumstances that are, at least in material terms, most resembling those assumed under the "traditional" male-as-breadwinner model.

## TRANSITIONING TO RETIREMENT

Conceptualized as a communicative process, retiring emphasizes overtime patterns of withdrawing from the labor force (Denton & Spencer, 2009; Gettings & Anderson, 2018; Szinovacz, 2003). The current project focuses on one particular chronological phase of this process: the transition to retirement. It is important to note that this language is not meant to suggest that processes of retiring are necessarily linear, as retiring has become an increasingly individualized experience for men and women (Kojola & Moen, 2016). Moreover, rather than use an a priori definition or cut-off to determine whether one is retired, participants in this study self-identified as retired.

### Adjusting to Retirement

To date, research that has explored the transition to retirement tended to focus on individual adjustment as evaluated by measuring a construct such as retirement satisfaction (e.g., Quick & Moen, 1998) or life satisfaction (e.g., Calasanti, 1996).

Findings have been heterogeneous in terms of how retiring influences well-being or successful aging outcomes, with some studies finding (a) slightly lower levels among retired people compared to those still working (e.g., Alpass et al., 2007), (b) no differences (e.g., Henning et al., 2016), and (c) somewhat higher levels (e.g., Gall et al., 1997). The quality of adjustment to retirement is influenced by a range of factors including individual attributes (e.g., age, Banerjee, 2016), situational characteristics (e.g., nature of pre-retirement work, Van Solinge & Henkens, 2008), psychosocial correlates (e.g., desire to engage in cognitive activity, Bye & Pushkar, 2009), and access to resources (e.g., financial, Calasanti, 1996). In these primarily quantitative studies, biological sex is typically considered as an individual attribute that mediates or moderates the association between retiring and well-being outcomes (Henning, et al., 2016). For example, job-related factors and income had a larger impact on males' well-being in retirement compared to females' well-being (e.g., Kim & Moen, 2002; Kubicek et al., 2011), but the reverse was true for social contacts (Kubicek et al., 2011) and marital quality (Kim & Moen, 2002). Although offering valuable insight, the design of these studies has tended to isolate factors instead of seeking a more holistic view of gendered life and career experiences. Using a life course perspective (Elder et al., 2003), the current study considers how the transition to retirement is situated within one's own trajectory as well as broader contexts.

## The Gendered Life Course and Retiring

A life course perspective emphasizes the ways that earlier life trajectories are linked to well-being later in life (Madero-Cabib & Fasang, 2016), and focuses on how life experiences accumulate to influence subsequent circumstances (Dannefer, 2003; DiPrete & Eirich, 2006). Scholars have convincingly argued that the life course, including work and career experiences, is inherently gendered (e.g., Moen, 2001; 2010). In terms of retirement, then, a starting point is to acknowledge that men and women frequently have different employment backgrounds and experiences including job type, compensation, career progression, and longevity, and that these factors influence broader work and career trajectories (Griffin et al., 2013). For example, women's work histories are more likely to be interrupted or discontinuous compared to men's (e.g., Duberley & Carmichael, 2016; Loretto & Vickerstaff, 2013). Often this is the result of women ceasing paid employment—either temporarily or permanently—to stay home and care for a family (one's own children but also one's parents, Garnick, 2016) and can mean that women have saved less money for retirement (National Institute on Retirement Security, 2016).

## Career Models and Retirement

Scholars have developed heuristics that reflect women's unique work-life experiences. Pringle and McCulloch Dixon (2003) offered a model of (women's) work lives that features four facets that can be arranged in any order, repeated, and/or experienced for any length of time. *Explore* is a period for pushing beyond one's boundaries and looking into new life possibilities. *Focus* means paying close attention to a particular life facet. *Rebalance* refers to a time when one attempts to re-align intellectual, emotional, physical, and spiritual concerns. Finally, *revive* involves a focus on one's own agency in terms of making decisions that revitalize and (re)energize passions. Although facets are not linked to age, retirement is referenced in the *revive* facet as offering a counter to traditional negative notions of aging associated with decline and preparation for death.

Mainiero and Sullivan's (2005) kaleidoscope model integrated *authenticity*, *balance*, and *challenge*, and posited that women's career histories are relational because women view their career choices in light of existing relationships and issues (rather than seeing careers as isolated). Foci may shift over time to foreground one aspect, which enables others to shift into the background. For instance, during the early years of one's career, a primary pattern for women may be to focus on challenges in one's career whereas balance and authenticity become lesser priorities. In later career periods, women may choose to focus on authenticity (balance and challenge shift to the background). The kaleidoscope career model offers a way of thinking about careers as inherently including both "work" and "non-work" demands, and accounts for the non-linear career trajectories often experienced by women. Notably, retirement is not explicitly mentioned in the initial descriptions of the model.

Despite limited treatment by these career models, it is logical that the aspects they highlight in work-life experiences continue to play out during the transition to retirement to create distinct, gendered retirement experiences (Sawyer & James, 2018). Indeed, researchers have started to explore women's retirement pathways. Duberley and colleagues' (2014) work provided insight into women's career and retirement trajectories in Britain, in particular underscoring the idea that retirement experiences are embedded in one's life course. Across all age groups of older adults (<50, >50, 50–64, 65–79, >80), females were less likely to be engaged in paid employment at all and less likely to be employed full-time (but more likely to be employed part-time) compared to their male counterparts. Some participants perceived retirement as a time of *continuity* in that they continued to fulfill their pre-retirement roles but to differing extents (e.g., remaining attached to an employer or type of work to a lesser degree, continuing role as caretaker). For others, retirement was a time of *change*, such as the opportunity to engage in new types of activities or the shock felt due to a lack of activity. Finally, Duberley et al. examined the choices and constraints that shaped participants' retirement experiences. For instance, women's retirement experiences were relational (e.g., influenced by husband's choices or the caretaking of others). Loe and Johnston (2016) identified a similar relational orientation among a sample of professional boomer women in the United States.

In addition, Duberley and Carmichael (2016) identified five trajectories among retired women in the United Kingdom that captured the combined influence of work and life decisions on retirement. For example, *professional* women typically retired gradually by engaging in part-time or bridge employment and were often financially secure, married property owners who felt confident and happy in retirement. There are likely similarities between the experiences of retiring women in the United Kingdom and United States given comparably aging populations and shifting financial landscapes (Slade, 2019), yet a life course emphasis on the situated nature of retirement suggests an overview of the retirement landscape for boomers in the United States is warranted.

## Retirement in the United States

Baby boomers in the United States are remaining in the labor force at the highest rates in over 50 years and the COVID-19 pandemic only had a modest impact on retirement timing (Thompson, 2022). According to the Pew Research Center (Fry, 2019), 66 % of boomers aged 54–64 were engaged in the paid labor force, and 29 % of all boomers aged 65–72 were engaged in paid labor or looking for work (compared to 21 % of the Silent Generation and 19 % of the Greatest Generation at this age). Boomers who remain in the labor force seemingly differ from those who retire. For instance, 38 % of boomers still in the labor force earned at least a bachelor's degree compared to 27 % of those not in the labor force, and individuals still in the labor force are more likely to be non-Hispanic White and live in a metropolitan area. Of Americans who retired in 2017, men retired at an average age of 59.62 years old and women at 60.11 years (DQYDJ, 2019). Retirees are expected to live an average of 20 years after retirement (USAGov, 2022).

In terms of retirement finances in the United States, the three most common savings options are plans offered by an employer, individual savings, and Social Security (a government program where all working individuals pay taxes that contribute to a fund that pays benefits to eligible individuals; USAGov, 2022). According to the National Institute on Retirement Security (2018), employers have moved away from offering traditional defined benefit pensions ("guarantee" a monthly income) to defined contribution plans such as 401(k)s (individuals manage own money). The current retirement savings picture in America is increasingly divided in the years following the Great Recession (Miller, 2018). Higher-income households with access to workplace retirement plans and money to invest have accumulated retirement wealth, whereas middle and lower-income households have remained the same or lost retirement wealth (Miller, 2018). The landscape for retiring Americans is shrouded in uncertainty in terms of factors such as timing, form, and finances, which necessitates sensemaking.

## A SENSEMAKING LENS

The impetus for sensemaking processes is a novel, confusing, or equivocal event about which individuals desire understanding (Weick, 1995). Sensemaking is of particular importance because of its connection to overall well-being, which is clearly related to successful aging (e.g., Koenig Kellas, 2017; Koenig Kellas & Trees, 2013). Narrative sensemaking (NSM) "helps individuals organize lived events—many of which are messy, multivocal, complicated, or confusing—into more manageable packages that make sense of the context of their lives and relationships" (Koenig Kellas, 2015, p. 254). NSM can be individual (the process of making meaning from personal experiences by creating stories) or communicated (shared with others; see communicated narrative sensemaking theory, CNSM), and empirical research supports connections between both forms of sensemaking and well-being (e.g., Koenig Kellas et al., 2010; Koenig Kellas & Manusov, 2003).

In the present context, individuals face challenges as they transition to retirement due to uncertainty around aspects of life such as new daily routines, shifting core identities, and changing patterns of interaction with close others, and they must contend with tensions emerging from differences between what they expected of retirement and retirement realities (Gettings, 2019). Retiring (older) adults who are better able to make sense of these experiences will likely enjoy higher well-being compared to those who face great difficulty in doing so. Indeed, older adults' communication about the meaning of work in their lives and preparing for retirement was positively associated with successful aging (Gettings & Kuang, 2022). It is with this background in mind that the present study was undertaken.

## THE PRESENT STUDY

Professional baby boomer women in the United States are simultaneously making sense of and (re)creating retirement processes. However, much of the literature on the retirement transition focuses on one-time individual adjustment and/or reflects a male-as-breadwinner norm. This study takes a life course perspective to explore sensemaking about the transition to retirement by asking: (RQ1) How do U.S. baby boomer professional women make sense of their transition to retirement?; and (RQ2) How does men's sensemaking about the transition to retirement (from a comparable sample) compare to women's?

## METHOD

### Participants

I recruited participants through personal networks and snowball sampling in two rounds of data collection. In the first round, inclusion criteria were identifying as a *woman* who retired in the past three years and had a partner, and in the second round were individuals who self-reported retiring in the past three years and had a partner (partner employment status could vary). I contacted those who responded to recruitment materials to schedule an interview and asked about the possibility of interviewing their partner. This study was part of a larger project aimed at understanding couples' transitions into retirement in the United States. As such, all participants who responded to recruitment calls were interviewed regardless of marital or employment status. However, only interviews from participants who were part of a dual-earner married couple who were both still living are included in the analysis for this chapter.

The final sample consisted of 40 participants (20 heterosexual married couples) who completed semi-structured interviews (at the time of the interviews, 18 of the women were retired and 17 of the men were). On average, women ($m$ = 64.15 years) were slightly younger than men ($m$ = 65.69 years), and most participants responded to an open-ended prompt as being White or Caucasian (1 woman as "Hispanic White" and 1 man as "Black"). In terms of the highest level of education completed, participants reported 16 MA/MS/MBA, 14 college graduates, 4 PhD/JD/MD, 1 some college/Associate Degree, and 2 high school (3 missing). The individual median pre-retirement annual income was $90,000 (range of $16,000–350,000), and the household was $155,000 ($63,000–400,000). Pre-retirement median income for women was $73,500 and for men was $81, 000 (6 participants did not report financial information). Of women, 17 reported taking time off during their career, 4 had not and 2 left the question blank. The primary reason women took time off was related to caring for children with some referring to longer periods of time like "didn't work until my children were in school" while others listed shorter timespans such as "3 months infant care leave." Of men, 8 reported taking time off during their career, 11 had not and 1 left the item blank. No men indicated childcare as a reason for a period of not working. Instead, men described breaks for time served in the military ("1971–1972 drafted to Vietnam"), medical issues, or for reasons of career exploration/additional schooling. Participants reported having, on average, 2.33 children (range 0 to 4) who were 36.18 years old (range 19–53). Participants resided in a variety of states in the Southern (e.g., TX, KY), Midwestern (e.g., IN, WI), and Eastern (e.g., NY, CT) United States.

## Procedure

I developed an interview protocol grounded in the retirement literature and based on the overarching research questions for the project. I then conducted pilot interviews with two married female retirees who had been retired for longer than three years to refine the protocol. The final protocol included questions such as: What does it mean to you to be retired? What have you found enjoyable/challenging about adjusting to retirement? Questions were adjusted to reflect employment status. Most partners were interviewed separately. Interviews were conducted face-to-face such as in the participant's home, a coffee shop, or a private room on campus ($n = 22$) or via phone ($n = 18$) and ranged in length from 22 to 121 minutes ($M = 59.65$). Interviews were audio recorded and transcribed. Participants also completed a short survey.

## Analysis

Analysis was an iterative process that was ongoing throughout data collection. To address RQ1, I first read through all transcripts several times and then engaged in open coding of the women's interviews with the goal to identify what was present in the data (Charmaz, 2006). To remain close to the data, I added a description to each sentence that described what was happening (e.g., "avoiding regular commitment" or "shortchanging relationships") with a focus on the transition to retirement. I also regularly wrote memos to capture my ideas about possible emerging themes. Owen's (1984) criteria of recurrence, repetition, and forcefulness guided this phase as these criteria helped determine frequently occurring issues and/or those discussed with intensity. Next, axial coding (Charmaz, 2006) facilitated reassembly of the fractured data and determined, in an abstract way, how threads of meaning could be woven across interviews. I wrote theoretical memos to describe category properties and compare themes. For instance, I reflected on the tension between a theme around participants not only "feeling compelled to stay busy" but also "feeling hesitant to make regular commitments." Ultimately, using life course and sensemaking perspectives as sensitizing concepts, I explored possible interpretations of how axial codes could be combined into a coherent whole. Together, these processes led me to develop a midlevel theory that was fully grounded in participants' experiences and provided a framework for understanding how women make sense of the transition to retirement. To address RQ2, I analyzed men's interviews using a similar process of open and axial coding. Next, I evaluated the extent to which men's sensemaking was similar to that of women's (i.e., my goal here was comparison).

I took additional steps to provide checks on the validity of the findings. First, a retired informant read the manuscript and offered suggestions. This individual fit study criteria but was not a participant. Additionally, I engaged in peer debriefing (Lincoln & Guba, 1985) by presenting study findings at multiple conferences and considering questions/feedback.

## FINDINGS AND INTERPRETATIONS

### Women's Sensemaking about the Transition to Retirement

In response to RQ1 that asked how U.S. baby boomer professional women make sense of their transition to retirement, I identified a framework that explicates how this sample articulated doing so in three phases (see Table 8.1): *pre-retirement*, *early retirement*, and the *future*.

### The Imbalance of Pre-retirement Life

Participants spoke positively about many features of their pre-retirement lives, but negatively about others. In terms of the former, participants took pride in their career success, had enjoyed their work, and appreciated the relationships they had developed throughout their working years. Lynn[1] (66, insurance agency owner) expressed that she "had worked so very hard to get that agency and now it was nice and I had it running lovely." Later she stated, "I loved what I was doing. My customers loved me…I had made so many good friends through the years. I started [in this career] when the kids were little babies and they came in for Halloween candy and then I'd be writing their car insurance and then writing them [insurance policies] when they got married and [bought] their first home."

Like Lynn, Betty (69, executive director of a healthcare organization) was proud of her career success (including financial rewards) and enjoyed her work: "So,

1 Pseudonyms are used in place of real names.

it was a very good career, I think. Very demanding. Good money. I made a lot of money. Some parts of it, I had a lot of fun…there were parts in those years when I thought I would never retire. I was like, *Retire? I'm having way too much fun. I love what I'm doing!*"

Despite these positive aspects of pre-retirement life, participants nevertheless felt frustrated by a sense of imbalance in that they were often not able to dedicate their time in ways they would have liked or to activities they felt were most important. The time requirements of a full-time job, in addition to other responsibilities, prevented participants in this sample from achieving the sense of balance they sought. Leslie (56, teacher) articulated that in pre-retirement, she believed she was "shortchanging my relationships, my family, because I have felt in the past with working full-time, that they did get pushed in the background at times. And it was something they just had to deal with. But it's not how I wanted life to go."

One reason for this "shortchanging" was that participants felt they were not fully in control of their pre-retirement time. They characterized work as an impediment to how they used or structured their time, as well as a limitation on the kinds of activities in which they could engage. Participants described feeling as though their time was "constrained" by work. For example, Megan (66, clothing business owner) explained that "for so many years…my whole life, really," she did not have "control of [her] time" due to "having to go to an office, or having deadlines, and that sort of thing." Rose (63, security awareness coordinator) also felt that she was not in control of how she spent her pre-retirement time, explaining that her employer had been wasting her time by not assigning her any particular tasks: "And I would go to work and I'm sitting going, 'I don't really have anything to do and this is a waste of time.' I mean this is my time. I'm working for you but you're not giving me anything to do."

Participants also explained that they were not able to engage in all the activities they wanted to in their pre-retirement lives because they lacked either the time or resources needed. Rachel (61, IT project manager) talked about her love of art, a passion that she "set aside for a really long time" because of "time constraints" and due to being "relatively ambitious and working hard to get to the next thing and wanting to do things really well so you're taking a little more time…And then had a house, a daughter, a husband who also wanted time. Family. So I just ran out of time." She acknowledged that these activities truly "enrich" her but explained that she did not have time for these "indulgences" in pre-retirement because "on a pragmatic level you're getting life done first." In addition to not having adequate time, some participants reported not having other resources needed to engage in desired activities, for instance, because they were drained by work. Courtney (66, secretary) explained that she was not able to read as much as she would have liked when she was working because her eyes were tired from spending time in front of the computer as part of her job.

### Opportunities for Balance in Early Retirement

Participants talked about their present retirement experience as one where they viewed many available options and were in control of those options (see Table 8.1, "Retirement"). They felt they had an opportunity to determine, or revisit, what was important to them and participate in activities accordingly. For many women, retirement ultimately meant a possibility to achieve the balance they lacked in their pre-retirement lives.

Mickey (59, insurance executive) put it succinctly: "It [retirement] is very much freelance. Every day, every week it's kind of whatever we [Mickey and her husband] feel like doing." Jill (67, professor) elaborated on this idea in describing what she saw as her new options:

> As a retired person, I feel like I have choice. I see roads open up in front of me…Now I see all kinds of choices. I could get more training and become something else…I can take…a very low-paying part-time job in the private sector … So retired to me … means I now have a substantial amount of control over my own destiny, lots of different types of choices, and very few expectations, other than the ones I deliver myself each morning when I wake up.

Being in control enabled some participants in this sample to work toward their desired balance in retirement. For Leslie, balance meant being able to invest her time and energy in all of her interests, which included work (part-time), relationships, and service (or, as she put it, "the best of all worlds"). In retirement, she suggested that "with a little bit of planning, you can have it all. You can have a balance of work or not work and exciting things to do."

Even though a number of these participants expressed a desire for a balanced life in retirement, some characterized it as illusory. In other words, there seemed to be an idealized view of a retirement where one can achieve the balance that proved elusive during one's pre-retirement life, but then there was the simultaneous realization that there will always be multiple things vying for one's time. Put succinctly, this sample of women sought balance but balance was still difficult to achieve.

For many participants, achieving balance in retirement meant accomplishing what they now—or still—viewed as their "work" before they engaged in pleasurable activities. Courtney described her struggle to manage her time so she can complete what she now described as her (unpaid) work, which included cleaning out the house, organizing items her daughters brought to the house, and prepping for holidays, while still having "time left to do things that she really likes to do."

Table 8.1: Professional women's retirement sensemaking framework

| | *Pre-Retirement* | *Early Retirement* | *Future* |
|---|---|---|---|
| *Time* | Past | Present/Short-Term | Long-Term |
| *Under Participants' Control?* | Out of Control | In Control | Impediments to One's Ability to be in Control (e.g., finances, health) |
| *Sense of Balance?* | Imbalanced | Opportunity to Seek/Create Balance | Unknown |
| *Degree of Uncertainty* | None (cannot change) | Certain | Uncertain |
| *Range of Choice* | Few Choices | Imperative of Doing vs. Reticence to Commit | (Likely) Constraints on Choice |
| *Awareness of Age* | Busy, "Work work work," Little time to focus on age | Recognition of Aging | End of Life/ Mortality |
| *Involvement in personal interests/ passions* | Couldn't focus on hobbies due to other commitments ("indulgences") | Time to pursue hobbies (although still, after "work" is done such as cleaning house) | Ability to participate might be negatively impacted (e.g., travel) |

Rachel clearly articulated the idea that achieving balance was a pre-retirement challenge and that it remained a challenge in her retired life:

> It's interesting that life balance was a challenge as a working person and I think it has been a challenge as a new retiree. Because you don't have the schedule to keep you out of things and yet there are things that I'm way far behind….So there's still this balance between doing stuff just for fun and doing the work of life that has to be done.

One explanation for the lingering challenge of achieving balance was that participants expressed an imperative to be doing (in retirement) and yet were reticent to commit. That is, participants voiced the idea that they—and all retirees—*should* be doing something. Betty (69, executive director of a healthcare organization) described a conversation she had in the past with her retired sister. At that point, Betty could not understand why her sister had not become involved in activities or why she was not "doing something." Betty stated, "I can't understand why she's retired and why she isn't *doing* something. I'm like—don't you want to consult? Don't you want to do something? And she's like 'no I really don't.'"

Greta (65, nurse anesthetist) explained that she prepared for retirement by starting a new hobby so that she would be able to keep herself busy in retirement.

> I made the decision that I was going to have to be able to entertain myself and keep myself busy…one of the first things I did when I retired was to buy a camera. And you know I've never done photography…but I need something like this to think about and to get me out. The first year [of retirement] I would say I spent, actually, the first 2 years feeling like: what should I be doing? But not wanting to yet. You know? Really embracing and loving that feeling of freedom.

As seen at the end of Greta's quotation, many participants articulated a second idea that is in tension with the initial "imperative of doing"—i.e., a reticence to commit. Although they felt compelled to be doing something and keeping themselves busy in retirement, they were hesitant to make regular commitments to any activity. Mickey clearly expressed her and her husband's reluctance to make commitments for a period of time after they retired:

> We just decided for a year we weren't going to commit—either one of us—to anything where we kind of had to be at a meeting or be involved. We're just going to kind of feel our way through it and decide what retirement means to us.

Betty said much the same thing. Before she retired, she could not understand why her sister wasn't "*doing* something" but now understood because she herself had retired.

> I couldn't get it until I retired. Then I got it. "Oh," I said. "Now I understand why you didn't want to do anything." So, she [my sister] did some volunteer work. I haven't done any volunteer work. Why? Because I don't want to commit to a schedule. Now, that could change. But so far, I'm like…I'd like to maybe work for the food pantry. There's a lot of volunteer jobs around that I could do. But I'm like, "Well, wait. Then I have to tell them I'll come every Wednesday? What if I want to do something else on Wednesday?"…So far it's been simpler not to get involved in anything.

Participants enjoyed having control over their schedules and activities in their early years of retirement and perceived that agreeing to any regular commitments would lessen this control. Several noted that they may be willing to make commitments again in a year or a few years but not so soon in their retirement. Thus, although many participants viewed (early) retirement as a time when they could achieve the balance that had eluded them during their working years (i.e., pre-retirement), few reported actually achieving this balance.

### The Time between the Parentheses: Envisioning the Future

Despite feeling in control and generally positive about life in the present, most participants were certain that bad things would happen in the future, but they were just uncertain about when. This tension between uncertainty and certainty played out in how participants explained their current behavior relative to their perceptions of the future. Jill viewed her current life as "the time between the parentheses." She revealed that her husband had a chronic disease and so believed that "at some point more will be asked of me. You know, in sickness and in health, for better or for worse." Much of Jill's current behavior was shaped by these negative future possibilities.

> So one of the things I wanted this retirement to be—this phase…I see it somewhat as the time between the parentheses. The one side of the parentheses representing the time before, when I was working, but the other side being the unknown, the what will happen. I wanted to make sure I had some of what that dream retirement is, where you get to have freedoms and travel… I'm in the parentheses. I don't know that I'm going to have this bad other side that involves me as a caregiver in ways that might not be pleasant at some point in the future. But I'm kind of storing up goodwill, joy, and happiness, so that when that day comes, I can take what is—I can take what is given to me, and I will never have the thought that I didn't live the life I could have or should have lived.

Jill articulated how her knowledge of what is likely to happen in the future influenced the way that she was constructing her current retirement experience. She made decisions that constituted her "dream retirement" where she was not constrained by anything, but with the knowledge that this period of time had an endpoint. Jill's comment also underscored the dyadic nature of the retirement trajectory. Although she acknowledged that she had some health issues, she seemed to believe that these would be a quick end to her life and she would "never know it." What seemed to be a more likely scenario in her view was that her husband's chronic illness would gradually encroach upon her ideal retirement and, hence, their ideal retirement together.

Similarly, Rose juxtaposed her current retirement experience with the unknown, yet likely, challenges of the future. She felt compelled to "grab it while I have all the things in alignment: my health, energy, the money" because she recognized the unpredictable constraints on the horizon.

> I'm really in the early process [of retirement]. I still have energy. I have good health. I want to travel. And as you go through there will be health concerns. There will probably be money issues maybe at some point that will prevent that. It's like grab it while I have all the things in alignment: my health, energy, the money. And do that because I do see a progression…and it's kind of like accepting it.

Taken together, women in this study made sense of retirement in three phases: *pre-retirement*, *early retirement*, and the *future*. Notably, this framework explains the normative way that women made sense of the retirement transition, although there were variations.

## Comparing Men and Women's Experiences of the Transition to Retirement

Men's sensemaking about the transition to retirement generally did not align with the women's sensemaking framework (RQ2). There are three notable points of contrast. First, men did not articulate the same sense of imbalance or shortchanging relationships/activities in their pre-retirement lives, nor did they report a desire to achieve balance in their early retirement years. It may be the case that men in this sample simply did not feel the same sense of imbalance that women described because men may have felt that they were doing what they were supposed to be doing (i.e., working full time) or what they had to do to support their families during their pre-retirement years. Women, on the other hand, may have felt more of a pull toward family life/motherhood *and* employment and, as a result, never quite felt as though every aspect of their life was getting the attention they wanted to give it.

Notably, women and men both reported feeling that they now had greater control over how they spend their time in retirement. Many of the men indicated that retirement meant freedom from work obligations, which included having control over how one spends time. For example, Timothy (61, nurse anesthetist) offered "freedom" as the only and "strongest" word he could think of to describe what retirement meant to him. He elaborated by saying "From work. From doing things I had to do and I knew I had to do." John (pharmaceutical lab technician) offered a similar explanation about the meaning of retirement and referenced sleeping patterns as an illustration of the control one has in retirement. He stated, "Well kind of the freedom to get up when you want, go to bed when you want … Your schedule is pretty much at your own discretion depending on what activities you get involved in."

As a second point of contrast, retirement for men represented an opportunity to *increase* involvement in passions, whereas retirement for women represented an opportunity to engage in the first place. That is, whereas women reported not having the time at all to "indulge" in passions during their pre-retirement years, men reported that they did not have *sufficient* time to engage in their passions in their pre-retirement lives but still did so to some extent. For example, Timothy explained that, in retirement, he has "an opportunity to really enjoy my passions. I have many passions." He described that this is something he had done when he was working but can now do more in retirement. For example, whereas he "used to go to a jazz festival in New Orleans every year. We'd go for usually one weekend. This year [in retirement], I went for 12 days." For Timothy, the difference between engaging in his passions before and during retirement is a matter of degree rather than an all or nothing issue.

Manuel (60, principal) talked about golfing in a similar way: "It was one of those 'you are retired' [moments] because I was out there [on the golf course] and it didn't matter how I was hitting the ball. It's like, I could do this, whereas before I retired, if I was out on the golf course, oftentimes I would be thinking about what I needed to do at school or what I needed to do at home." Men in the sample described that they were able to participate in their passions during their working years but that these events were often impeded by work commitments or thoughts. In retirement, they are fully able to engage in these activities.

A third point of contrast is that men did not express the same imperative of doing. That is, women reported feeling obligated to be doing something during their retirement. And, although men certainly remained busy during retirement and some even suggested that staying engaged is important to well-being, for the most part they did not subscribe to the same imperative. Rather, a meaning that emerged across men in the sample (but not across women in the sample) is that retirement can mean relaxation. Luke (56, vice president for operations at a gas and oil company) exemplified this idea by describing retirement as: "Hopefully relaxing. Low stress. Enjoyable." Another participant, TJ (62, pressroom foreman), chose "relax" as one of his three words to describe retirement and elaborated by comparing himself to a dog.

> I'm very dog-like. I can sit still and kind of watch the trees and the breeze blow by for two or three hours at a time and then jump up and do something. Pretty much what dogs do. They lay around until somebody gives them a ball to play with or a stick.

Moreover, men did not express a reticence to commit. The idea of committing or not committing in retirement did not emerge as part of the meaning of retirement for men (not that it is not mentioned at all but just not nearly as often as in the women's interviews). In sum, men's sensemaking about the transition to retirement did not resemble the three-phase process articulated by the women in this study.

## CONCLUSION

Although baby boomer women's career experiences have been marked as unique compared to those of previous generations (e.g., Bialik & Fry, 2019), their transitions into retirement have not yet been fully explored (Duberley & Carmichael, 2016; Sawyer & James, 2018). The study reported in this chapter addressed this issue by exploring how recently retired boomer women in the United States made sense of their transitions to retirement. Analyses identified three phases—pre-retirement, early retirement, and the future—that shed light on the role that communication about work/retirement plays in how women perceive their everyday retirement experiences. This framework did not explain professional men's transitions into retirement, which supports the notion of the gendered life course.

## REFERENCES

Alpass, F., Towers, A., Stephens, C., Fitzgerald, E., Stevenson, B., & Davey, J. (2007). Independence, well-being, and social participation in an aging population. *Annals of the New York Academy of Sciences*, *114*, 241–250. <https://doi.org/10.1196/annals.1396.009>

Banerjee, S. (April 1, 2016). Trends in retirement satisfaction in the United States: Fewer having a great time. *EBRI Notes*, *37*(4). <https://ssrn.com/abstract=2772072>

Bialik, K., & Fry, R. (2019, February 14). Millennial life: How young adulthood today compares with prior generations. Retrieved from <https://www.pewsocialtrends.org/essay/millennial-life-how-young-adulthood-today-compares-with-prior-generations/>

Birkett, H. (2013). *The embedded nature of the retirement experience: A life course study*. University of Birmingham.

Bye, D., & Pushkar, D. (2009). How need for cognition and perceived control are differentially linked to emotional outcomes in the transition to retirement. *Motivation and Emotion*, *33*(3), 320–332. <https://doi.org/10.1007/s11031-009-9135-3>

Calasanti, T. M. (1996). Gender and life satisfaction in retirement: An assessment of the male model. *The Journals of Gerontology Series B: Psychological Sciences and Social Sciences*, *51*(1), S18–S29. <https://doi.org/10.1093/geronb/51B.1.S18>

Charmaz, K. (2006). *Constructing grounded theory: A practical guide through qualitative analysis*. Sage.

Denton, F. T., & Spencer, B. G. (2009). What is retirement? A review and assessment of alternative concepts and measures. *Canadian Journal on Aging*, *28*(1), 63–76. <https://doi.org/10.1017/S0714980809090047>

Dannefer, D. (2003). Cumulative advantage/disadvantage and the life course: Cross-fertilizing age and social science theory. *The Journals of Gerontology Series B: Psychological Sciences and Social Sciences*, *58*(6), S327–S337. <https://doi.org/10.1093/geronb/58.6.S327>

DiPrete, T. A., & Eirich, G. M. (2006). Cumulative advantage as a mechanism for inequality: A review of theoretical and empirical developments. *Annual Review of Sociology*, 32, 271–297. <http://www.jstor.org/stable/29737740>

Duberley, J., & Carmichael, F. (2016). Career pathways into retirement in the UK: Linking older women's pasts to the present. *Gender, Work & Organization*, *23*(6), 582–599. <https://doi.org/10.1111/gwao.12144>

Duberley, J., Carmichael, F., & Szmigin, I. (2014). Exploring women's retirement: Continuity, context and career transition. *Gender, Work & Organization*, *21*(1), 71–90. <https://doi.org/10.1111/gwao.12013>

DQYDJ. (2019, November 14). Average retirement age in the United States. Retrieved from <https://dqydj.com/average-retirement-age-in-the-united-states/>

Elder, G. H., Johnson, M. K., & Crosnoe, R. (2003). The emergence and development of life course theory. In J. T. Mortimer & M. J. Shanahan (Eds.), *Handbook of the life course* (pp. 3–19). Kluwer Academic Publishers

Fry, R. (2019, July 24). *Baby boomers are staying in the labor force at rates not seen in generations for people their age*. Pew Research. <https://www.pewresearch.org/fact-tank/2019/07/24/baby-boomers-us-labor-force/>

Gall, T. L., Evans, D. R., & Howard, J. (1997). The retirement adjustment process: Changes in the well-being of male retirees across time. *The Journals of Gerontology: Psychological Sciences and Social Sciences, 52B*(3), S110–S117. <https://doi.org/10.1093/geronb/52B.3.P110>

Garnick, D. (2016, October). *Income insights: Gender retirement gap*. SSRN. <https://papers.ssrn.com/sol3/papers.cfm?abstract_id=2888911>

Gettings, P. E. (2019). Meanings of talk about the transition to retirement: Connecting macro and micro discourses. *Communication Monographs, 86*(4), 479–500. <https://doi.org/10.1080/03637751.2019.1614203>

Gettings, P.E. & Anderson, L.B. (2018) Applying a life course perspective to retirement: A literature review and research agenda for communication scholars. *Annals of the International Communication Association, 42*(3), 224–241. <https://doi.org/10.1080/23808985.2018.1497453>

Gettings, P. E., & Kuang, K. (2022). Extending the communicative ecology model of successful aging using talk about careers and retirement. *Communication Monographs, 89*(4), 493–514. <https://doi.org/10.1080/03637751.2021.2025410>

Griffin, B., Loh, V., & Hesketh, B., (2013). Age, gender, and the retirement process. In M. Wang (Ed.), *The Oxford handbook of retirement* (pp. 202–214). Oxford University Press.

Henning, G., Lindwall, M., & Johansson, B. (2016). Continuity in well-being in the transition to retirement. *GeroPsych, 29*(4), 225–237. <https://doi.org/10.1024/1662-9647/a000155>

Kim, J. E., & Moen, P. (2002). Retirement transitions, gender, and psychological well-being: A life-course, ecological model. *The Journals of Gerontology Series B: Psychological Sciences and Social Sciences, 57*(3), P212–P222. <https://doi.org/10.1093/geronb/57.3.P212>

Koenig Kellas, J. (2015). Narrative theories: Making sense of interpersonal communication. In D. O. Braithwaite & P. Schrodt (Eds.), *Engaging theories in interpersonal communication: Multiple perspectives* (2nd ed.), (pp. 253–266). Sage.

Koenig Kellas, J. K. (2017). Communicated narrative sense-making theory: Linking storytelling and well-being. In D. O. Braithwaite, E. A. Suter, & K. Floyd (Eds.), *Engaging theories in family communication* (pp. 62–74). Routledge.

Koenig Kellas, J., & Manusov, V. (2003). What's in a story? The relationship between narrative completeness and adjustment to relationship dissolution. *Journal of Social and Personal Relationships, 20*, 285–307. <https://doi.org/10.1177/0265407503020003002>

Koenig Kellas, J., & Trees, A. R. (2006). Finding meaning in difficult family experiences: Sense-making and interaction processes during joint family storytelling. *Journal of Family Communication, 6*(1), 49–76. <https://doi.org/10.1207/s15327698jfc0601_4>

Koenig Kellas, J., & Trees, A. (2013). Family stories and storytelling: Windows into the family soul. In A. L. Vangelisti (Ed.), *Routledge handbook of family communication* (pp. 391–406). Routledge.

Koenig Kellas, J., Trees, A. R., Schrodt, P., LeClair-Underberg, C., & Willer, E. K. (2010). Exploring links between well-being and interactional sense-making in married couples' jointly told stories of stress. *Journal of Family Communication, 10*, 174–193. <https://doi.org/10.1080/15267431.2010.489217>

Kojola, E., & Moen, P. (2016). No more lock-step retirement: Boomers' shifting meanings of work and retirement. *Journal of Aging Studies, 36*, 59–70. <https://doi.org/10.1016/j.jaging.2015.12.003>

Kubicek, B., Korunka, C., Raymo, J. M., & Hoonakker, P. (2011). Psychological well-being in retirement: The effects of personal and gendered contextual resources. *Journal of Occupational Health Psychology*, *16*(2), 230–246. <https://doi.org/10.1037/a0022334>

Lincoln, Y., & Guba, E. (1985). *Naturalistic inquiry*. Sage.

Loe, M., & Johnston, D. K. (2016). Professional women "rebalancing" in retirement: Time, relationships, and body. *Journal of Women & Aging*, *28*(5), 418–430. <https://doi.org/10.1080/08952841.2015.1018047>

Loretto, W., & Vickerstaff, S. (2013). The domestic and gendered context for retirement. *Human Relations*, *66*(1), 65–86. <https://doi.org/10.1177/0018726712455832>

Madero-Cabib, I., & Fasang, A. E. (2016). Gendered work–family life courses and financial well-being in retirement. *Advances in Life Course Research*, *27*, 43–60. <https://doi.org/10.1016/j.alcr.2015.11.003>

Miller, M. (2018). *Ten years after onset of Great Recession, how are U.S. retirees doing?* Reuters. <https://www.reuters.com/article/us-column-miller-retirement/ten-years-after-onset-of-great-recession-how-are-u-s-retirees-doing-idUSKCN1M7165>

Moen, P. (2001). Constructing a life course. *Marriage & Family Review*, *30*(4), 97–109. <https://doi.org/10.1300/J002v30n04_06>

Moen, P. (2010). From "work-family" to the "gendered life course" and "fit": Five challenges to the field. SSG Sozialwissenschaften, USB Köln. <https://nbn-resolving.org/urn:nbn:de:0168-ssoar-130461>

Mainiero, L. A., & Sullivan, S. E. (2005). Kaleidoscope careers: An alternate explanation for the "opt-out "revolution. *Academy of Management Perspectives*, *19*(1), 106–123. <https://doi.org/10.5465/ame.2005.15841962>

National Institute on Retirement Security. (2016). *Women 80% more likely to be impoverished in retirement.* <https://www.nirsonline.org/2016/03/women-80-more-likely-to-be-impoverished-in-retirement/>

National Institute on Retirement Security. (2018). *Retirement in America: Out of reach for working Americans.* <https://www.nirsonline.org/wp-content/uploads/2018/09/FINAL-Report-.pdf>

Owen, W. F. (1984). Interpretive themes in relational communication. *Quarterly Journal of Speech*, *70*(3), 274–287. <https://doi.org/10.1080/00335638409383697>

Pringle, J. K., & Dixon, K. M. (2003). Re-incarnating life in the careers of women. *Career Development International*, *8(6)*, 291–300. <https://doi.org/10.1108/13620430310496107>

Quick, H. E., & Moen, P. (1998). Gender, employment and retirement quality: A life course approach to the differential experiences of men and women. *Journal of Occupational Health Psychology*, *3*(1), 44–64. <https://doi.org/10.1037/1076-8998.3.1.44>

Sawyer, A. M., & James, S. (2018). Are baby boomer women redefining retirement?. *Sociology Compass*, *12*(10), e12625. <https://doi.org/10.1111/soc4.12625>

Slade, F. (2019, March 21). *How does the United States retirement system compare to other countries?* Benefits Pro. <https://www.benefitspro.com/2019/03/21/how-does-the-united-states-retirement-system-compare-to-other-countries/?slreturn=20221122102839>

Szinovacz, M. E. 2003. Contexts and pathways: Retirement as institution, process, and experience. In G. A. Adams & T. A. Beehr (Eds.), *Retirement: Reasons, processes, and results* (pp. 6–52). Springer.

Thompson, D. (2022, September 19). *Pandemic disrupted labor markets but had modest impact on retirement timing*. U.S. Census Bureau. <https://www.census.gov/library/stories/2022/09/did-covid-19-change-retirement-timing.html#:~:text=The%20COVID%2D19%20pandemic's%20disruption,and%20Program%20Participation%20(SIPP)>.

U.S. Census Bureau. (2015, July). *International database.* <http://www.census.gov/population/international/data/idb/informationGateway.php>

USAGov (2022). *Retirement.* <https://www.usa.gov/retirement>

Van Solinge, H., & Henkens, K. (2008). Adjustment to and satisfaction with retirement: Two of a kind? *Psychology and Aging*, *23*(2), 422–434. <https://doi.org/10.1037/0882-7974.23.2.422>

Weick, K. E. (1992). Agenda setting in organizational behavior: A theory-focused approach. *Journal of Management Inquiry,* 1(3), 171–182. <https://doi.org/10.1177/105649269213>

Weick, K. E. (1995). *Sensemaking in organizations.* Sage.

CHAPTER NINE

# The Portrayal of Aging Spaces from a Public Relations Perspective

LINDSEY B. ANDERSON AND VICTORIA MCDERMOTT

Aging is a complex process that is made meaningful through communication. As the population continues to become more age diverse given improved health initiatives and longer life expectancies, it becomes increasingly important to understand the nuances of aging. One area of communication scholarship that contributes to larger discourses of aging is public relations.

Public relations, as its name suggests, highlights the communicative construction of relationships between organizations and publics or stakeholders (Edwards, 2012). Through the lens of public relations, communicative activity can be used to establish legitimacy (Golant & Sillince, 2007; Patel et al., 2005), facilitate dialogue (Taylor & Kent, 2014), and create advocacy (Ciszek, 2015). These concepts have been theorized to contribute to a fully functioning society (Heath, 2006), which is the space in which discourse created through public relations can enhance decision-making.

It would then follow that public relations scholarship and practice would also play an important role in the communication construction of aging spaces as people look toward organizations to guide their understanding of age/aging. However, past research in this area shows that the depiction of aging in public relations relies heavily on age-based stereotypes that ultimately benefit an organization (e.g., showing older people as vulnerable and then selling them a device to mitigate this portrayal) (see Anderson, 2018). The field of public relations theory, scholarship, and practice provides many potentially rich areas of inquiry for changing age-based stereotypes in meaningful ways. This piece specifically situates public relations concepts (e.g., legitimacy, dialogue, and advocacy) as a way to create a fully functioning society, i.e., a framework for changing experiences of equity and accessibility for aging populations through dialogic communicative practices. Indeed, the fully functioning society framework "draws on the norms of exchange whereby community members seek to maximize outcomes and minimize costs of personal and collective association and (this) decision making process" (Heath, 2006, p. 96). In this decision-making process, individuals (individually and collectively) seek to make rewarding decisions in the face of risks posed by uncertainties that require enlightened decision-making by obtaining information (facts), opinions, and policy recommendations from various sources. Given this background, the fully functioning society framework would have important implications for aging populations. We begin with an overview of portrayals of aging. We then provide an overview of public relations and consider the potential intersection of three key concepts in public relations literature with aging research, as well as how this can contribute to a fully functioning society. We close with a discussion of the value of researching aging spaces from the perspective of public relations and provide avenues for future research.

## PORTRAYALS OF AGING

Primarily, depictions of age/aging have been shown to highlight aging in a binary, as either unsuccessful or successful aging. These messages tend to be based on age-based stereotypes (Hummert, et al., 1994) and are used to support an organization's outcomes (e.g., product sales, increased membership). In this section, we review existing public relations scholarship that depict aging in negative and positive ways through the portrayal of age-based stereotypes.

### Age-Based Stereotypes

Stereotypes can be both positive and negative (Fiske et al., 2002). For example, one persistent age-based stereotype is that older adults are warm, yet incompetent (Cuddy et al., 2005). Hummert and colleagues (1994) completed early work that categorized common age-based stereotypes, which included five negatively oriented categories (severely impaired, shrew/curmudgeon, recluse, despondent, and vulnerable) and three positively oriented categories (John Wayne conservative, liberal matriarch/patriarch, and perfect grandparent). Although an update may be needed to this typology, the categories still reflect the communication surrounding the topics of age and aging as organizational messages continue to perpetuate age-based stereotypes.

## Depictions of Unsuccessful Aging

Some of the most predominant messages related to aging use negative age-based stereotypes (e.g., declines in health, cognition, increased isolation) to depict unsuccessful aging. In doing so, this type of public relations messaging uses fear appeals associated with markers of unsuccessful aging, such as declines in health, financial uncertainty, and isolation to "sell" organizational goods/services (see Anderson, 2018). Further, colloquial terms used in popular culture can also work in tandem with organizational messages to reinforce age-based stereotypes (e.g., geezer, old-timer, blue or gray hairs).

Many organizations can and have used the depictions of unsuccessful aging for their benefit. For example, BMW used the aging workforce to justify its redesign of factory lines. Anderson (2013) identified the frames BMW used to present the organization as proactively preparing for an aging workforce, a problem rife with health concerns for workplaces, especially those that require physical labor. In order to counter the expected reductions in efficiency and productivity as well as the assumed increase in absences and injuries, BMW instituted dozens of updates to an experimental production line (e.g., magnifying glasses, stretching station, wooden floors, and ergonomic standing chairs) that were intended to help older workers continue to work at a high level over time. The ultimate effect of these changes was to reinforce perceptions of older people as being weak and vulnerable. Similarly, AARP (formerly known as the American Association of Retired Persons) capitalized on negative health stereotypes regarding older adults during the COVID pandemic. AARP created a series of TeleTown halls that positioned older adults as a "vulnerable" population and in doing so, perpetuated concerns about health and aging (Anderson, 2021).

From the depictions of aging presented by organizations, we can see an effect on the conceptualization of age in popular culture. One example is the communication work completed on the phrase, "OK Boomer" (Anderson, 2022). This disparaging retort has been used by non-members of the Baby Boomer generation (born between 1946 and 1964) to emphasize an "out of touch" stereotype of older people and has been repeated by media organizations (Pew Research Center, 2019). Indeed, an analysis of media outlets reporting on the phrase uncovered that the use of "OK Boomer" was grounded in a unidimensional stereotype that older adults were removed from the values (e.g., acceptance of lifestyles that do not fall in line with heteronormativity) accepted and promoted by today's culture. This communication not only reinforced generational divides, but it ultimately created an "us versus them" mentality that reinforced a sense of acceptance around ageist communicative behaviors and problematic intergenerational interactions. "OK Boomer" continues to be used as a form of insult and dismissal for older adults, especially in organizational settings.

Ultimately, past scholarship that explores aging from a public relations perspective demonstrates the ways that age-based stereotypes have been used for organizational gains. However, not all depictions of aging show unsuccessful aging. Public relations work related to aging continues to broaden and show a wider range of aging experiences.

## Depictions of Successful Aging

In contrast with unsuccessful aging, depictions of successful aging portrayed by and enacted in certain organizations draw on positive stereotypes to emphasize beneficial aspects of aging and potential life milestones that accompany chronological age (e.g., experience, retirement, family). In doing so, they often challenge assumptions about age/aging. For instance, Anderson (2015) examined how AARP has challenged the story of retirement by crafting and presenting strategic narratives that highlight the strengths that come along with an aging workforce; specifically the accounts of work after the age of 50 centered on the experience that older adults bring to the workplace through continued work or the shift to "encore" careers. This work highlights the benefits of aging, challenging negative assumptions that aging makes you severely impaired or despondent, and thus unable to contribute valuably to the workforce. Following the success of the campaign in 2015, in 2018 AARP launched the #DisruptAging campaign which sought to upend logic about age/aging by presenting messages that countered commonly held age-based stereotypes. For example, the campaign depicted older adults as athletes through photos and testimonials of older adults playing softball, biking, and running. In so doing, it emphasized existing identity anchors from the featured person's youth as a way to emphasize the older adults' activity level and health (Anderson & Guo, 2021).

Interestingly, organizations are able to use depictions of successful aging to their benefit. For instance, Lim and Lee (2022) completed a case study in which they explored the public relations practices of Yuhan-Kimberly South Korea, a health and hygiene company, to understand how these efforts can benefit an aging population as well as produce a competitive advantage for the organization. Their findings demonstrate that in order to create a sense of shared values among its public, Yuhan-Kimberly created job opportunities for older adults and attempted to challenge negative assumptions held about aging by highlighting older adults' capabilities and efficacy in the workplace and community through relationship cultivation strategies. Although organizations used these positive portrayals of aging for a self-serving purpose, they did provide an alternative narrative to the traditional conceptualization of older workers as a hindrance in the workplace.

Another example of how organizations can draw on the positive depictions of aging was demonstrated through an analysis of marketing materials produced by Pulte Homes (a brand of 55 and older communities) (Anderson, 2019). The materials portrayed its residents as "successful ager" who (1) proactively planned for future needs, (2) expressed optimism about aging, (3) actively resisted age-based stereotypes, and (4) minimized the role of communication technology. These depictions were intended to encourage other older adults to buy into Pulte's brand if they wanted to "successfully" age. However, the depictions of residents were partial and only showed the positives of age (e.g., an image of a couple with their grandchildren sitting on a porch).

Overall, there are a multitude of ways that public relations can enhance understanding of age/aging. Traditionally, organizations have taken an "either-or" approach to portray age/aging in a negative or positive light. Ultimately, however, aging is a multifaceted process that public relations has the potential to positively affect through the co-creation of narratives with publics, stakeholders, and organizations alike.

## THE INTERSECTION OF PUBLIC RELATIONS AND AGING

### Defining Public Relations

Public relations is both a social science field and professional practice (Vasquez & Taylor, 2001). Although there are a variety of ways in which scholars have conceptualized the definition of public relations, we define public relations as the flow of strategic communication between an organization and others in the management of relationships (Edwards, 2012). Specifically for this piece, we define "others" as stakeholders, e.g., an influencer, beneficiary, or risk bearer to an organization's "wealth-creating capacity and activities" (Smith, 2012, p. 6). Within the public relations literature, stakeholders differ from other terms used to describe publics as stakeholders may take on more responsibility with the organization than other groups of publics. However, those who view themselves as stakeholders and who the organization views as stakeholders can vary. Ultimately, how an organization determines its stakeholders and communicates with said stakeholders can then have an effect on how the organization is perceived by others. Another important point to note related to our conceptualization of public relations is that similar to Curtin and Gaither (2005), we view public relations as more than just a tool to serve organizational goals, and instead, consider the value of public relations for creating space for dialogue, encouraging diverse viewpoints, acting in public interest, and offering honest steps toward recommendations that advocate for public interest while also advancing organizational goals (Brunner & Smallwood, 2019).

## Three Concepts for Considering the Intersection of Public Relations and Aging

From these conceptualizations of public relations, organizations, and stakeholders, three important concepts may provide important avenues for inquiry regarding public relations and aging: legitimacy, dialogue, and advocacy. The section below begins with an explanation of the public relations theory or concept, followed by a connection to the aging literature and suggestions for future research.

### Legitimacy

Legitimacy is a central concept in public relations (Deephouse & Carter, 2005). Legitimacy is "a generalized perception or assumption that the actions of an entity are desirable, proper or appropriate within some socially constructed system of norms, values, beliefs, and definitions" (Suchman, 1995, p. 574). Thus, legitimacy is the result of social adherence to regulative, normative, or cognitive norms and expectations (Deephouse & Carter, 2005). Legitimacy is often constructed through communication and language, such as organizational storytelling and the identification of dominant narratives (Golant & Sillince, 2007). In this construction of legitimacy through discourse, organizations and publics or stakeholders play an important role in the process of defining and (re)creating societal norms and values. Therefore, organizations could in fact disrupt socially constructed norms in their communication with stakeholders.

In terms of aging, public relations practice and scholarship should explore how organizations communicate legitimacy in terms of how organizations address and engage with aging issues (e.g., retirement). This examination should seek to create more holistic portrayals of age as it identifies partial portrayals through the overreliance on unidimensional stereotypes. More holistic portrayals of aging could open up new relationships with new groups of stakeholders who may feel excluded from dominant discourse; thus impacting who interacts with an organization and encouraging multivocal and inclusive communication practices (e.g., two-way communication). Furthermore, communicating legitimacy related to aging may increase people's efficacy and expectations related to the aging process by informing and (re)shaping societal norms and values. Future research should consider how the expectations of aging promoted by organizations can in turn affect societal norms and trends like the "OK Boomer," as well as how potentially harmful these stereotypes can be.

### Dialogue

Similar to legitimacy, dialogue plays an important role in organization–stakeholder relationships. Traditionally, Grunig and Grunig (1992) characterized dialogue through a two-way symmetrical model of communication that encourages direct and transparent communication between organizations and their publics. This, however, is an idealistic, albeit normative version of dialogue that is not always possible to achieve (Davidson, 2016). Kent and Taylor (2002) took a broader approach to dialogue in the public relations context when they defined it as "a product of ongoing communication and relationships" (p. 24). Therefore, dialogue can change the nature of a relationship by placing emphasis on the relationship and allowing for opportunities for dissent, open debate, and the creation of possibilities. Dialogic theory, which underscores the potential of dialogue in relationship building, has five tenets. Mutuality refers to the notion that organizations and publics are inextricably tied together. Propinquity describes temporality and spontaneity of interactions with publics (Kent & Taylor, 2002). Empathy defines the supportiveness and confirmation of public goals. Risk is characterized by vulnerability and the willingness to engage with publics on their own terms. Finally, commitment is the "extent to which an organization gives itself over to dialogue, interpretation, and understanding in its interactions with publics" (Kent & Taylor, 2002, p. 25). Using the five tenets of dialogue (e.g., mutuality, propinquity, empathy, risk, and commitment), a dialogic orientation can increase the likelihood that publics and organizations will better understand each other. Dialogue has also been known to play a key role in engagement. Engagement is both an orientation that influences interactions and an approach that guides the process of interactions among groups (Taylor & Kent, 2014). Engagement is a foundational concept and necessary for public relations contributions to a fully functioning society (Taylor & Kent, 2014), as organizations and publics can make decisions that create social capital through engagement with each other.

In terms of aging, it is becoming increasingly important to include older adults' voices into communication about aging. As the population continues to age, more stakeholders will join this group. With current stereotypical portrayals of older adults in public relations messaging, many feel ignored by the "either-or" representation. Dialogue may provide an important space for active engagement in which the conceptualization of aging can be co-created between organizations and stakeholders. In this shift from one-dimensional representation, a genuine effort to engage with older adults in meaningful ways can create important dialogue to reconceptualize our understanding of aging, as well as begin to effectively tackle many of the complex issues associated with aging, (e.g., gaps in the current healthcare system). Thus, we propose future research should examine dialogue about age/aging using a multi-level approach that examines how messages from organizations, media, publics/stakeholders, communities, and individuals come together to create resilient aging spaces (see Buzzanell & Houston, 2018). This research should seek to identify archetypes of productive dialogue that can be implemented to enhance the aging process.

### Advocacy/Activism

From dialogue, we can also consider the role of activism in organization–stakeholder communication and relationships. From a more traditional functionalist perspective, activists have been seen as obstacles an organization must navigate or manage in order to achieve organizational success (Botan & Taylor, 2004). In contrast, however, Curtin and Gaither (2005) argue that moving away from theorizing public relations as an organizational function and toward a conceptualization that is inclusive of social, cultural, and political contexts expands the space of public relations to include activism. As defined by Smith (2005), "activism is a process by which a group of people exert pressure on organizations or other institutions to change policies, practices, or conditions that they find problematic" (p. 6). Further, Ciszek (2015) argues, "Many of the tactics used by activists are public relations tactics and their motives can be viewed as public relations strategies" (p. 447). Thus, from this definition activists engage in the facilitation and management of relationships as public relations practitioners. The role of activists and the mission of activism inherently seek to identify power. From this identification of power, activists may seek to raise awareness, shift attitudes, and change certain actions oftentimes through public relations theory and practice (Ciszek, 2015).

Advocacy is a place where public relations scholarship and practice can make significant contributions to aging discourses. It is important for organizations to advocate for older adults in a variety of contexts (e.g., the workplace, healthcare settings), which could make more inclusive and supportive communication spaces that facilitate successful aging. Advocacy may also be helpful for breaking steadfast stereotypes related to portrayals of aging, as well as for driving important changes to systems that may situate older adults as impediments rather than beneficial members of society. We propose that future research examines how public relations contributes to and/or challenges *rhetorics of vulnerability* surrounding age/aging. Older adults have long had to counter assumptions about vulnerability (in terms of health and susceptibility to scams). During COVID-19 the positioning of older adults as a "vulnerable population" further cemented this discourse (Anderson & Gettings, 2022). It would be worthwhile to uncover the ways in which organizations contribute to these discourses or challenge them as they seek to disrupt assumptions about age/aging and decline and seek to promote ways to enhance the messaging to support successful aging processes.

### A Fully Functioning Society through Public Relations in Aging Spaces

Used separately or in conjunction these three different public relations frameworks (i.e., legitimacy, dialogue, advocacy) can seek to move us toward a fully functioning society in which inclusion and equity are prioritized through the communicative co-construction of shared values. The fully functioning society framework reflects a complex and non-linear approach to public relations (Holtzhausen, 2011) that is grounded in eight fundamental principles: (1) organizational effort to transform uncertainty into order (i.e., to impose order over a complicated issue); (2) corporate responsibility (i.e., the role that organizations play in civil discourse); (3) power resource management (i.e., the use of influence responsibility); (4) community as conflicting and conjoined interests and expectations (i.e., the reality that different groups have multiple and complex interests that converge and diverge); (5) relationship as symmetry (i.e., reflects the fit between societal actors); (6) organizational communication (i.e., positions organizations as responsible rhetors in civic discourse); (7) responsible advocacy (i.e., reliance of facts and evidence that is non-partisan); and (8) narrative and rhetoric leading to enlightened choice (i.e., communication that informs expectations, preferences, and enactment) (Heath, 2006).

From these principles, we can seek to challenge current portrayals and stereotypes related to aging and aging spaces to improve the lived experiences of older adults, especially for those who are excluded from or stigmatized by current societal discourses related to aging. It has been argued that public relations can be used to facilitate the building and sustaining of a fully functioning society as organizations are modern rhetors, acting as a steward of multiple interests (Anderson & Guo, 2021). Thus, because "public relations supplies advocacy, narratives, and other forms of rhetoric through messages, images, campaigns, and events in multiple media channels" (Anderson & Guo, 2021, p. 25), public relations can be used to co-create meaning and discourse in society. Specifically, using a fully function society approach, public relations can be used to foster community collaboration and meaning-making through the facilitation of legitimacy, dialogue, and advocacy to challenge and shift our current conceptualizations of age/aging.

## CONCLUSION

Past scholarship has identified ways that public relations messages have reinforced or challenged commonly held age-based stereotypes through communication for organizational benefits. However, public relations is an area that can make significant strides toward building productive aging spaces that facilitate successful aging through establishing legitimacy, engaging in meaningful dialogue, advocacy, and the development of a fully functioning society. Indeed, the intersection of public relations and aging could be a place to build and support aging processes. Through legitimacy, we can seek to disrupt social norms and expectations surrounding aging. Instead of taking a binary approach to aging, organizations are challenged to show the many complexities that surround aging to create more holistic/realistic portrayals. Through dialogue, organizations are encouraged to engage aging populations in genuine give-and-take to learn from aging stakeholders. Creating the space for engagement can help to identify the role resilience may be able to play in aging spaces. Finally, through activism and advocacy, we can counter stereotypical assumptions related to aging. Moreover, through activism, stakeholders and organizations are challenged to consider how to create more equitable and accessible experiences for older adults in the workplace and healthcare settings, which may currently not be serving this population to the best of its ability. In all, the intersection of public relations and aging is an important area of scholarship and practice that has the potential to create aging spaces that facilitate and inhibit successful aging.

## REFERENCES


Anderson, L. B. (2013). How frames present BMW as embracing an aging workforce. *Public Relations Review, 39*(5), 484–490. <https://doi.org/10.1016/j.pubrev.2013.02.003>

Anderson, L. B. (2015). Changing the story of retirement: How AARP utilizes a strategic narrative to advocate for the aging workforce. *Public Relations Review, 41*(3), 357–364. <https://doi.org/10.1016/j.pubrev.2015.02.004>

Anderson, L. B. (2018). Merging risk and financial communication: Understanding how Prudential creates and resolves the retirement risk. *Public Relations Inquiry, 7*(1), 63–82. <https://doi.org/10.1177/2046147X17736792>

Anderson, L. B. (2019). Communicating legitimacy through portrayals of successful aging: An examination of Pulte Homes' online communication strategies. *Public Relations Inquiry, 9*(1), 27–46. <https://doi.org/10.1177/2046147X19840072>

Anderson, L. B. (2021). Serving public interests and enacting organizational values: An examination of public interest relations through AARP's tele-town halls. *Public Relations Review, 47*(5), 102–109. <https://doi.org/10.1016/j.pubrev.2021.102109>

Anderson, L. B. (2022). "OK Boomer": Demagogic discourse and intergenerational communication. *Journal of Intergenerational Relationships, 21*(2), 253–268. <https://doi.org/10.1080/15350770.2022.2030846>

Anderson, L. B. & Gettings, P. E. (2022). "Old age scares me": Exploring young adults' feelings about aging before and during COVID-19. *Journal of Aging Studies, 60,* <https://doi.org/10.1016/j.jaging.2022.100998>

Anderson, L. B., & Guo, J. S. (2021). Communicating stakeholder resilience: understanding how resilience discourse can build a fully functioning society. *Journal of Public Relations Research, 33*(1), 23–38. <https://doi.org/10.1080/1062726X.2020.1867986>

Botan, C. & Taylor, M. (2004). Public relations: State of the field. *Journal of Communication, 54*(4), 645–661. <https://doi.org/10.1111/j.1460-2466.2004.tb02649.x>

Brunner, B. R., & Smallwood, A. M. (2019). Prioritizing public interest in public relations: Public interest relations. *Public Relations Inquiry, 8*(3), 245–264. <https://doi.org/10.1177/2046147X19870275>

Buzzanell, P. M., & Houston, J. B. (2018). Communication and resilience: Multilevel applications and insights – A Journal of Applied Communication Research forum. *Journal of Applied Communication Research, 46(1)*, 1–4. <https://doi.org/10.1080/00909882.2017.1412086>

Ciszek, E. L. (2015). Bridging the gap: Mapping the relationship between activism and public relations. *Public Relations Review, 41*(4), 447–455. <https://doi.org/10.1016/j.pubrev.2015.05.016>

Cuddy, A. J. C., Norton, M. I., & Fiske, S. T. (2005). This old stereotype: The pervasiveness and persistence of the elderly stereotype. *Journal of Social Issues, 61*(2), 267–285. <https://doi.org/10.1111/j.1540-4560.2005.00405.x>

Curtin, P. A. & Gaither, T. K. (2005). Privileging identity, difference and power: The circuit of culture as a basis for public relations theory. *Journal of Public Relations Research, 17*(2), 91–115. <https://doi.org/10.1207/s1532754xjprr1702_3>

Davidson, S. (2016). Public relations theory: An agonistic critique of the turns to dialogue and symmetry. *Public Relations Inquiry, 5*(2), 145–167. <https://doi.org/10.1177/2046147X16649007>

Deephouse, D. L., & Carter, S. M. (2005). An examination of differences between organizational legitimacy and organizational reputation. *Journal of Management Studies, 42*(2), 329–360. <https://doi.org/10.1111/j.1467-6486.2005.00499.x>

Fiske, S. T., Cuddy, A. J. C., Glick, P., & Xu, J. (2002). A model of (often mixed) stereotype content: Competence and warmth respectively follow from perceived status and competition. *Journal of Personality and Social Psychology, 82*(6), 878–902. <https://doi.org/10.1037/0022-3514.82.6.878>

Edwards, L. (2012). Defining the "object" of public relations research: A new starting point. *Public Relations Inquiry, 1*(1), 7–30. <https://doi.org/10.1177/2046147X11422149>

Golant, B. D., & Sillince, J. A. (2007). The constitution of organizational legitimacy: A narrative perspective. *Organization Studies, 28*(8), 1149–1167. <https://doi.org/10.1177/0170840607075671>

Grunig, J. E., & Grunig, L. A. (1992). Models of public relations and communication. In J. E. Grunig (Ed.), *Excellence in public relations and communication management* (pp. 285–325). Routledge.

Heath, R. L. (2006). Onward into more fog: Thoughts on public relations' research directions. *Journal of Public Relations Research, 18*(2), 93–114. <https://doi.org/10.1207/s1532754xjprr1802_2>

Holtzhausen, D. R. (2011). The need for a postmodern turn in global public relations. In N. Bardhan, & C. K. Weaver (Eds.), *Public relations in global contexts: Multi-paradigmatic perspectives* (pp. 140–166). Routledge.

Hummert, M. L., Garstka, T. A., Shaner, J. L., & Strahm, S. (1994). Stereotypes of the elderly held by young, middle-aged, and elderly adults. *Journal of Gerontology, 49*(5), P240–P249. <https://doi.org/10.1093/geronj/49.5.P240>

Kent, M. L., & Taylor, M. (2002). Toward a dialogic theory of public relations. *Public Relations Review, 28*(1), 21–37. <https://doi.org/10.1016/S0363-8111(02)00108-X>

Lim, J-K, R. & Lee S. Y. (2022). Creating shared value (CSV) and mutually beneficial relationships to address societal issues and develop corporate competitive advantage: A case study of Yuhan-Kimberly and an aging population. *Public Relations Review, 48*(4). <https://doi.org/10.1016/j.pubrev.2022.102225>

Patel, A. M., Xavier, R. J., & Broom, G. (2005). Toward a model of organizational legitimacy in public relations theory and practice. In *Proceedings of the International Communication Association Conference* (pp. 1–22). <https://eprints.qut.edu.au/10132/1/10132.pdf>

Pew Research Center (2019). Defining generations: Where Millennials end and Generation Z begins. <https://www.pewresearch.org/fact-tank/2019/01/17/where-millennials-end-and-generation-z-begins/>

Smith, B. G. (2012). Public relations identity and the stakeholder–organization relationship: A revised theoretical position for public relations scholarship. *Public Relations Review, 38*(5), 838–845. <https://doi.org/10.1016/j.pubrev.2012.06.011>

Smith, M. F. (2005). Activism. In R. L. Heath & W. T. Coombs (Eds.), *Encyclopedia of public relations* (pp. 5–10). Sage.

Suchman, M. C. (1995). Managing legitimacy: Strategic and institutional approaches. *Academy of Management Review, 20*(3), 571–610. <https://doi.org/10.5465/amr.1995.9508080331>

Taylor, M., & Kent, M. L. (2014). Dialogic engagement: Clarifying foundational concepts. *Journal of Public Relations Research, 26*(5), 384–398. <https://doi.org/10.1080/1062726X.2014.956106>

Vasquez, G. & Taylor, M. (2001). Research perspectives on "the public." In R. L. Heath (Ed.), *Handbook of public relations* (pp. 139–154). Sage.

PART FOUR

# Translational Communication and Health

CHAPTER TEN

# Communication, Community, and Co-design: Using Precision Messages to Enhance Health Equity

JANICE L. KRIEGER AND AANTAKI RAISA

The goal of this part is to provide an overview of the importance of translational communication in health contexts. Both chapters in this part focus on the importance of place-based cultural identity in shaping the way individuals think, behave, and communicate about health and well-being. The goal of the current chapter is to apply a cultural identity lens to the development of digital health interventions. The second chapter (Palmer-Wackerly and Wahed) describes academic-community partnerships and qualitative research methods as effective strategies for developing a deep understanding of community as both the locus of the problem and the solution for addressing well-being.

The perspective presented in this chapter on designing, implementing, and evaluating culturally tailored interventions that utilize precision messaging techniques to enhance health equity began over twenty years ago when I (JK) collected my dissertation data with rural, low-income women living in rural Appalachia. Nearly all participants asked me the same question: "Why are you doing this research in this community?" What they really wanted to know was simply this: "Who are you and why do you care about cancer in Appalachia?" Many of the women articulated concerns that people outside the region stereotype them as low-income, uneducated, and at fault for the health problems they experience. Some only agreed to participate after learning that I was also from Appalachia and wanted to conduct research to benefit the people living there.

The positionality of scientists conducting certain types of research is an issue that is too easily dismissed in the sciences. Often, scientists are trained to believe that their culture, family background, and life experiences are irrelevant to their work. In my experience, my culture has had a profound influence on who I am and how I relate to others. My family (in a variety of forms) are central to my motivation and focus. My experiences shape my ability to empathize with others and enable me to nurture others from diverse backgrounds in their career.

In my view, the mentoring we receive as scientists is part of our culture. Just as my family of origin shaped my career, so too has my academic family. I am honored to coauthor this book with my forever mentor and friend, Professor Jon Nussbaum, and my academic siblings who also benefitted from his mentorship. At a time when many scholars were focused on "convenient samples," Jon Nussbaum persuaded his mentees of the importance of studying communication processes at every age and stage of life. He taught us to be curious and humble about how much we had to learn from our participants. I have been fortunate to share this knowledge with my mentees and begin my own twig on our academic family tree. Chapter 11 is co-authored by one of my first mentees from Ohio State (Angela Palmer-Wackerly). I am equally privileged to co-author this chapter with one of my last mentees from the University of Florida (Aantaki Raisa). I am bonded to these women through a passion to use our voice—as scholars, as women, and as friends to leave this world better than we found it.

An important cultural element of my academic family is the importance of boundary spanning. Boundary spanners are people who move knowledge from one place to another within an organization and/or in society. My earliest models of this approach to health communication scholarship included individuals that sought to connect to other disciplines and ground their work in different contexts. One example of this is Roxanne Parrott's research with the Georgia Cancer Control Program working within migrant farm communities to develop cancer prevention campaigns. Another is Michael Hecht and Michelle Miller-Day's partnership with substance use prevention specialists, educators, and experts in child development in elementary, middle, and high schools to develop communication strategies that could be used competently in different relationships in early life. And, of course, Jon Nussbaum's collaboration with geriatricians in retirement communities to improve communication with the elderly to promote healthy aging.

Boundary spanners often find themselves at the intersection of disciplines, cultures, and ways of being. While sometimes exhilarating, it can also be uncomfortable because it demands learning new vocabulary, methods, norms, and values. Fortunately, Collins Airhihenbuwa drilled the idea of "getting comfortable being uncomfortable" into my consciousness. Boundary spanning, or advancing knowledge through the intersection of disciplines, is a core feature of what the National Institute of Health refers to as translational sciences. The term "translation" has two formal meanings. The first is the process of converting words from one language to another. However, a broader definition is to convert something into a different form. Applied to the field of communication, translational communication refers to converting ideas from one cultural perspective to another to enable connection with an intended audience.

A key component of culture, and cultural identity, is language. For this reason, science (and scientists) represents a culture. Too often, the process of translating science for lay audiences is characterized as "dumbing down" information. However, true translation is not simplification. It transforms how one group of individuals engage in sensemaking into a new entity that empowers another group to understand the rationality of another experience or perspective. For this reason, translational communication should be bidirectional. In other words, it is equally important to translate cultural knowledge and ways of being to scientific audiences as it is for scientific audiences to translate information grounded in scientific approaches for other cultural identity groups.

The future is bright for the next generation of translational communication scientists. The need for translational approaches to health and well-being is endless, and there will always be new audiences, new topics, and new technologies to investigate. In this chapter, we weave together health communication, intergroup communication, and language to examine health messages from the perspective of geographic and cultural space. We will provide an overview of the foundational arguments for translational communication approaches, the connection of intergroup identities with space and place, and an example from an ongoing program of research demonstrating how these principles are being integrated into knowledge translation interventions in digital environments. Next, we address our positionality in this chapter by providing a brief overview of how culture, family, and experiences have influenced our work.

## OUR JOURNEYS TO ACADEMIA

### Meet Janice

As many scholars who study translational science will attest, the biggest scientific gaps are not between what we know and what we do not know, but between what we know (i.e., cognition) and what we do (i.e., behavior). As a communication scientist interested in translational science issues, I have been fascinated by the role of language in cognition and behavior. One example of this is my interest in metaphors, and how culture shapes the interpretation of metaphors in health and science contexts. However, as the COVID-19 pandemic taught us, translating science is more than just an academic exercise. It can be the difference between life and death. While I have spent my career striving for academic excellence in the traditional venues, such as publications, I have also focused much of time and effort being an ambassador for the discipline outside my discipline and advocating for the value of communication in public health efforts.

I have always been intrigued by the role of geography in how we make sense of information about health. I am a first-generation college student born and reared in a rural part of Appalachia. I remember realizing during my first graduate seminar on health communication that none of the readings presented a perspective on communication in family or clinical care that reflected my own experiences. At that point, I realized that either (a) I was a unicorn or (b) the literature did not reflect the lived experiences of individuals with my background. It turned out that both were true. While I am an individual with unique thoughts, experiences, and perspectives, some of those characteristics are shaped by my cultural identity. This realization has shaped the trajectory of my career, which is to engage in research, writing, mentoring, and community service that elevates the voices of individuals and communities who need to be engaged in dialogue about addressing the healthcare challenges of our time.

## Meet Aantaki

I am a transplant from Bangladesh and have lived in the United States for a decade. My interest in academia ignited while working as a community reporter in the Bangladeshi immigrant community in Queens, New York and then as an interpreter at a medical malpractice law firm in Manhattan. Both these experiences gave me a front-row seat to observe how cultural and linguistic differences can result in adverse health outcomes. This practical experience at the intersection of health communication and culture was pivotal in my decision to start graduate school at the University of Florida under the mentorship of Janice Krieger.

Driven by the motto of "where you live should not determine whether you live," my academic goal has been to utilize my knowledge, skills, and access to resources to conduct research for health equity and justice. This drives my passion to conduct rigorous scientific research in the field of health intervention development to meet the needs of underrepresented populations, such as immigrants, and citizens of the Global South. My work focuses on using appropriate language and framing when talking about individuals and communities who are from backgrounds other than Western, White, English-speaking, and other characteristics that are disproportionately represented in behavioral science research.

My training has also made me very aware of the disconnect between health intervention goals and unintended consequences. I have found that actively integrating the perspectives and voices of the people for whom the interventions are designed can reduce the risk of unintended negative consequences. Using the principles of cultural grounding, community-based participatory research, and culture-centered approach, my goal is to continue my research on how to translate between the scientific community and underrepresented populations to diversify the data that guide public health policy. Next, we provide an overview of the theoretical approaches that underpin these professional goals.

## OVERVIEW OF TRANSLATIONAL COMMUNICATION SCIENCE

The disconnect between what available scientific evidence suggests should happen and what happens in practice is known as the knowledge-practice gap (Pablos-Mendez & Shademani, 2006). For example, many of us know how we should communicate with others, but how often do we fail to behave in that way? Communication is not alone in this problem. In the context of healthcare, it is oft lamented that it can take 17 years for innovations in basic medical research to be translated to the clinic in a way that improves the healthcare patients receive (Trochim, 2010). To address this problem, the National Institutes of Health (NIH) launched the *NIH Roadmap* to increase the speed at which a scientific discovery can have a meaningful influence on clinical care (Collins et al., 2014). In 2011, the Public Health Service Act was amended to create The National Center for Advancing Translational Sciences (NCATS) to promote research translation, meaning the process of turning observations in the laboratory, clinic, and community into interventions that improve the health of individuals and the public (Collins, 2011).

While the creation of NCATS is often credited as a catalyst for translational research, it is important to note that the communication discipline was explicitly focused on research translation a few years earlier. For example, there was a preconference to the annual meeting of the National Communication Association (NCA) focused on translational scholarship in 1998 (Petronio, 2007). Since this preconference, translational scholarship has remained a central feature in our discipline as represented by a variety of journals, conferences, and divisions within our national and international organizations. An important part of the growth of translational scholarship is the increasing partnerships between communication scientists and researchers from other disciplines (Treise et al., 2016). Funding agencies such as the National Institutes of Health are increasing the number of funding announcements that focus on communication science and Healthy People 2030 includes a national aim to improve health communication (*Stakeholder Engagement and Communication for Healthy People 2030*, n.d.). Next, we turn to the importance of communication as a key scientific component of our national efforts around translational science.

## THE ROLE OF LANGUAGE AND COMMUNICATION IN TRANSLATIONAL SCIENCE

Communication is central to the larger translational science mission in two important ways. The first and most obvious way is through making findings from basic research useful to the public. Like many other domains in science and humanities, there is much work to be done to transform scholarship appearing in academic outlets like journals and conferences so that it is accessible and useful for improving the well-being of people in day-to-day life. Indeed, for the knowledge translation process to work, individuals with expertise in basic theory and research must communicate findings to individuals who can integrate those ideas in practice and evaluate effectiveness by increasing external validity. For knowledge to move from basic to translational to implementation, the lifecycle of discovery must be intentionally curated.

The second way is equally important, but less obvious. One of the main barriers to science translation is poor communication. An example is the term *knowledge translation* itself. Most scholars agree that it is important to bridge the knowledge-practice gap. However, they disagree on how to define what that means. Even the term "knowledge" is problematic. Critiques have focused on the nature of what does and does not count as knowledge based on what is considered scientific "evidence" (Greenhalgh & Wieringa, 2011). Another critique is that there is unequal power between scientists and other stakeholders in prioritizing certain types of "knowledge" for translation (Estabrooks et al., 2006). The term *translation* is also potentially problematic because it assumes that knowledge can be effectively utilized in a new context if it is simply summarized, packaged, and presented appropriately (Engebretsen et al., 2017).

From a communication perspective, these critiques can be viewed as a tension between mental models of knowledge translation grounded in an information deficit model versus a dialogic model of communication (Krieger & Gallois, 2017). An information deficit approach consists of a source having a resource (i.e., information) that a recipient needs, hence unequal status. Furthermore, the needs of the "recipient" will be met through a transactional transfer of the information. Within this mental model, knowledge translation is a process that decreases the accuracy or specificity of information in favor of comprehensibility.

Conversely, the dialogic model approaches knowledge translation as knowledge co-creation. Knowledge co-creation is a complex process that requires bi-directional message exchange that contextualizes knowledge for an intended audience within a specific culture. From this perspective, medicine is a cultural context complete with linguistic and cultural symbols used by a given speech community. As such, the translation process benefits from the expertise of trained communication scholars who can serve as boundary spanners with knowledge of the culture of science and of other speech communities.

The challenges in knowledge translation discussed so far represent macro-level issues in communication science. Challenges exist on a more micro-level, also. This is apparent in the language choices healthcare providers make when communicating information to patients. Given that many patient populations experience low health literacy, healthcare providers are often advised to use plain language, meaning literal language free of technical jargon and simple grammatical structure (Stableford & Mettger, 2007). Although reducing the amount of overly technical or difficult terms seems like a simple solution, it may not be sufficient for establishing shared meaning. In such cases, other translational strategies are warranted. An alternate strategy to plain language is metaphor. Metaphors are linguistic devices that compare well-known relationships to help explain new, unknown connections intended to facilitate information processing (Kendall-Taylor & Haydon, 2016). In certain cases, metaphors can be more effective for explaining complex information than plain language (Krieger et al., 2010).

Humans naturally use metaphors as tools for creating shared meaning. The COVID-19 pandemic provided a case study of the ubiquity of metaphors for explaining new scientific information to the public (Semino, 2021). To compare the advantages of plain language and metaphorical communication strategies, consider the widespread scientific concern about "R0" (pronounced R-naught) during the pandemic. R0 was explained by ABC News as an indicator of how contagious a disease is, or how easily it spreads from person to person in a community. This plain language approach seems clear. But, compare it to a more metaphorical approach. The website Medscape framed it this way: "Think of COVID-19 as a fire burning in a forest. All of us are trees. The R0 is the wind speed. The higher it is, the faster the fire tears through the forest. But just like a forest fire, COVID-19 needs fuel to keep going. We're the fuel" (*COVID-19 Death Predictions*, n.d.).

Metaphors also became popular for addressing COVID-19 vaccine hesitancy. One approach used by some healthcare providers was to compare the COVID-19 vaccine to disabling the landing gear on an airplane. In this metaphor, the goal of an airplane (i.e., virus) is to land (i.e., enter the cell). Receiving the COVID-19 vaccine could be explained as disabling the "landing gear" on an airplane, meaning that the vaccine prevents the virus from entering the cell. While metaphorical approaches such as this have intuitive appeal, many popular medical metaphorical strategies remain untested with diverse populations. This is problematic because metaphors rely on cultural knowledge to be successful; thus, shared cultural knowledge of the connections between the metaphor ground and the vehicle cannot simply be assumed (Krieger, 2014).

Whether using metaphors or not, cultural competence is key for achieving translational goals in health and science communication. While interpersonal interactions are ideally suited to dialogic approaches, the reality of the modern healthcare environment requires that much of the knowledge translation occurs via technology. In our work, we refer to the process of developing health interventions with evidence-based data about the communication partner as *precision messaging*. This term evolved as a companion to precision medicine, a term introduced in 2015 to refer to precise treatments utilizing biological and psychosocial characteristics of a given patient that distinguish them from other patients with the same clinical condition (Scherr et al., 2017). Next, we define precision messaging and describe ways it can be applied.

## TRANSLATIONAL COMMUNICATION, CULTURAL IDENTITY, AND GEOGRAPHIC CONTEXT

Just as precision medicine seeks to deliver therapies customized to the individual, the goal of precision messaging is to identify meaningful characteristics within a population that will affect message processing and adapt messages based on these characteristics to facilitate attention, comprehension, and evidence-based decision-making. While certain sociodemographic characteristics are commonly incorporated in messaging efforts such as ethnicity, age, and gender, others are just beginning to be considered. Geography is one such factor of interest in this section. Despite awareness that health inequities often follow geographic boundaries, the role of place in health communication is understudied. While physical *place* can influence health via long distances to receive healthcare or reduced access to healthy foods, the corresponding social *space* refers to the ways in which individuals socially construct geography as part of their social identity. The next section explores how and when place functions as a salient social identity in translational health communication contexts.

## Rural Place and Social Categorization

The economic and political landscape in many industrialized countries is such that more lucrative positions (e.g., high-tech, administrative headquarters) are typically located in urban centers with employment in rural areas tending to offer employment in sectors that are considered less prestigious or require less skill (Dickens, 2000). Although the number of individuals living in non-metro areas has declined in recent years, over 46 million Americans consider rural (or non-metro) areas home, and these areas constitute 72 % of the United States' surface geography (J. C. Davis et al., 2022). Rural areas in the United States are locations with low population density (i.e., few people per land unit area) and are geographically separated from urban metropolitan centers. Importantly, this is not universal. In densely populated countries such as Bangladesh, rurality is associated with access to amenities, not population density per se.

Importantly, residing in rural (or urban) areas is associated with cultural meanings well beyond mere physical geography. Place identity refers to circumstances in which the physical environment and the corresponding cultural values associated with a given space function as important to sense of self (i.e., avowed identity) or a salient social group membership of others (i.e., ascribed identity) (Twigger-Ross & Uzzell, 1996). Place identity focuses on the environmental and social characteristics that promote avowed urban or rural identities (Belanche et al., 2021). However, there is limited research on how and when place identity influences health and health outcomes. One way to understand this phenomenon is through the lens of social identity and communication.

## Communication Accommodation Theory (CAT)

Communication accommodation theory (CAT) proposed by Howard Giles in the 1970s addresses, explores, and explains the variety of communicative adjustments made by individuals interacting with others based on perceived social group memberships. When interacting with individuals from other groups, people naturally make assumptions, based on their sociohistorical, interpersonal, and individual experiences, about the other's needs, knowledge, or background. Those assumptions drive the communicator's pace of speaking, choice of words, paralinguistic usage, and nonverbal gestures (Giles, 2016). These adjustments and the assumptions that drive them can be intentional or unintentional. The purpose of such adjustments is to establish the communicator's similarity or dissimilarity with the interactant or to help or hinder a communication partner's understanding of what is being said. If the assumptions made about the partner are correct, the purpose of the adjustments is likely to be accomplished. If not, the adjustments are likely to result in unintended consequences (Gasiorek, 2016).

Intergroup communication is defined as interactions where at least one interactant accesses and applies a social category (e.g., age, ethnicity, gender, sexual orientation, social class, education level, occupation, nationality, political affiliation, religion, health status) to that interaction (Giles & Maass, 2016). For example, when a clinician in the United States perceives a patient to be an immigrant, the clinician assigns themselves to the "non-immigrant American" category. This categorization activates the pertinent beliefs about either group that are already held by the clinician, and those beliefs are then reflected, consciously or unconsciously, in their verbal and nonverbal communication with the patient.

In situations where clinicians come from different racial, ethnic, or national cultures than their patients, CAT effectively explains the accommodative strategies that clinicians apply in the hopes of being perceived as convergent by their patients. For clinicians who are immigrants to the United States, for example, such strategies include learning American slang, practicing American pronunciation, and changing their speech rate (Jain & Krieger, 2011). Indeed, there are numerous skill training programs to improve intercultural communication competence, especially among clinicians (Watson et al., 2016).

## CAT Applied to Patient–Clinician Interactions

A significant contribution of CAT in the context of patient–clinician interactions is its ability to empirically examine communication outcomes in intergroup contexts (Watson et al., 2016). For example, a healthcare professional may increase their volume of speech in response to a patient with gray hair and visibly aging skin based on the social stereotype that older adults are hard of hearing. If that assumption is correct, the increased volume may be perceived as helpful. If that assumption is incorrect, the patient may feel offended and be less inclined to engage in meaningful dialogue about their health. Adjusting communication based on social stereotypes, rather than need, is considered overaccommodation. Overaccommodation can result in patients perceiving healthcare providers as patronizing. When patients feel stereotyped by healthcare providers, they can react with their own strategies that prevent satisfaction with the medical encounter (Lagacé et al., 2012).

Despite the increasing number of communication skill training programs, empirical evidence points to continuing racial disparities related to communication competence, regardless of socioeconomic background (Hamel et al., 2022). For example, a literature review on implicit bias held by clinicians found significant positive bias toward White or light-skinned patients and against Black, Hispanic, American Indian, or dark-skinned patients, such bias leads to poorer patient–clinician communication and disparities in treatment recommendations (Maina et al., 2018). CAT helps explain how unconscious biases resulting from intergroup stereotypes can have deleterious outcomes for groups that experience health inequities. In the following section, we briefly describe the established cultural accommodation approaches to health message and health intervention design.

## Cultural Targeting, Tailoring, and Grounding.

*Cultural targeting* refers to customizing health messages for specific cultural groups, such as first-generation immigrants from a specific country (e.g., Bangladesh) or a specific cultural origin (e.g., South Asia), while *cultural tailoring* refers to customizing health messages for a specific individual, and requires a higher level of precision (Kreuter & McClure, 2004). *Linguistic targeting* refers to language concordance or "matching." Linguistic targeting strategies are considered the "lowest common denominator of cultural sensitivity" as it only requires translating the messages of an intervention to the native language of the target audience (Rogler et al., 1987). *Cultural grounding* is a strategy in which members of the target audience actively participate in the development and implementation of the health intervention, and thus their own group-specific norms, values, beliefs, and concerns (i.e., deep structures of culture), as related to the health issue of concern, are addressed in the health message (Hecht & Krieger, 2006).

## Culture-Centered Approach.

A culture-centered approach adds another layer to cultural grounding. In all the approaches to cultural communication accommodation discussed earlier, the health issue of concern is identified by experts outside of a cultural group (e.g., U.S.-born scientists identifying a health issue among a specific immigrant population and trying to find a solution to that issue). The culture-centered approach argues that in addition to active participation by members of the target audience members in the development and implementation of a health message or intervention, the health issue of concern should be identified or brought up by members of the group themselves. Thus, that cultural group is granted the power and agency to decide which or what health issues they need or want to be resolved at the time (Dutta, 2007).

## Cultural Variance Framework

The cultural variance framework, like cultural grounding and the culture-centered approach, acknowledges the dynamic nature of cultural affiliations. It ties the idea of group and individual identities relevant to culture into the message design. This framework identifies three routes through which culture influences individuals' health behaviors: identity affiliation, cultural attributes, and contextual specificity. One or a combination of these routes can be used in message design (Davis & Resnicow, 2012).

*Identity affiliation* refers to the subjective culture(s) with which individuals self-identify and draw upon when enacting beliefs, behaviors, norms, roles, values, and assumptions. Two prominent examples of identity affiliations that vary at an individual level are ethnic/racial identity and acculturation. While ethnic/racial identity affiliations are relevant when developing health messages within a national culture, acculturation is often most relevant for immigrants. When an individual is both an immigrant and a member of an ethnic/racial minority (e.g., South Asian immigrants), both ethnic/racial identity and acculturation need to be considered in determining the individual's identity affiliations.

*Cultural attributes* are defined as the combination of specific beliefs, norms, values, and behaviors that form an individual's subjective culture(s). For example, although South Asian culture is often associated with collectivism, South Asians differ in their involvement in practices pertaining to collectivism (e.g., prioritizing the family's needs over the self). Members of subcultures within South Asian culture also vary in their personal endorsement of and engagement in the specific beliefs, behaviors, and assumptions which constitute their culture(s).

Finally, *contextual specificity* is defined as the degree of influence of the contextual cues to which a particular identity affiliation or cultural attribute is salient to an individual in a specific context. Some identity affiliations and cultural attributes can be considered an overall subjective cultural identity for an individual, while others are specific only to certain contexts. For example, a Bangladeshi might identify themselves as a secular, nonreligious person, even while their religious upbringing in a Muslim family might influence their food habits (e.g., not consuming alcohol or pork). In this case, the individual's overall salient identity is secular/nonreligious, but in the context of food consumption, their religious identity becomes salient.

As these perspectives and examples demonstrate, culture is pervasive in human attitudes and behaviors related to health. As a result, many interactions in healthcare have high potential to become intergroup in nature. The challenges of managing intergroup communication are not limited to face-to-face interaction. Health campaigns and even human-machine interaction can be viewed through intergroup lenses as well (Lee et al., 2014). In the following section, we briefly describe the established cultural accommodation approaches to health message and health intervention design in contexts that do not include face-to-face interaction.

## ACCOMMODATING CULTURE IN HEALTH INTERVENTION DEVELOPMENT

Based on a synthesis of the different approaches for cultural communication accommodation, one common strategy can be identified as permeating all approaches. That is, when developing heath messages for a cultural group, ask or involve the group members in decisions about how, where, and when they want to receive the message, and from whom. Culturally accommodating interventions can be of two types: developed from scratch for a particular cultural group, or adapted from an intervention that was originally developed for another cultural group (Marsiglia & Booth, 2015). The latter approach involves an adaptation process that starts with the need-based, surface-level structures of the intervention, which is defined as the imagery, language, and colors used in the intervention. The necessary changes can then be achieved by interviewing the members of the intended audience or cultural group, conducting focus group discussions, applying think-aloud methods, or doing usability testing (Creswell & Poth, 2018).

Based on feedback from the participants, the researchers may then realize that certain deep structure changes need to be made in the adapted versions of the intervention. Such changes may include framing the message differently (e.g., collectivist vs. individualistic; negative vs. positive), incorporating new constructs (e.g., fear reduction), or discarding some constructs (e.g., uncertainty). No matter what changes are made, the reasons for those changes need to be empirically justified and the effect of those changes need to be tested before mass implementation of the adaptation. Advances in technology are making it increasingly feasible to adapt interventions for different cultural groups. Next, we examine virtual humans as one avenue for delivering culturally adapted health interventions.

## TECHNOLOGY: EHEALTH INNOVATIONS TO IMPROVE COMMUNICATION ACCOMMODATION

One strategy for reducing racial and ethnic biases in clinician-patient communication has been the use of eHealth technologies, which can be tailored to patients' specific needs. Virtual interactions are increasingly used in numerous aspects of healthcare, such as psychological and psychiatric consultation, suicide prevention, palliative cancer care, diet and fitness coaching, and pain management (Laranjo et al., 2018). Developing virtual humans to deliver messages is more effective in some circumstances than traditional messaging techniques, such as written text (Krieger et al., 2021). Virtual humans are an innovative eHealth technology that can be easily customized to address diverse cultural aspects of a health topic (Vilaro, Wilson-Howard, et al., 2020; Zalake et al., 2019). Next, we discuss different types of virtual technology used in healthcare settings and the various ways that culture, acculturation, and communication accommodations can be mobilized to develop more effective ehealth interventions.

### Virtual Assistants

Virtual assistants (VAs) are computer-generated entities, with or without an animated appearance, that can emulate human behaviors such as physical gestures, linguistic and paralinguistic behaviors, and interpersonal communication (Provoost et al., 2017). Depending on the type of computer program that controls their interactions, VAs can be divided into two categories. First, VAs based on machine learning algorithms can generate live responses to comments made by a human interactant (Allouch et al., 2021). VAs use natural language processing to understand verbal or written human communication. Common examples of this include Siri (responding to verbal communication) and chatbots (responding to written communication). The second type is VAs based on dialogue management algorithms (Mohamad Suhaili et al., 2021). This type of VA is programmed to generate a predetermined, limited set of responses based on inputs from human users. These VAs do not use natural language processing and provide interactants with finite options of communication. Examples of such VAs include automated voice assistants that provide limited options to the user (e.g., banking service voice bots) and are unable to respond to queries not already programmed into the VA's system.

VAs can also be categorized based on the modality of communication, namely, voice only (e.g., Alexa), text only (e.g., website chatbots), or embodied. Embodied VAs—visual digital entities that mimic human-like body language—have an anthropomorphized presence and are also known as embodied conversational agents (Provoost et al., 2017). This type of VA can communicate both verbally through voice and/or text and nonverbally through body language, unlike the other types of VA, which communicate only verbally.

## Virtual Assistants in Healthcare

VAs have been used in healthcare since the 1960s. ELIZA provided text-based psychotherapy counseling with limited, preprogrammed responses starting in 1966 (Milne-Ives et al., 2020), and the idea of virtual patients was first proposed in the 1970s (Cendan & Lok, 2012). VAs started being used in healthcare much more frequently in the 2000s. In 2006, VAs were developed as simulated patients to help standardize patient responses and teach medical students information-taking and communication skills (Stevens et al., 2006). Use of VAs to help patients has mostly been seen in mental healthcare, but also in care provided for physical health, neurodivergence, language impairment, sexual health, substance abuse, sleep apnea, diabetes, and hypertension (Laranjo et al., 2018).

More recently, VAs are also being used in cancer care. The CDC launched the VA Linda in 2019 to interact with and answer questions from cancer survivors (Bartley, 2019). Tina was launched in 2018 by the CDC Foundation to improve cancer patient–provider communication (Stinson, 2018), while research scholars in cancer prevention from the University of Florida developed their own VA-based tools, such as ALEX (Agent Leveraging Empathy for eXams; Krieger et al., 2021). Commercial companies are also entering the space, as exemplified by the WellBe VA, which has been described as an "Alexa for health care" (McDonald, 2020).

VAs can be especially advantageous in cancer prevention through raising awareness of and educating patients about preventative measures. This is due to the VAs' ease of access: Anyone with internet access on a computer or smartphone can take advantage of them. They can be customized based on the users' cancer literacy and tailored with different languages, accents, and levels of informational detail (Vilaro, Wilson-Howard, et al., 2020). Cancer prevention VAs can thus be used to reduce health inequities by serving patients in rural areas with limited clinic access, patients from linguistic or cultural minority groups, and patients with limited educational backgrounds (O'Leary et al., 2020; Vilaro et al., 2022). VAs may be especially useful in addressing geographic cancer health inequities. In one study, participants with a higher rural identity had a more positive impression of a VA recommending colorectal cancer than those with lower rural identity (Cooks et al., 2022).

VAs combine the benefits of eHealth technologies (e.g., they can be accessed from anywhere) and the interactivity of human-to-human communication. Moreover, VAs can be tailored to any degree of precision based on the target audience's needs. They can be matched demographically with the patient (e.g., in voice, name, gender, skin tone, clothes). They can be programmed in any language or accent. Their message content can be tailored to the target audience's literacy level, informational needs, and cancer literacy.

However, VAs developed without empirical evidence or risks of biases in mind can also increase the digital divide and produce adverse health outcomes. In fact, with the rise of VAs and machine learning technologies, numerous commercial apps became available with promises of mental healthcare, weight loss, and cancer care. Most of these apps are not scientifically evaluated, and their development lacks transparency and scientific rigor (Szinay et al., 2021). Such technologies, developed without inputs from pluralistic perspectives, reinforce existing inequities (Buolamwini & Gebru, 2018). Hence, it is important to systematically evaluate the development of VAs, especially those intended to address chronic and serious health issues. Next, we apply the lessons learned about accommodation, culture, health intervention design, and technology to a case study of developing a VA to address cancer screening.

## CASE STUDY: DEVELOPING A VA FOR CANCER SCREENING AMONG IMMIGRANT POPULATIONS

Asian Americans are the fastest-growing racial and ethnic group in the United States (Budiman & Ruiz, 2021). They are also one of the largest immigrant groups that hold cultural beliefs about cancer that act as barriers to preventing or reducing cancer-related morbidity and mortality. Fear of cancer is pervasive among multiple Asian populations, manifesting itself in cancer fatalism (i.e., nothing can be done if diagnosed with cancer); reluctance to screen for fear of positive diagnosis; fear of treatment, pain, and cost; and fear of being abandoned by family, friends, and the community (Wong-Kim et al., 2003). In many Asian cultures, cancer is bad karma or punishment for sins (Steiness et al., 2018). For example, studies have shown that some Chinese Americans believe cancer is contagious (Wong-Kim et al., 2003), and some Indian American women do not believe cancer is a serious disease (Wu et al., 2006).

New or recent immigrants tend to adhere to the health-related beliefs and behaviors of their country of origin (Lee et al., 2021). Some immigrants, despite having lived in their host country for years, do not adapt to the host country's culture and socialize only with people from the same background, beliefs, values, and health behaviors (Wong-Kim et al., 2003). Thus, they adhere to their root country's cancer-related beliefs. Immigrants who develop more integrated or assimilated identities may adapt to their host country's culture surrounding cancer care.

## Acculturated Identities and Health Outcomes

Long-term observations in U.S. medical and social research about immigrants' health have identified an "immigrant paradox." This paradox is that despite living in low socioeconomic status and underserved communities, immigrants display better health outcomes than members of the host culture. However, a longer duration of residence in the host country tends to result in more detrimental health outcomes among new immigrant populations (Alcántara et al., 2017). Acculturation is one possible explanation for the relationship between immigrants' longevity in the United States and the subsequent deterioration of their health outcomes.

A systematic review of acculturation's influence on Asian Americans found that immigrants more adherent to their root cultures showed less propensity toward alcohol use, while immigrants with a stronger propensity toward American culture had significantly higher levels of alcohol consumption (Lui & Zamboanga, 2018). A meta-analysis of tobacco use among Asian Americans found that men had decreasing levels of tobacco use as they acculturated more toward mainstream American culture, while women and adolescents increased their tobacco consumption as they acculturated more toward mainstream culture (Choi et al., 2008). In contrast to the negative effects of acculturation toward the U.S. mainstream on Asian Americans' tobacco and alcohol consumption, cancer screening behaviors among Asian Americans have been found to be positively related to higher levels of acculturation toward their host culture (Lee et al., 2014).

However, most studies discussing the effects of acculturation on health outcomes have used unidimensional models of acculturation that reject an individual's ability to independently adhere to both their root and host cultures. Such models assume that when an individual acculturates toward their host culture, they automatically reject their root culture, and vice versa. This, despite empirical data, has shown these two cultural affiliations to be independent of each other (Schwartz & Unger, 2017). This has potentially profound implications for cancer screening among immigrant populations. We became very interested in how to accommodate for different levels of acculturation in cancer screening interventions. This became the focus of AR's dissertation research (Raisa, 2023).

## Formative Research on Developing a VA for Bangladeshi Immigrants

In many South Asian cultures, the word "cancer" is taboo, and in some South Asian languages, there is no word for cancer at all. Some persistent myths among South Asians include cancer being a result of the evil eye or God's curse, and people being social outcasts if diagnosed with this "curse." Other cultural norms, such as talking about certain body parts (e.g., breasts, genitals) being taboo or inappropriate in the public sphere or even with clinicians, or the fear of being a social outcast or being abandoned by cancer, influence cancer-related behaviors indirectly (Story et al., 2011). A scoping review of cancer prevention education programs conducted in Bangladesh found that Bangladeshis reported high levels of fear of cancer but low levels of feelings of vulnerability to cancer, which led to a lack of preventive behaviors such as regular screening (Raisa et al., 2020).

Specific cultural norms among South Asian immigrants in the United States have in fact been found to be prime inhibitors of taking preventative measures of CRC, such as regular screening under the guidelines. For example, South Asian immigrants have low rates of CRC screening due to feelings of shame regarding invasive screening processes like colonoscopy, or to modesty that prohibits them from talking about private body parts (Ivey et al., 2018).

In fact, South Asians have reported reservations even with non-invasive CRC screening procedures like FIT. For example, a study of South Asian Muslims found that the community perception of using FIT was that one had to touch one's feces, which is considered unholy and would void their *wadu*, a cleansing ritual Muslims perform before prater (Kazi et al., 2020). The study also found a lack of motivation to disseminate CRC-related information in the community through social or semi-private (extended family) get-togethers and discussions, since the topic of cancer invoked discomfort and fear along with other stigma and taboo.

Given the taboo around cancer and cancer screening in Bangladeshi culture, we were interested in whether a VA would be a feasible strategy to translate the importance of cancer screening in a culturally sensitive manner for this community. We conducted in-depth interviews with thirty individuals who immigrated to the United States from Bangladesh. During the interviews, we asked questions about their immigration experience, and their perceptions of cancer, and asked them to interact with a prototype of a VA that we developed. After the interview, we asked participants to complete a short survey on their experience with the VA.

The full results of this study are published in AR's doctoral dissertation (Raisa, 2023). However, there are a few key findings relevant to the focus of this chapter. Bangladeshi immigrant participants were open to using a VA for cancer prevention information. They felt that a VA would be convenient to use because they would not have to go to a healthcare provider for the information. However, findings around appearance and preferred language were complex.

In the interviews, participants stated that they had no preference for gender, race/ethnicity, but then they preferred a VA with a South Asian/Bengali ethnicity. However, when participants could choose between VAs of diverse ethnicities and genders, clear preferences emerged. Participants exhibited a strong preference for a white, male VA followed by a brown, female VA. This finding alludes to the necessity of data triangulation using self-reported qualitative and quantitative data along with behavioral observations for behavioral intervention development.

The participants in this study were all bilingual (English and Bangla). The prototype was developed in English. All participants preferred the English version of the intervention for themselves. The reasons participants preferred English included their own proficiency, an expectation that medical encounters would be in English, and a lack of standardization of Bangla language for medical terminology. However, most participants felt that offering a cancer screening app in Bangla would be more appropriate for the larger Bangladeshi immigrant community, specifically the elderly members. This finding has interesting implications. Even though members of the intended population were included in the adaptation process, they tended to report that their communication needs diverged from "other" immigrants.

The results of the formative research indicated that VAs have the potential to improve communication on stigmatized health issues among immigrant populations. Based on these (and additional findings), we developed several VAs to represent various degrees of the cultural accommodation participants recommended. Currently, we are working on experimentally evaluating how and when cultural accommodations influence communication outcomes compared to standard messaging. There is a need for further translational communication scholarship on how to accommodate the various levels of acculturation in immigrant communities to achieve health equity.

## CONCLUSION

The goal of this book is to contextualize health communication as inextricably linked to language and social interaction. This chapter addresses this larger challenge by introducing principles and practices of translational communication and linking these concepts to cultural identity. The next chapter will delve into the role of academic-community partnerships in the translational communication process as well as photovoice as a tool for doing translational work. Together, these chapters emphasize the importance of culture, community, language, and identity for creating frames by which humans create meaning about their health.

## REFERENCES


Alcántara, C., Estevez, C. D., & Alegría, M. (2017). Latino and Asian immigrant adult health: Paradoxes and explanations. In *The Oxford handbook of acculturation and health* (pp. 197–220). Oxford University Press.

Allouch, M., Azaria, A., & Azoulay, R. (2021). Conversational agents: Goals, tchnologies, vision and challenges. *Sensors (Basel, Switzerland)*, *21*(24), 8448. <https://doi.org/10.3390/s21248448>

Bartley, S. (2019, October 24). *Linda answers cancer survivors' questions about healthy living.* Centers for Disease Control and Prevention. <https://blogs.cdc.gov/cancer/2019/10/24/linda-answers-cancer-survivors-questions-about-healthy-living/>

Belanche, D., Casaló Ariño, L., & Rubio, M. (2021). Local place identity: A comparison between residents of rural and urban communities. *Journal of Rural Studies*, *82*, 242–252. <https://doi.org/10.1016/j.jrurstud.2021.01.003>

Budiman, A., & Ruiz, N. G. (2021). *Asian Americans are the fastest-growing racial or ethnic group in the U.S.* <https://policycommons.net/artifacts/1501578/asian-americans-are-the-fastest-growing-racial-or-ethnic-group-in-the-us/2160516/>

Buolamwini, J., & Gebru, T. (2018). Gender shades: Intersectional accuracy disparities in commercial gender classification. *Proceedings of the 1st Conference on Fairness, Accountability and Transparency*, 77–91. <https://proceedings.mlr.press/v81/buolamwini18a.html>

Cendan, J., & Lok, B. (2012). The use of virtual patients in medical school curricula. *Advances in Physiology Education*, *36*(1), 48–53. <https://doi.org/10.1152/advan.00054.2011>

Choi, S., Rankin, S., Stewart, A., & Oka, R. (2008). Effects of acculturation on smoking behavior in Asian Americans: A meta-analysis. *Journal of Cardiovascular Nursing*, *23*(1), 67–73. <https://doi.org/10.1097/01.JCN.0000305057.96247.f2>

Collins, F. S. (2011). Reengineering translational science: The time is right. *Science Translational Medicine*, *3*(90), 90cm17–90cm17. <https://doi.org/10.1126/scitranslmed.3002747>

Collins, F. S., Wilder, E. L., & Zerhouni, E. (2014). Funding transdisciplinary research. NIH Roadmap/Common Fund at 10 years. *Science (New York, N.Y.)*, *345*(6194), 274–276. <https://doi.org/10.1126/science.1255860>

Cooks, E. J., Duke, K. A., Flood-Grady, E., Vilaro, M. J., Ghosh, R., Parker, N., Te, P., George, T. J., Lok, B. C., Williams, M., Carek, P., & Krieger, J. L. (2022). Can virtual human clinicians help close the gap in colorectal cancer screening for rural adults in the United States? The influence of rural identity on perceptions of virtual human clinicians. *Preventive Medicine Reports*, *30*, 102034. <https://doi.org/10.1016/j.pmedr.2022.102034>

*COVID-19 Death Predictions: What Do We Need to Know?* (n.d.). Medscape. Retrieved January 28, 2023, from <https://www.medscape.com/viewarticle/927791>

Creswell, J. W., & Poth, C. N. (2018). *Qualitative inquiry & research design: Choosing among five approaches* (Fourth edition). Sage.

Davis, J. C., Rupasingha, A., Cromartie, J., & Sanders, A. (2022). *Rural America at a Glance: 2022 Edition*. <http://www.ers.usda.gov/publications/pub-details/?pubid=105154>

Davis, R. E., & Resnicow, K. (2012). The cultural variance framework for tailoring health messages. In H. Cho (Ed.) *Health communication message design: theory and practice* (pp. 115–136). SAGE Publications.

Dickens, P. (2000). Society, space and the biotic level: An urban and rural sociology for the new millennium. *Sociology*, *34*(1), 147–164. <https://doi.org/10.1177/S0038038500000109>

Dutta, M. J. (2007). Communicating about culture and health: Theorizing culture-centered and cultural sensitivity approaches. *Communication Theory*, *17*(3), 304–328. <https://doi.org/10.1111/j.1468-2885.2007.00297.x>

Engebretsen, E., Sandset, T. J., & Ødemark, J. (2017). Expanding the knowledge translation metaphor. *Health Research Policy and Systems*, *15*(1), 19. <https://doi.org/10.1186/s12961-017-0184-x>

Estabrooks, C. A., Thompson, D. S., Lovely, J. J. E., & Hofmeyer, A. (2006). A guide to knowledge translation theory. *The Journal of Continuing Education in the Health Professions*, *26*(1), 25–36. <https://doi.org/10.1002/chp.48>

Gasiorek, J. (2016). Theoretical perspectives on interpersonal adjustments in language and communication. In H. Giles (Ed.) *Communication Accommodation Theory: Negotiating Personal Relationships and Social Identities across Contexts*, (pp. 13–35). Cambridge University Press.

Giles, H. (2016). Communication Accommodation Theory. In *The international encyclopedia of communication theory and philosophy* (pp. 1–7). John Wiley & Sons, Ltd. <https://doi.org/10.1002/9781118766804.wbiect056>

Giles, H., & Maass, A. (2016). Advances in and prospects for intergroup communication: Prologue. In H. Giles & E. Maass (Eds.) *Advances in intergroup communication* (pp. 1–15). Peter Lang Publishing. <https://doi.org/10.3726/b10467>

Greenberg, A. L., Brand, N. R., Zambeli-Ljepović, A., Barnes, K. E., Chiou, S. H., Rhoads, K. F., Adam, M. A., & Sarin, A. (2023). Exploring the complexity and spectrum of racial/ethnic disparities in colon cancer management. *International Journal for Equity in Health*, *22*(1), 68. <https://doi.org/10.1186/s12939-023-01883-w>

Greenhalgh, T., & Wieringa, S. (2011). Is it time to drop the "knowledge translation" metaphor? A critical literature review. *Journal of the Royal Society of Medicine*, *104*(12), 501–509. <https://doi.org/10.1258/jrsm.2011.110285>

Hamel, L. M., Moulder, R., Ramseyer, F. T., Penner, L. A., Albrecht, T. L., Boker, S., & Eggly, S. (2022). Nonverbal synchrony: An indicator of clinical communication quality in racially-concordant and racially-discordant oncology interactions. *Cancer Control*, *29*. <https://doi.org/10.1177/10732748221113905>

Hecht, M. L., & Krieger, J. L. R. (2006). The principle of cultural grounding in school-based substance abuse prevention: The drug resistance strategies project. *Journal of Language and Social Psychology*, *25*(3), 301–319. <https://doi.org/10.1177/0261927X06289476>

Ivey, S. L., Mukherjea, A., Patel, A., Kapoor, N., Rau, S., Kazi, E., Bhatia, J., Somsouk, M., & Tseng, W. (2018). Colorectal cancer screening among South Asians: Focus group findings on attitudes, knowledge, barriers and facilitators. *Journal of Health Care for the Poor and Underserved*, *29*(4), 1416–1437.

Jain, P., & Krieger, J. L. (2011). Moving beyond the language barrier: The communication strategies used by international medical graduates in intercultural medical encounters. *Patient Education and Counseling*, *84*(1), 98–104. <https://doi.org/10.1016/j.pec.2010.06.022>

Kazi, E., Sareshwala, S., Ansari, Z., Sahota, D., Katyal, T., Tseng, W., & Ivey, S. L. (2020). Promoting colorectal cancer screening in South Asian Muslims living in the USA. *Journal of Cancer Education*, *36*(4), 865–873. <https://doi.org/10.1007/s13187-020-01715-3>

Kendall-Taylor, N., & Haydon, A. (2016). Using metaphor to translate the science of resilience and developmental outcomes. *Public Understanding of Science*, *25*(5), 576–587. <https://doi.org/10.1177/0963662514564918>

Kreuter, M. W., & McClure, S. M. (2004). The role of culture in health communication. *Annual Review of Public Health*, *25*(1), 439–455. <https://doi.org/10.1146/annurev.publhealth.25.101802.123000>

Krieger, J. L. (2014). Last resort or roll of the die? Exploring the role of metaphors in cancer clinical trials education among medically underserved populations. *Journal of Health Communication*, *19*(10), 1161–1177. <https://doi.org/10.1080/10810730.2013.801537>

Krieger, J. L., & Gallois, C. (2017). Translating science: Using the science of language to explicate the language of science. *Journal of Language and Social Psychology*, *36*(1), 3–13. <https://doi.org/10.1177/0261927X16663256>

Krieger, J. L., Neil, J. M., Duke, K. A., Zalake, M. S., Tavassoli, F., Vilaro, M. J., Wilson-Howard, D. S., Chavez, S. Y., Laber, E. B., Davidian, M., George, T. J., Modave, F. P., Odedina, F. T., & Lok, B. C. (2021). A pilot study examining the efficacy of delivering colorectal cancer screening messages via virtual health assistants. *American Journal of Preventive Medicine*, *61*(2), 251–255. <https://doi.org/10.1016/j.amepre.2021.01.014>

Krieger, J. L., Parrott, R. L., & Nussbaum, J. F. (2010). Metaphor use and health literacy: A pilot study of strategies to explain randomization in cancer clinical trials. *Journal of Health Communication*, *16*(1), 3–16. <https://doi.org/10.1080/10810730.2010.529494>

Lagacé, M., Tanguay, A., Lavallée, M.-L., Laplante, J., & Robichaud, S. (2012). The silent impact of ageist communication in long term care facilities: Elders' perspectives on quality of life and coping strategies. *Journal of Aging Studies*, *26*(3), 335–342. <https://doi.org/10.1016/j.jaging.2012.03.002>

Laranjo, L., Dunn, A., Tong, H. L., Kocaballi, A. B., Chen, J., Bashir, R., Surian, D., Gallego, B., Magrabi, F., Lau, A., & Coiera, E. (2018). Conversational agents in healthcare: A systematic review. *Journal of the American Medical Informatics Association*, *0*. <https://doi.org/10.1093/jamia/ocy072>

Lee, J.-E. R., Nass, C. I., & Bailenson, J. N. (2014). Does the mask govern the mind?: Effects of arbitrary gender representation on quantitative task performance in avatar-represented virtual groups. *Cyberpsychology, Behavior, and Social Networking*, *17*(4), 248–254. https://doi.org/10.1089/cyber.2013.0358

Lee, R. J., Madan, R. A., Kim, J., Posadas, E. M., & Yu, E. Y. (2021). Disparities in Cancer Care and the Asian American Population. *The Oncologist*, *26*, 453–460. https://doi.org/10.1002/onco.13748

Lee, S., Chen, L., Jung, M. Y., Baezconde-Garbanati, L., & Juon, H.-S. (2014). Acculturation and cancer screening among Asian Americans: Role of health insurance and having a regular physician. *Journal of Community Health*, *39*(2), 201–212. <https://doi.org/10.1007/s10900-013-9763-0>

Lui, P. P., & Zamboanga, B. L. (2018). Acculturation and alcohol use among Asian Americans: A meta-analytic review. *Psychology of Addictive Behaviors*, *32*(2), 173–186. <https://doi.org/10.1037/adb0000340>

Maina, I. W., Belton, T. D., Ginzberg, S., Singh, A., & Johnson, T. J. (2018). A decade of studying implicit racial/ethnic bias in healthcare providers using the implicit association test. *Social Science & Medicine*, *199*, 219–229. <https://doi.org/10.1016/j.socscimed.2017.05.009>

Marsiglia, F. F., & Booth, J. M. (2015). Cultural adaptation of interventions in real practice settings. *Research on Social Work Practice*, *25*(4), 423–432. <https://doi.org/10.1177/1049731514535989>

McDonald, R. (2020, August 7). *"Alexa for health care": new virtual assistant helps patients with cancer at home*. CURE; MJH Life Sciences. <https://www.curetoday.com/view/alexa-for-health-care-new-virtual-assistant-helps-patients-with-cancer-at-home>

Milne-Ives, M., Cock, C. de, Lim, E., Shehadeh, M. H., Pennington, N. de, Mole, G., Normando, E., & Meinert, E. (2020). The effectiveness of artificial intelligence conversational agents in health care: systematic review. *Journal of Medical Internet Research, 22*(10), e20346. <https://doi.org/10.2196/20346>

Mohamad Suhaili, S., Salim, N., & Jambli, M. N. (2021). Service chatbots: A systematic review. *Expert Systems with Applications, 184*, 115461. <https://doi.org/10.1016/j.eswa.2021.115461>

O'Leary, T. K., Stowell, E., Kimani, E., Parmar, D., Olafsson, S., Hoffman, J., Parker, A. G., Paasche-Orlow, M. K., & Bickmore, T. (2020). Community-based cultural tailoring of virtual agents. *Proceedings of the 20th ACM International Conference on Intelligent Virtual Agents, IVA 2020*. <https://doi.org/10.1145/3383652.3423875>

Pablos-Mendez, A., & Shademani, R. (2006). Knowledge translation in global health. *Journal of Continuing Education in the Health Professions, 26*(1), 81–86. <https://doi.org/10.1002/chp.54>

Petronio, S. (2007). JACR commentaries on translating research into practice: Introduction. *Journal of Applied Communication Research, 35*(3), 215–217. <https://doi.org/10.1080/00909880701434190>

Provoost, S., Lau, H. M., Ruwaard, J., & Riper, H. (2017). Embodied conversational agents in clinical psychology: A scoping review. *Journal of Medical Internet Research, 19*(5), e151. <https://doi.org/10.2196/jmir.6553>

Quinn, S. C., Garza, M. A., Butler, J., Fryer, C. S., Casper, E. T., Thomas, S. B., Barnard, D., & Kim, K. H. (2012). Improving informed consent with minority participants: Results from researcher and community surveys. *Journal of Empirical Research on Human Research Ethics : JERHRE, 7*(5), 44–55. <https://doi.org/10.1525/jer.2012.7.5.44>

Raisa. (2023). *Tailoring Digital Interventions for Acculturating Individuals*. University of Florida.

Raisa, A., Bylund, C., Islam, S., & Krieger, J. (2020). A systematic scoping review of cancer communication about prevention and detection in bangladesh. In B. Watson & J. Krieger (Eds.), *Expanding horizons in health communication* (Vol. 6, pp. 223–248). Springer Singapore. https://doi.org/10.1007/978-981-15-4389-0_11

Rogler, L. H., Malgady, R. G., Costantino, G., & Blumenthal, R. (1987). What do culturally sensitive mental health services mean? The case of Hispanics. *American Psychologist, 42*(6), 565–570. <https://doi.org/10.1037/0003-066X.42.6.565>

Schwartz, S. J., & Unger, J. (2017). *The oxford handbook of acculturation and health*. Oxford University Press.

Semino, E. (2021). "Not soldiers but fire-fighters" – metaphors and covid-19. *Health Communication, 36*(1), 50–58. <https://doi.org/10.1080/10410236.2020.1844989>

Stableford, S., & Mettger, W. (2007). Plain language: A strategic response to the health literacy challenge. *Journal of Public Health Policy, 28*(1), 71–93. <https://doi.org/10.1057/palgrave.jphp.3200102>

SAC (2018). Stakeholder engagement and communication for Healthy People 2030. Report 5. Washington, DC: Department of Health and Human Services.

Steiness, H. S., Villegas-Gold, M., Parveen, H., Ferdousy, T., & Ginsburg, O. (2018). Barriers to care for women with breast cancer symptoms in rural Bangladesh. *Health Care for Women International, 39*(5), 536–554. <https://doi.org/10.1080/07399332.2018.1446958>

Stevens, A., Hernandez, J., Johnsen, K., Dickerson, R., Raij, A., Harrison, C., DiPietro, M., Allen, B., Ferdig, R., Foti, S., Jackson, J., Shin, M., Cendan, J., Watson, R., Duerson, M., Lok, B., Cohen,

M., Wagner, P., & Lind, D. S. (2006). The use of virtual patients to teach medical students history taking and communication skills. *The American Journal of Surgery*, *191*(6), 806–811. <https://doi.org/10.1016/j.amjsurg.2006.03.002>

Stinson, C. (2018, November 29). *CDC Foundation launches TINA, an innovative virtual tool to improve cancer patient-provider conversations about infection risk | CDC foundation.*. CDC Foundation. <https://www.cdcfoundation.org/pr/2018/preventing-infections-cancer-patients-program-TINA-tool>

Story, H. L., Love, R. R., Salim, R., Roberto, A. J., Krieger, J. L., & Ginsburg, O. M. (2011). Improving outcomes from breast cancer in a low-income country: Lessons from Bangladesh. *International Journal of Breast Cancer*, *2012*. <https://doi.org/10.1155/2012/423562>

Szinay, D., Perski, O., Jones, A., Chadborn, T., Brown, J., & Naughton, F. (2021). Influences on the uptake of health and well-being apps and curated app portals: Think-aloud and interview study. *JMIR mHealth and uHealth*, *9*(4), e27173. <https://doi.org/10.2196/27173>

Treise, D., Baralt, C., Birnbrauer, K., Krieger, J., & Neil, J. (2016). Establishing the need for health communication research: Best practices model for building transdisciplinary collaborations. *Journal of Applied Communication Research*, *44*(2), 194–198. <https://doi.org/10.1080/00909882.2016.1155729>

Trochim, W. (2010). Translation won't happen without dissemination and implementation: Some measurement and evaluation issues. *3rd Annual Conference on the Science of Dissemination and Implementation*, 581–629.

Twigger-Ross, C., & Uzzell, D. (1996). Place and identity processes. *Journal of Environmental Psychology – J ENVIRON PSYCHOL*, *16*, 205–220. <https://doi.org/10.1006/jevp.1996.0017>

Vilaro, M. J., Wilson-Howard, D. S., Griffin, L. N., Tavassoli, F., Zalake, M. S., Lok, B. C., Modave, F. P., George, T. J., Carek, P. J., & Krieger, J. L. (2020). Tailoring virtual human-delivered interventions: A digital intervention promoting colorectal cancer screening for Black women. *Psycho-Oncology*, *29*(12), 2048–2056. <https://doi.org/10.1002/pon.5538>

Vilaro, M. J., Wilson-Howard, D. S., Griffin, L. N., Tavassoli, F., Zalake, M. S., Lok, B. C., Modave, F. P., George, T. J., Carek, P. J., & Krieger, J. L. (2020). Tailoring virtual human-delivered interventions: A digital intervention promoting colorectal cancer screening for Black women. *Psycho-Oncology*, *29*(12), 2048–2056. <https://doi.org/10.1002/pon.5538>

Vilaro, M. J., Wilson-Howard, D. S., Neil, J. M., Tavassoli, F., Zalake, M. S., Lok, B. C., Modave, F. P., George, T. J., Odedina, F. T., Carek, P. J., Mys, A. M., & Krieger, J. L. (2022). A subjective culture approach to cancer prevention: Rural black and white adults' perceptions of using virtual health assistants to promote colorectal cancer screening. *Health Communication*, *37*(8), 1–12.

Wang, J., Moehring, J., Stuhr, S., & Krug, M. (2013). Barriers to colorectal cancer screening in Hispanics in the United States: An integrative review. *Applied Nursing Research: ANR*, *26*(4), 218–224. <https://doi.org/10.1016/j.apnr.2013.08.005>

Watson, B. M., Jones, L., & Hewett, D. G. (2016). Accommodating health. In H. Giles (Ed.), *Communication accommodation theory* (1st ed., pp. 152–168). Cambridge University Press. <https://doi.org/10.1017/CBO9781316226537.008>

Wong-Kim, E., Sun, A., & Demattos, M. C. (2003). Assessing cancer beliefs in a Chinese immigrant community. *Cancer Control*, *10*(5_suppl), 22–28. <https://doi.org/10.1177/107327480301005s04>

Wu, T.-Y., West, B., Chen, Y.-W., & Hergert, C. (2006). Health beliefs and practices related to breast cancer screening in Filipino, Chinese and Asian-Indian women. *Cancer Detection and Prevention*, *30*(1), 58–66. <https://doi.org/10.1016/j.cdp.2005.06.013>

Zalake, M., Tavassoli, F., Duke, K., George, T., Modave, F., Neil, J., Krieger, J., & Lok, B. (2021). Internet-based tailored virtual human health intervention to promote colorectal cancer screening: Design guidelines from two user studies. *Journal on Multimodal User Interfaces*, *15*(2), 147–162. <https://doi.org/10.1007/s12193-020-00357-5>

Zalake, M., Tavassoli, F., Griffin, L., Krieger, J., & Lok, B. (2019). Internet-based tailored virtual human health intervention to promote colorectal cancer screening: Design guidelines from two user studies. *Proceedings of the 19th ACM International Conference on Intelligent Virtual Agents – IVA '19*, 73–80. <https://doi.org/10.1145/3308532.3329471>

CHAPTER ELEVEN

# Rooted in "Places and Spaces": Sensemaking about Identity, Culture, and Health in the Rural Midwest

ANGELA L. PALMER-WACKERLY AND KAZI HANEEYA WAHED
Department of Communication Studies,
University of Nebraska-Lincoln

We are told that power lies in the truth of our stories. But, as academics, we often focus on *others'* stories, not our own. We think about our students' stories, to which we listen frequently and feel honored when they share them with us, beginning to understand them more as "whole" people, seeing their hopes, struggles, and vulnerabilities. We think about the stories we have researched, stories of heartbreak and resilience because of fertility problems, cancer, chronic illness, (im) migration, and deportation. And, we also think of the stories we assign in our courses, stories that come alive through qualitative research, podcasts, and short films. With our students, advisees, and sometimes colleagues, we share snippets of our stories, but in finding our academic voices, we often sideline our own stories, worrying that they will not be accepted in our academic culture, which upholds words and phrases like "gold standard research" and objectivity, while discouraging "navel-gazing," "me-search," and "fluffy writing." Thus, we learn to sideline our stories and focus on others. It is only recently that both of us have started to increasingly share our stories, full of hope, challenges, and vulnerabilities, with our students and colleagues inside and outside of academia. As a result, we see the way it has helped deepen our connection to each other, and our students and research partners, especially in health equity. We find that within our sensemaking and vulnerability, we have a deeper connection to the work that we do as well as with whom we work, keeping us motivated even when the work seems daunting. Our storytelling, combined with the storytelling of our participants, focuses not only on interpersonal communication but also on structural change to enhance access to resources. Thus, we focus on language, culture, and identity in not only the micro-sense but also the macro-sense. We share our stories here in hopes that it encourages all of us to (continue to) share our stories with our students, colleagues, research partners, and perhaps even policy makers, to find a deeper connection to each other and our work, with the goal of advocating with others for structural inclusion, both in academia and within our communities.

To accomplish this goal, we give more details below about our nontraditional journeys to academia and how we became interested in culture, identity, health, and place. Next, we provide a narrative account of two research studies that sought to center the voices of immigrants living in rural Nebraska as well as the key theories that currently inform our work. We conclude with what we would like ourselves as well as other researchers to think about as they work to improve health equity within immigrant communities, particularly in rural areas.

## NAVIGATING PLACE AND SPACE AS OUTSIDERS

Each person's story is unique, and telling our stories allows us to relate to each other more deeply and empathetically, understanding why and how we center our values within our work. Though our stories have distinct differences (e.g., Angela was born and raised in the United States and Hanee in Bangladesh), we also share commonalities in that we both have moved several times; navigated diverse cultural contexts, including witnessing the strengths and challenges of living in rural areas; and managing stigma that occurs with health and relational experiences. We also worked for several years outside of academia before returning and navigating the culture of higher education, noticing that we did not fit the "typical" student model. Thus, in our work, we try to be purposeful in including diverse others who also experience structural barriers when trying to succeed within higher education.

### Meet Angela

#### Navigating Place

The longest thread linking my various experiences—living in 20 different "homes" in my 45 years of living—is that my experiences often felt different from those I was surrounded by. Before I graduated high school, I moved with my family to three different communities in two states—each, though only 8 hours away from each other, vastly different from the last. Both of my parents grew up in poverty in Youngstown, Ohio, and my grandparents struggled with alcohol with one who died by suicide. I knew of only three people in my parents' generation who went to college. Until the age of 7, I, too, grew up in poverty, living on food stamps, but I did not know until much later in my life as it seemed that everyone else struggled as much as we did, so it seemed normal. We were also surrounded by a lot of love from a very large Italian, Catholic family and had a strong sense of community support. But, I also grew up when the culture of Youngstown as a place was changing. In 1977, the year I was born, on a September day known as "Black Monday," the steel mills shut down. What was once among America's most populous 50 cities has become one of the fastest shrinking cities with a current population of 65,000. With its mafia influence, political racketeering, and high crime rates, it was once dubbed "Crime City USA." Our house was broken into twice, once when we were sleeping. After that, when I was 10, we moved 8 hours away to the suburbs of York, Pennsylvania, which delivered a culture shock from my under-resourced, racially and ethnically diverse, urban upbringing to a largely homogeneous, suburban, middle-class community.

I had moved from a city where it felt like everyone was connected through expansive networks to an area where people and neighbors felt disconnected and family groups were much smaller. While growing up in Youngstown, I knew very few families who weren't Catholic. All my friends were now either Protestant or Jewish. According to my friends, the closest person resembling my dad was Saddam Hussein. I was invited to my friends' bar and bat mitzvahs that were larger and more expensive than weddings I had ever attended (and, I'm Italian and Catholic). Poverty and alcoholism, which were rampant in Youngstown, seemed distant in my now predominantly White suburban school. But, my family eventually created long-lasting friendships, some continuing to this day. At home, though, my mom and dad were struggling to raise four kids by themselves without family nearby, and so, when I was 15, we moved back to Ohio, three hours from Youngstown.

Not only was I angry about leaving a place I loved—for the second time—I now lived in a community, though in Ohio, that couldn't be more different from either of the first two places I lived. The village of Lexington was a small, rural suburb of Mansfield. Our neighborhood had well water, no streetlights, and was surrounded by farm fields. I saw my first deer (of my life) about a year later. But, the relationships and cultural identity were also different here: It seemed like *everyone*, though not related, knew each other and talked about each other—*allll* the time. Suddenly, everyone seemed open and friendly, eager to meet us, yet also eager to fill us in on the gossip of everyone else. Within three months, before I even started 10th grade, I knew who had mental health issues, who had family history problems, who the nice kids were, and who I should stay away from. My school was predominantly White but this time, evangelical Christianity (which I had never heard of) was prominent, even in school. In Math class, a friend told me I was going to hell because I was Catholic and she was "concerned for my salvation." People took off school to hunt and harvest with one neighboring school hosting a "drive your tractor to school day." Shocked as I was with these cultural changes, I eventually grew to love the people here, as did three of my four siblings, who all, including me, married someone from there. I still text daily with my high school best friends.

After high school, I went to the branch of Ohio State University in my town for a year to save money, eventually moving to Columbus, Ohio to attend the main campus. The majority of my classes had over 400 people in them and were in an auditorium. I worked nearly 40 hours a week to take out as few student loans as possible. I almost dropped out as I went from straight As to Cs and Ds. Eventually, I found my friends and my footing, working in the Ohio Senate and at an after-school program with youth from under-resourced communities. After five years, I graduated from college, moved to Washington D.C. to work on Capitol Hill, then Boston to earn an MA in Journalism and work for a local lifestyle magazine company, and then back to Columbus, Ohio to work for a business magazine. I fell in love with writing, storytelling, and research.

### Navigating Space

In 2007, as the Great Recession was looming and journalism was fundamentally transforming (and tanking), I began teaching an evening writing course at a local technical college. I loved it and also my students. Most of them had full-time jobs and were first-generation college students from either rural or urban environments. I immediately related to them. In 2010, after three years of teaching, I went back to Ohio State to earn a research Master's and PhD to combine my love of writing with my newfound love of teaching—especially to students from under-resourced backgrounds. Though I loved learning, I was approximately 10 years older than most of the 70+ graduate students in our program, I did not know how to use PowerPoint, and I wanted to conduct only qualitative research (in a largely quantitative department) because of the ability to examine in-depth, nuanced experiences and stories that didn't seem to "fit" the general population. I remember asking in one graduate seminar, "What is the difference between concept and construct?" and felt that the language and culture of academia were outside of my grasp.

I also experienced discrimination when it became clear that my experiences did not map onto academia's traditional graduate student population. In 2014, my husband and I adopted our infant son, and I was given only three weeks of maternity leave instead of the six weeks my other graduate student colleagues received because I was not a "biological mom and didn't need six weeks of recovery" (though state law prohibited children from entering daycare until six weeks old). I was told by HR that I was "lucky to get 3 weeks" and that if they "gave me 6 weeks, they would have to give 6 weeks to all parents, including dads and gay and lesbian parents who did not give birth to a child, and they could not do that. And, couldn't my mother or mother-in-law help out?" Arguing for equitable parental leave practices (with research to support my argument), I unsuccessfully appealed to the department, college, and university. Eventually, through the university's graduate student council, I helped to change that policy to allow an equitable six weeks for all new graduate student parents, whether through biology or adoption. Though the policy change occurred 18 months later while in my current job, I was thrilled that it would benefit others after me. At the same time, I worked as a project manager for a study funded by the National Cancer Institute, examining cancer clinical trial decision-making in the Ohio Appalachian region. For one year, I traveled several times and hours a week to patients' and families' homes interviewing them about how communication affected their decision-making about clinical trials. I immediately related to the Appalachian communities, which resembled a mix of my hometowns. By then, Youngstown had been officially designated as part of the Ohio Appalachian region and the other Appalachian communities were mostly rural, economically distressed, largely White communities with large and closely knit families, substance abuse, and a fierce loyalty to place. As intellectually, emotionally, and logistically difficult as this research was, I knew this was the work for me. I wanted to advocate with people who exist outside our traditional social structures to promote inclusion and belonging for all.

## MEET HANEE

### Navigating Place

I am an international student from Bangladesh, a densely populated country with over 170 million people. I am in the third year of my PhD program, studying interpersonal, family, and health communication at the University of Nebraska-Lincoln. I was born and raised in a very diverse family. My mother is from India, and my father is from Bangladesh. My mother speaks a different language (Hindi) but can also speak Bangla, while my father speaks only Bangla. I have been raised with two cultures and languages and now am fluent in 5 languages: Bangla, Hindi, Urdu, English, and Japanese.

I was born in Dhaka, the capital city of Bangladesh. When I was 1, we moved to Chittagong, Bangladesh's chief Indian Ocean port. When I was 12, we moved back to Dhaka because my father worked in a governmental job at the Power

Development Board. However, in 2013, my family moved to New York City with a family visa for permanent residency, sponsored by my uncle who had been living in the United States since 1985. I was working in Japan so I could not move with my parents. In 2020, they moved to Buffalo and bought a house because of the large Bangladeshi community there.

In 2013, after I finished my undergraduate degree in Marketing from Southeast University in Bangladesh, I moved to Japan to work for a laundry company as a marketing executive. Japan is well known for its rich culture and generosity. But it is also known for its high suicide rates, ranking seventh in the world. People are in mental health crises, reluctant to engage in mental health conversations due to stigma. Because they do not want to be seen as weak, many people do not seek help or go to a counselor. In my company, I was the only foreign employee; therefore, I had many Japanese friends and colleagues. Many of them thought that self-harm was easier than having a mental health conversation. Consequently, they had a culture of silence with their friends and family around their mental health issues. As a result, they chose suicide attempts. My Japanese experience made me think about the impact of effective mental health communication. Like Japan, mental health is stigmatized in Bangladesh and people avoid talking about their mental health. They rarely go to mental health counselors, and if they do, they don't share it with anyone. But it is not only mental health stigma that exists; I have also experienced social and relational stigma.

Divorce is seen negatively in our country, mainly for women. Divorced women are seen as infected and cursed. Divorce can negatively impact family prestige and even impair the possibility of getting a potential groom for divorced women's sisters. I am a divorced woman. I was very young (24 yrs.) when I got divorced. I was in Japan when I got married; then after my divorce, I returned to Bangladesh. The journey after divorce was not easy for me. I was not invited to one of my relative's weddings because they believed I would bring unhappiness to the newlywed couple. Thus, the first thing that families tell their divorced daughters and sisters is to keep their divorced identity secret. I have been told to keep it secret by my closest relatives because it could be a problem for their family prestige and children's marriages. Sadly, women like me in my country deal with it alone. This solo struggle leads us to immense depression, and we don't see a counselor because of mental health stigma. So we are facing the double stigma of mental health stigma and social/relational stigma, which enormously increases our mental health distress. As a result, I decided to focus my research on cultural stigma and mental health and well-being in communities. As a communication scholar, I can share untold stories, discuss stigmatized topics, and find ways to mitigate the stigma and psychological distress among minoritized individuals and communities.

## Navigating Space

In 2018, I came to the United States as an international student. In 2020, I earned my masters in Communication Studies from Murray State University in Kentucky. Murray is a tiny city with only 2,000 people, and the university's land area covers 80% of the town. I was the only Bangladeshi student there. There were other students with other nationalities, like Indian, Asian, and Pakistanis, but most of the students were White Americans. The city was tiny, and access to resources was limited. We had one Walmart, a few restaurants, and only one clinic for medical services. However, the clinic only offered primary services like medication for fever and flu. So, to see a doctor or go to a hospital, we had to drive two hours to Nashville. It was time consuming and inconvenient, especially when suffering from illness.

During the second year of my master's program, I suffered from a severe ear infection. The infection was so intense that I could not sleep due to my pain. I went to the nearby clinic, but my infection was severe, so I had to drive to the hospital, which was 2 hours away in excruciating pain. I was lucky that I had friends who took me to the hospital during that time. But I have seen many international and immigrant friends in Murray who preferred taking medication from the store rather than seeing a doctor due to the limited availability of medical services.

In 2020, my mother was diagnosed with cancer. My mother cannot speak English well, so I had to translate for her whenever we saw a doctor. At the hospital, a nurse asked her if she wanted an interpreter, but she wanted someone from the family to interpret because she felt very comfortable and relaxed with her family. Usually with an interpreter, a patient needs to maintain formal conversation and my mom feels pressure at that moment. However, due to hospital policy, the hospital had to provide an interpreter who could explain the forms before going through the surgery. I was with my mother while the interpreter translated the conversation between the doctor and my mother. Throughout the process, I noticed two things. First, the hospital did not provide an in-person interpreter (they were using a phone in the room), which made the conversation difficult for my mother because she sometimes uses nonverbal signals (gestures/hand movements) to express her problems. These signals were not visible to the interpreter; consequently, my mother felt even more stressed after the phone interpretation. Second, the quality of the interpreter needed to be better. I noticed a moment when the interpreter struggled to translate some Bangla words into English. At that time, I had to step in and help to translate it. What's the point of using an interpreter service if I have to do it anyway? As a result, my mother distrusted and was dissatisfied with the service, and she was concerned that she needed to be provided with more adequate information.

Every immigrant's experiences, including struggles with health equity, are different. My mother's struggles and health experiences were mainly related to language proficiency and healthcare services. But, many immigrants face other health experiences that restrict them from receiving healthcare resources. A year later, I started my PhD program at the University of Nebraska, focusing on stigma communication and mental health well-being among minoritized people and communities. Through my research, I hope to create a bridge to unveil many immigrants' stories and health experiences and help mitigate the health disparities experienced by immigrants, minoritized populations, and communities.

In conclusion, by making sense of our stories and sharing them with others, we have realized that in all these experiences, our social identities, which include our academic identities, have crystallized by merging all of the cultural experiences from our lives—from urban to suburban to rural—to understand, navigate, and, when necessary, resist norms and expectations to find our own way forward.

## USING ARTS-BASED RESEARCH TO CENTER IMMIGRANT IDENTITIES AND VOICES

In the following section, we describe two projects that have informed and transformed our way of doing research with marginalized populations. As per the Culture-Centered Approach, both projects were focused on communication within the local context, placing participants at the center of the research (Dutta, 2008). Both projects occurred within Nebraska in diverse, rural communities in different parts of the state, yet share a history of migration for safety and better economic opportunities. To center participants' voices, we used arts-based research methods to collect their stories. Thus, first, we give an overview of arts-based research, followed by an overview of each project, in which we outline the local context, theories that have informed our work, the need for academic-community partnership, and a summary of important results.

### Storytelling through Arts-Based Research

One culturally centered and effective way to create and share stories is through art. Arts-based research is a mode of formal qualitative inquiry that uses artistic processes to understand and articulate the subjectivity of human experience. According to McNiff (2007), "art-based research can be defined as the systematic use of the artistic process, the actual making of artistic expressions in all the different forms of the arts, as a primary way of understanding and examining experience by both researchers and the people that they involve in their studies" (p. 29). Art-making is an embodied research and sensemaking process and outcome (Harter, 2013; Vacchelli, 2018) that can take the form of a collage (Vacchelli, 2018) or mural (Harter, 2013), photo exhibit (i.e., Photovoice) (Palmer-Wackerly et al., 2021), drawings and paintings (Mulongo et al., 2021), poetry, dancing, singing, and/or drumming (Lu & Yuen, 2012), among other art forms, such as carving, quilting, painting, narrative writing, filmmaking, and theater (McNiff, 2007). Specifically among individuals struggling with mental health issues, art-making not only creates a space for processing and healing within individuals and as a group, but it can also create mutual respect and trust between researchers and participants (Van Lith, 2014), gather important information about mental health needs and access (Vacchelli, 2018), and strengthen social capital within a group (Jay et al., 2021). In particular, visual arts-based narrative research has been shown to be effective in documenting and sharing the marginalized identities and complex, emotionally distressing experiences of people who are refugees from non-Western cultures (Mulongo et al., 2021, p. 237).

Arts-based research is a mode of formal qualitative inquiry that uses artistic processes to understand and articulate the subjectivity of human experience. Traditionally, arts-based research (ABR) methods have been applied either as data collection or dissemination techniques (Coemans et al., 2015). When art forms are considered research data, images, sculptures, or collages can replace or complement the traditional data (interviews, observations, surveys) and support the interpretation process of the researcher. Research participants may use art as a conduit to communicate with researchers about their daily life situations, experiences, concerns, challenges, or obstacles. Additionally, ABR methods translate an outcome of a particular research project, replacing or complementing a traditional research report and moving away from the traditional sole focus on textual accounts of phenomena under investigation (Foster, 2012). In this case, the art form is considered the vehicle for disseminating research findings. The findings may be presented as a drama or dance performance, an exhibition of images or visual representation, an artifact, or a collage (Coemans et al., 2015).

One popular method that combines both art as research and dissemination is photovoice. Photovoice is a visual research method applied to understanding the social world through the lens of those experiencing it. Photovoice involves participatory photography and the integration of photographs into the research process (Wang & Burris, 1997). By placing the cameras into the hands of the research participants, they can oversee how they document their reality, and in doing so amplify their voices for all to better witness how they understand and navigate their worlds (Wagner et al., 2016). By documenting their reality through photographs, they may be better able to capture audiences' attention by engaging them cognitively and emotionally and putting a "human face on the data" (Wang et al., 1996, p. 1395). Scholars consider narratives to be effective in conveying messages because narratives are intuitive forms of communication that people comprehend easily. Below, we give details into how we incorporated arts-based research, including Photovoice, into two studies in rural Nebraska.

## HealthVoiceVision

### The Local Context

HealthVoiceVision was a two-year (2016–2018), interdisciplinary research project consisting of three phases in Lexington, NE, a rural community consisting of approximately 10,300 people (U.S. Census Bureau, 2021a). Funded by a grant through the Rural Futures Institute, which is affiliated with the University of Nebraska-Lincoln (UNL), HealthVoiceVision brought together three sets of partners: the local hospital, the local community members, and academic researchers affiliated with the Minority Health Disparities Initiative (MHDI) at UNL. Located three hours from Lincoln, NE, the state's capital, Lexington has seen dramatic growth in racial/ethnic population diversity because of its nearby meatpacking and agricultural opportunities, which attract (im)migrant and refugee individuals and families. For decades, Hispanic immigrants had migrated to Lexington while Somali refugees had resettled there more recently in the past 5–10 years. Currently, Lexington's ethnic racial population estimates are 63.3 % Hispanic; 13.6 % Black or African, and 21.1 % White (non-Hispanic), while 41.4 % are estimated to be foreign-born (U.S. Census Bureau, 2021b).

### Desire for Academic-Community Partnership

As a result of these demographic changes, Lexington's local hospital, the Lexington Regional Health Center, and UNL's MHDI had met to discuss health needs based on these demographic shifts and how research might help. One of the needs identified by hospital administration, informed by the perspectives of their community health workers who served both their Hispanic/Latinx and Somali communities, was a city-specific, community-wide survey to document the needs of the diverse community members, whose voices were often not included in the county-wide health assessments. As the hospital explained, these health assessments typically reflect the health needs at a county level, rather than at a city level. In other words, even though Lexington is the county seat of Dawson County, the health needs of the majority White population within the county were broadly reflected instead of the majority Hispanic/Latinx and Somali populations living specifically within the city of Lexington. Thus, the health needs of the diverse populations living in Lexington are largely undocumented because 56 % of Dawson County's approximately 24,000 people identify as White (non-Hispanic) only (U.S. Census Bureau, 2021b). With the help of university researchers, the regional hospital and other community partners, such as community organizers, wanted to use this future city-level data to attract future grant funding to meet the needs of the local populations. The MHDI academic research team created a mixed-methods research proposal with 3 phases: (1) a photovoice project to center the voices and perspectives of the Hispanic and Somali community members; (2) a community-wide survey to quantitatively assess the types and prevalence of health needs; and (3) a public exhibit and cultural celebration, showcasing the photos from Phase 1.

## Theories That Informed This Project

To examine the influence of structures on participants' health experiences, we centered the project on the Social Ecological Model (SEM), Social Determinants of Health (SDOH), and the Culture-Centered Approach (CCA).

*Social Ecological Model.* First, within the SEM, McLeroy et al. (1988) outlined five levels of communication and behavior that influence health: (1) *intrapersonal or individual factors* (i.e., attitudes, knowledge, skills, personality traits), (2) *interpersonal factors* (i.e., families, friends, relationships), (3) *organizational or institutional factors* (i.e., rules, regulations, policies, and informal structures which may constrain or promote recommended behaviors), (4) *community factors* (i.e., social networks and norms that exists within a community between groups and organizations), and (5) *public policy* (e.g., local, state, and federal policies and laws that create barriers and facilitators around healthcare prevention and treatment).

*Social Determinants of Health.* The SDOH works seamlessly with the SEM in that it illustrates five structural elements that influence how and why people experience different health (in)equities across the micro-, meso-, and macro-levels of human behavior (USDHHS, n.d.). These elements include (1) economic stability (i.e., income, job opportunities), (2) education access and quality (i.e., school and educational opportunities), (3) healthcare access and quality (i.e., health insurance, screening and prevention), (4) neighborhood and built environment (i.e., safe housing, transportation, pollution), and (5) social and community context (i.e., social support, social capital, health literacy).

*The Culture-Centered Approach.* Within communication, one theory that co-exists alongside the SEM and SDOH and has allowed us to connect micro-communication to macro-communication is the Culture-Centered Approach (CCA). According to Dutta (2008), the CCA is a metatheoretical framework that explores the meanings and experiences of health in marginalized populations through the concepts of culture, structure, and agency. Dutta (2018) defines *culture* as "the shared values, practices, and meanings that are negotiated in communities" (p. 241), recognizing that communities are constituted by heterogeneous identities, perspectives, and therefore voices. *Structure* refers to the socially organized set of rules, policies, and procedures that constrain and enable cultural groups' communication and behavior. These social, political, and economic structures are created by communication and reflect the "flow of power within social systems" (p. 241). *Agency* within the CCA refers to both the daily experiences of decision-making that people must negotiate within these structures and also the transformative practices that people engage in to resist these structures (p. 241). While CCA is complementary to a community-based participatory research (CBPR) approach, it differs in that through CCA, the co-creation of knowledge is meant to transform the structural inequities through a local-national-global system of power (p. 240).

## Results

*Phase 1: Photovoice.* Phase 1 had three purposes: (1) to hear about the health experiences of the community members themselves; (2) to build trust between all research partners; and (3) to showcase and increase awareness of the diverse cultural values and experiences in a public forum to a larger public audience. More specific details about this project's methods and findings can be found in Palmer-Wackerly et al. (2021); however, a brief summary is included here. Phase 1 occurred over 10 weeks in Spring 2017, during which 13 participants described their health experiences in focus groups through photos they took in answer to a weekly prompt (e.g., *What is health and wellness to you? Where do you feel that you are in-/excluded within your community? Where and from whom do you seek support?*).

The project partners originally designed the Hispanic and Somali focus groups, led by community health workers (CHWs) who could speak in Spanish and Somali, to meet and share their photos separately. About midway through the data collection, however, both groups asked to combine to learn more about each other's cultural experiences. What followed was an exciting intercultural space where photos, experiences, and languages were exchanged. To help with intercultural understanding, CHWs translated to all participants who could not understand English, Somali, or Spanish. Participants began to relate with each other, recognizing similarities in not only their experiences but also their differences. For example, intercultural similarities included challenges with affordable housing, and feeling invisible to city leaders. Intercultural differences included access to healthcare, with Somali participants—who are refugees—surprised to hear that some Hispanic participants did not have access to health insurance.

Meanwhile, Hispanic participants were surprised to learn that Somali participants felt excluded in youth sports because they did not know how to access these activities and that some Somali employees had difficulty receiving work breaks so that they could honor their religious values and pray. Each week, participants collectively selected the photos they felt best captured their experiences while also writing a caption (which if necessary was translated to English) to explain why this photo was important to their experience. Phase 1 ended with participants acknowledging that because they share so many similarities in their experiences, they should interact more to help each other with their differences. For example, a research partner and Hispanic CHW said that she would notify the Somali community leader when it was time to sign up for future sports seasons so that he could share it with others while a local meatpacking plant began offering more prayer breaks to employees who were Muslims.

*Phase 2: Community Survey.* Phase 2 consisted of a survey of 325 participants, conducted through respondent-driven sampling over 10 days in October 2017. Originally the research design included random spatial sampling, where researchers sample every fifth house in a clockwise direction on randomly selected neighborhood blocks. However, because of the 2016 Presidential election, CHWs reported community member fears of deportation and a general mistrust of researchers or documentation. Thus, CHWs used respondent-driven sampling (RDS), which has been shown to be effective in "hard-to-reach" populations (Dombrowski et al., 2013). CHWs became the sole recruiters; they knocked on doors, made reminder calls, and offered $25 to community members if they took the survey and an additional $10 for each referral. The survey was stationed at a fitness center (run by the hospital), a Spanish-speaking church, and the Somali Community Center. CHWs explained that no identifying information would be taken, and participants could confidentially participate through a self-administered survey in English, Somali, or Spanish using audio-computer-assisted self-interview (ACASI) software. The research team projected three months for survey data collection; because of the trusted relationships between CHWs and community members, within a span of 10 days, 325 people had participated and the survey closed (see Chaidez et al., 2021; Palmer-Wackerly et al., 2021; Tippens et al., 2020 for more details). In response to our community partners' request for information about the current health status of its rapidly changing rural population, our team conducted two analyses from the survey data: (1) a comparative analysis of health, happiness, and hope as they relate to the social determinants of health between Hispanic, Somali, and White populations (Chaidez et al., 2021); and (2) an examination of emotional support and mental health among Somali men (Tippens et al., 2020).

*Health and Happiness.* Participants in this study (Chaidez et al., 2021) were largely Hispanic (*n*=204, 74.7 %) or Somali (*n*=57, 20.9 %), and most individuals were foreign-born (*n*=199, 73.4 %). White participants comprised 4.4 % of the sample (*n*=12), and our CHW research partner said the majority of White participants moved *to* Lexington to be closer to medical care for health reasons such as disability service access. People who identified as more than one ethnic/racial category were eliminated from analysis for comparative population purposes. Monthly household incomes were also in the lowest income bracket for a majority of participants across all ethnic/racial groups, ranging from $0 to $1,750 (59 % of Hispanic, 93 % of Somali, and 58 % of White households).

Results from Chaidez et al. (2021) showed that while most participants reported high levels of happiness, in comparison with Somali and White participants, Hispanic participants reported significantly less health, happiness, and hope and more variation with Somali participants reporting feeling less hopeful about the future of their community. Additionally, while all ethnic/racial groups reported a high sense of belonging in their community overall, variation was evident among Somali participants with 36 % reporting that they do not feel a sense of community belonging. A majority of all participants across ethnic/racial groups reported that they are moderately or very worried about their finances. Work-related injuries were also a concern with 35 % of Hispanics, 19 % Somalis, and 25 % of Whites being injured while working. A majority of these injuries occurred while working in Lexington, and about 10 % of participants said they did not report their injury to their employer for fear of losing their jobs. Of those who sought medical attention, a significant proportion said their employer covered none ($0) of their medical expenses (24.5 % of Hispanics (*n*=49), 50 % of Somalis (*n*=8), and 50 % of Whites (*n*=2)). In regard to workplace safety training, significantly fewer Somali participants (22 %) received training in comparison to Hispanic (76.3 %) and White (90.9 %) participants.

*Emotional Support and Mental Health among Somali Men.* Participants in this study included 49 Somali men. Men were the focus of this study because of their under-researched intersectional identity concerns, which include a "triple jeopardy" of discrimination in post-migration settings based on social identities of being refugees, racialized as Black, and predominantly Muslim as well as self-perceptions of loss of masculinity and dignity as they increasingly rely on the "welfare state" (Tippens et al., 2020, p. 172). A majority of research among post-migration Somali participants involves women and children. Most participants (65 %) reported living in Lexington for approximately one year. Among participants, nearly all (98 %) reported being "happy" or "very happy" while 22 % reported experiencing moderate levels of distress and 10 % reported experiencing high levels of distress. Nearly one-third of participants reported relying on informal support (i.e., elder family/clan member, family/clan member own age, friend) when feeling sad, stressed, or worried while approximately one-fourth of participants reported relying on formal support (i.e., doctor, healer, community health worker, mental health professional, religious leader, community leader) when feeling sad, stressed, or worried. As expected, participants who experienced significantly higher distress sought more of either/both informal and formal support than participants who did not seek support.

*Phase 3: Photovoice Exhibits.* Phase 3 included a photography exhibit, based on the photos participants collectively chose in their Photovoice focus groups, and were aimed at reaching broad audiences including local residents and policymakers. The exhibit, *Looking Past Skin*, included 48 curated photos displayed in vintage windowpanes, which served as frames. The exhibit was on display in the Dawson County Historical Society Museum in Lexington in Fall 2017 and moved to Lincoln in Spring 2018 to the Nebraska History Museum. Both exhibits focused on historical to present immigration in the state of Nebraska, with Dawson County connecting the area's rich immigration history involving German and Scandinavian immigrants to its current amalgamation of Hispanic and Somali immigrants while the state's history museum created an immigration timeline beginning 10,000+ years ago to showcase our collective immigrant identity as human beings living in the United States. Both exhibits included a special "Ask a Doctor" simulation, which allowed museum goers to experience first-hand the difficulty of visiting a doctor who speaks another language. Both exhibits kicked off their showcases with a preview event: Dawson County hosted an intercultural celebration of both Hispanic and Somali food and dance, inviting community members and the city policymakers while the state history museum hosted a reception for community members, city and state policymakers, and educators. At the Dawson County event, the Somali and Hispanic research partners spoke, discussing how much they learned through this process, including how much they have in common with each other.

In conclusion, HealthVoiceVision was a project of enormous collaboration, creativity, and effort occurring across multiple phases, academic disciplines, cultural groups, and community members. Below, we offer another example of arts-based research among Latinx participants in a rural, Midwest community.

## Narrative Mapping with Rural, Latinx Adolescent Voices

### The Local Context

Our study took place in a small Nebraskan rural town with a population of approximately 2000 people according to the U.S. Census (U.S. Census Bureau, 2021c). Approximately 50 % of the town's population is Hispanic. Much like other rural areas across Nebraska, the town's local meat processing plant attracts immigrants and refugees looking for stable work opportunities in safe communities.

### Desire for Academic-Community Partnership

On an outreach visit led by the University of Nebraska-Lincoln Extension Program, members of our research team met with an extension educator, who leads a local after-school program dedicated to the academic success of high school students in the region. The extension member is bilingual in Spanish and English and identifies as Hispanic/Latinx. He expressed an interest in wanting to expose his students to the process of research to educate them on its importance in the creation of knowledge. He also wanted to create closer ties with faculty members to begin to familiarize his students, all of whom are to be first-generation college students, with academic culture. He said many are stressed about their futures. Because the community desire for partnership was broadly defined, our research team decided to center adolescents' voices by using an arts-based research method, Narrative Mapping, to allow them to tell us about the topics that they think are most important to their lives. To give some direction, based on the extension educator's experience working with them, we asked them to think about experiences and feelings around stress, education, and health.

Narrative mapping asks participants to draw "maps" of real and temporal places depicting any story or stories they would like to express (Thompson, 2021). The process involves two steps: (1) *intra*personal sensemaking when the participant draws the map itself, and (2) *inter*personal sensemaking when the participant explains the map to another person. Narrative mapping is particularly helpful when participants experience stress (Thompson, 2021) and can help process overwhelming thoughts and feelings about identities, relationships, and difficulties through "communicated sense-making," or communicating the meaning of those events to themselves and others (Koenig Kellas & Kranstuber Horstman, 2015). The study was supposed to occur across both high school programs; however, the Covid-19 pandemic occurred a week after recruiting at one high school and all community research was put on hold. After community research was allowed to begin again, we recruited 20 adolescent students from a local high school, where Hispanic youth make up 73 % of the total high school enrollment of 169 students

(Nebraska Education Profile, n.d.). Although we were required by University Covid-19 protocol to conduct virtual research, our extension educator team member recruited participants in-person because of county health protocols and his role within the school and community (for more details, see Palmer-Wackerly et al., 2022).

### Theory That Informed This Project

*Communicated Narrative Sense-Making.* In addition to the theories, especially the Culture-Centered Approach, another theory informed this second project: Communicated Narrative Sense-Making (CNSM). CNSM theory empirically examines the links between storytelling and individual and relational health and well-being (Koenig Kellas, 2022). Within CNSM theory, there are three heuristics that examine the narrative processes researchers have used: retrospective, interactional, and translational storytelling. *Retrospective storytelling* focuses on how the content or type of narratives may reveal individual or relational meanings, values, and beliefs (Koenig Kellas, 2022). *Interactional storytelling* is concerned with how the process of storytelling among people can help explain sensemaking and relational well-being. It focuses on the interactions among storytellers and listeners by examining verbal and nonverbal behaviors such as perspective-taking, levels of engagement, turn-taking, and story coherence (Koenig Kellas, 2022). Lastly, *translational storytelling* focuses on the design and implementation of interventions, building on findings from retrospective and interactional storytelling studies, to help participants make sense of difficult experiences to improve relational health and well-being (Koenig Kellas, 2022). In health contexts, narratives are particularly powerful in that they can help vulnerable individuals create and share stories that can improve healing and coping, including helping people mobilize resources for resilience and social awareness (Harter et al., 2013). We communicate stories (and sensemaking in general) intrapersonally, interpersonally, and/or communally. Sharing and processing stories can alleviate suffering and make "circumstances more bearable" (Harter et al., 2013, p. 164) by functioning as both a "mirror," or a reflection of individuals as they are, and a "lamp" that creates a path toward the possible (Fine, 2002, p. 238; Harter et al., 2013, p. 152).

Within relationships, the communicated perspective-taking (CPT) aspect of CNSM is particularly important. When we engage in CPT, we communicate not only that we both understand another individual's perspective through cognitive empathy but also that we have the capacity to feel what they are feeling and express compassion through affective empathy (Koenig Kellas & Kranstuber Horstman, 2015). By jointly processing, creating, and communicating that meaning-making with each other, we achieve individual and relational well-being (Horstman &

Holman, 2018), particularly in relation to stressful events, illness, or health concerns (Koenig Kellas et al., 2020).

## Results

Because this was participants' first time engaging in research, we wanted participants to tell us what mattered most to them. A benefit of narrative mapping is that it gives creative control to participants to tell their story how *they* want to. The participants made sense of their experiences in three ways: *Linear Journeys as Redemptive Narratives*, *Nature Scenes as Metaphorical Narratives*, and *Visual Snapshots as Chaotic Narratives.* Some students who drew linear, redemptive journeys highlighted a few significant details (e.g., birth, move to the U.S., school); whereas, others created very detailed maps with numerous additional details (e.g., family trauma, such as deportation, incarceration, death, illness) (see Figure 11.1).

Students who used metaphors to narratively make sense of their experiences focused on wanting to feel calm and relaxed. They focused on current stressors and what would comfort them, places such as a park, a beach, or trees and water. Finally, those who engaged in Snapshots told chaotic narratives that communicated a sense of what their lives looked and felt like at that moment in several different areas of their lives, like a big-picture view of several chaotic moments occurring at one time. Common themes across the sensemaking vehicles were (1) stress related to family pressure and expectations concerning work; (2) educational uncertainties, especially concerning finances; and (3) mental health concerns, including anxiety, loneliness, and not enough downtime. Although some students

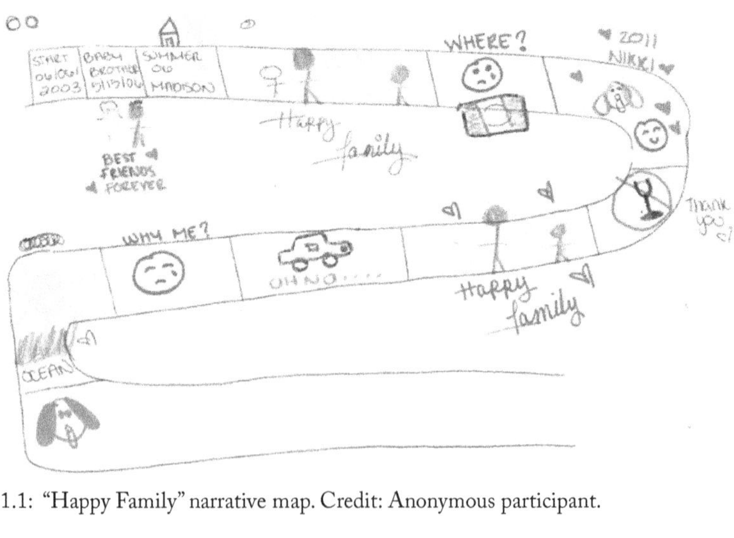


Figure 11.1: "Happy Family" narrative map. Credit: Anonymous participant.

were initially hesitant to engage in this activity because of fear of vulnerability, all but one student reported that they enjoyed it, even if some were surprised that they did. Students reported liking that they could create coherence and perspective around events they hadn't previously connected. They also enjoyed both giving and receiving empathetic perspective-taking about experiences that were important to them (with one participant saying she knew her best friend since four years old and they hadn't talked before about the experiences reflected in their maps). Students also found the activity relaxing and empowering. Several students struggled with vulnerability, but eventually became more comfortable especially as they realized they could control what and how they disclosed their information.

## MOVING FORWARD: IMPROVING CULTURE-CENTERED HEALTH COMMUNICATION IN THE RURAL MIDWEST

Based on our experiences trying to improve health equity for marginalized individuals, especially immigrant and refugee populations, living in rural spaces, we consider three main priorities for researchers moving forward: (1) consideration and alleviation of structural barriers within health communication interventions and research; (2) a need to focus explicitly on sustainability of research partner relationships and project outcomes; and (3) inclusion of scholars on the research team who share identities with community members whenever possible.

### Addressing Community Members' Structural Barriers in our Research

While firmly believing that we as researchers should not be striving to do "everything" in one research project, we believe we have a long-term ethical obligation to also center a community's needs within the focus, not the periphery, of our projects. Because health equity is rooted within the social-structural determinants of health, these determinants must be addressed within our communication research in order to produce meaningful change. For example, in our HealthVoiceVision project, although we met a community need (i.e., a request for data documenting the health status of the diverse population living within the city of Lexington, Nebraska, as opposed to the larger and Whiter population in Dawson County), the community health workers explained to us that the two ongoing needs for health and safety were (1) affordable housing, and (2) access to mental health services (Palmer-Wackerly et al., 2021). Some MHDI faculty who facilitated HealthVoiceVision have tried to meet this need by applying for grant funding to implement programs in Lexington, but so far have not been successful. MHDI, itself a grant-funded mechanism at the university, is asking for more hard funding from our university in order to support more community-based health equity projects, but until this request is realized, MHDI has to focus on the projects where they have received grant funding in order to continue existing within the university.

Another example that we know from our rural health equity work is that the community health workers, whom we rely on to bridge the access gap between minoritized ethnic/racial populations and healthcare services, face considerable structural barriers in their work (Toney et al., 2022). For example, many CHWs are grant-funded and so their work is funded on a temporary basis, and even those who work at hospitals or clinics, which may have more stable pay, are underpaid for the work they are expected to do. Additionally, many CHWs told us that their hospitals and clinics are woefully understaffed for interpreters and resorted to using cleaning staff to fulfill their interpreting needs (Palmer-Wackerly et al., 2019). Thus, the ethical question becomes if we are trying to improve health equity among diverse ethnic/racial populations, why are we exploiting and using the labor from the (mostly women) health workers in order to accomplish this goal? Thus, we support Dutta's (2008) argument that if we are not centering our population's needs and desires (including those of community health workers) in our goal of improving health equity, we are instead "using" them because we aren't listening to their desires for help in raising their pay, creating more stable hours, and advocating in a meaningful, impactful way to be included in state and national healthcare policies that include their services but not their voices (Palmer-Wackerly et al., 2019).

A health communication concern involving language that has been a long-term structural barrier to healthcare access is availability and use of translation services (Schlange et al., 2022). Federally assisted programs are required by Title VI of the Civil Rights Act of 1964 to offer all individuals meaningful access to their services, regardless of patients' ability to speak English (U.S. DHHS, 2020). However, "meaningful access" is not clear and thus Title VI has been considered an "unfunded mandate" (Dunker, 2022). For example, in Spring 2022, both Medicaid and a major insurance provider in the state of Nebraska said that it is no longer reimbursing healthcare providers for in-person translation services. According to federal law, healthcare providers who receive federal funding for their healthcare services are responsible for providing these translation services, but the Nebraska Department of Health & Human Services has reported that neither insurance plans nor Medicaid is responsible for reimbursing those *providers* for those services. Instead, the healthcare providers need to directly pay the translators (Dunker, 2022). In a narrative review of U.S. research studies examining translation mode and effectiveness (Schlange et al., 2022), we found that providers chronically underused professionally trained interpreters, preferring to use in-person, particularly ad hoc translation services, because of ease of use and avoiding barriers such as waiting times and lack of training in how to include interpreters. The review also suggested that providers relied more heavily on professional in-person translators when they were reimbursed by a third party, whereas ad hoc translators were more likely to be used in rural areas. Some studies also suggested that providers were satisfied with translation via videoconferencing, and the authors concluded that videoconferencing should be used if in-person professional translation is not available (Nápoles et al., 2010). In our review, results indicated that any type of professionally trained translation service generally has better health outcomes, including patient satisfaction, in comparison with ad hoc translation (e.g., translation from another employee or family member), though some patients prefer to rely on family members over others because of mistrust and comfortability. Regardless of mode, addressing the language and communication needs of people who have low-proficiency English and/or a preference for a language other than English is vital to addressing their health needs, or health inequities such as a higher number of emergency department visits, poorer health status, and higher likelihood of missing work and not seeking healthcare in comparison with the general White population, will remain (Schlange et al., 2022). Thus, we have an ethical responsibility to consider, and we argue address, the structural barriers to health equity that exist for the populations with whom we are working. If we do not, then we are continuing to serve mostly ourselves and our careers rather than the populations with whom we're partnering.

## Addressing Academia's Structural Barriers in Our Research

While the purpose of the chapter was to write about language, identity, and culture in our research, we must also consider how the predominant language, identity, and culture of academia effect our rural health equity goals. In considering academia's structural barriers to health equity work, we address two key areas for which we would like to encourage communication-focused academics to advocate/change to move our work from the academic-centered, community-based participatory efforts to the more participant-centered, advocacy research efforts (Dutta, 2018): (1) structural support for community partner relationship development, which includes time and money; and (2) flexible tenure requirements, which recognize the importance and impact of community-based participatory, and particularly culturally centered, research.

### Structural Academic Research Support

Research support from other sources than grant funding agencies and foundations is key to sustainable relationship building with community partners. Relationship development requires considerable time and effort before trust is created and maintained by all academic and community partners (Harter et al., 2011). As we learned from HealthVoiceVision, trust needs to also be created and maintained *within* academic partnerships (Palmer-Wackerly et al., 2021). Because the culture of academia is growing in its desire and outcome of reflecting a private business, focus has increasingly been put on "outcomes," which most often privilege higher quantity over quality in student numbers, in grant applications, and in publications. This pressure for "more" creates a "scarcity mindset" (Mazak, 2020) that we don't have enough time, energy, or resources to accomplish university goals for its students, staff, and faculty. An implicit and sometimes explicit message for graduate students and early career faculty from well-meaning mentors is to focus on "getting tenure" by doing work that allows us to "crank out publications." Community-based work can still be part of scholars' tenure portfolios, but to not make their tenure file solely about community-based work because it's too slow moving and risky in terms of the types of outcomes that the academic institution values (e.g., publications, grants, etc.). Then after tenure, or even better after full professorship, scholars can focus their work solely on community-based work. This message, founded upon the values of the academic system for quantity over quality, is intended to be an objective barometer of academic success, one that can allow tenure committees and institutions to compare and evaluate all faculty.

However, structural health equity work involves a lot of time, money, and effort, much of which is messy and difficult to quantify. We suggest that universities and tenure committees can and should value quality over quantity, allowing for researchers to focus on *impact* of their work as valued in the community in terms of improving health equity (Warren et al., 2018), as well as impact of their work in creating more connection with the university, especially for land-grant institutions, whose mission is to serve and educate the state's population. This effort is particularly important in rural states, like Nebraska, where the urban populations of Lincoln and Omaha are half the state's population but only a very small part of the land distribution. Thus, we propose that the university support positions that are specifically meant to build partnerships with the community and academia. These positions could be part of university extension; however, in reality, extension positions meant to improve health equity are usually focused on a health promotion particular area, like nutrition or soil quality, and not the general healthcare access concerns of its marginalized populations. One way to address the healthcare access needs within extension is to add an extension team who serves health equity and healthcare access needs specifically for certain regions around the state.

For example, we like the model that the University of Nebraska uses in Extension for education. Our research partner in our Narrative Mapping study works in rural school districts, and his main responsibility is to increase higher education access for rural, first-generation, immigrant students from under-resourced households. He reviews their homework, guides them in their college essays, and helps them apply for scholarships. If not for his work, it is unlikely all of his students would have gone onto college, given the barriers they face in terms of financial aid, sometimes lack of parental support, and challenges in understanding expectations of college entrance requirements. Just as with HealthVoiceVision, participants communicated to us in this study that above all, they want help with mental health and coping with stress. So while we can and want to work toward helping them with psychosocial support as well as mental healthcare access, we can't ignore the structural pressures they are facing that are causing some of this stress, such as their household income level and family member immigration status. We have an ethical responsibility to include advocacy efforts addressing these structural barriers in any project we have moving forward involving their health. Thus, much like our extension educator research team member connects marginalized youth to the larger goal of higher education access, a health equity extension team could focus on connecting marginalized populations to healthcare, especially mental healthcare services.

Another aspect of needed structural academic support would be an entire office of Community Engagement at the University that is supported with hard money from the university, not via a research center that depends on soft money. Thus, an entire office could sustainably focus on connecting faculty, staff, and students to each other and the communities they want to serve. The ongoing relationship building that is needed to occur to maintain that trust and consistent face time overtime could occur because faculty members wouldn't be solely responsible for developing and maintaining these partnerships while also balancing grant- and research writing in addition to increasing teaching and service loads.

## Inclusion of and Support for Academic Researchers with Diverse Ethnic/Racial Identities

While much organizational messaging of colleges and universities has been to focus on the "individual resilience" of students, staff, and faculty, *collective resilience* would be most helpful (Ahn et al., 2021). Colleges and universities could implement policies that could help build resilience, such as (1) remote work opportunities, which allow for more time to travel to communities for engaged research; and (2) extra pay for bilingual research team members, from undergraduate researchers to faculty members who provide these services for nominal fees. Often, research that requires language translation could not take place without these extra services from research team members; however, the amount of effort and time put into these services is often poorly understood and/or underappreciated and thus underpaid by those asking for these services.

As higher education institutions increasingly place value on diversity, equity, and inclusion, we strongly argue for structural supports to be in place to support underrepresented scholars (Johnson, 2020), including international scholars, many of whom face different challenges than their peers. First, more service is often asked of scholars with diverse ethnic and racial identities. This additional service, or "service tax," occurs for at least two reasons. First, faculty and administration ask racially and ethnically diverse students and faculty to become more involved in diversity, equity, and inclusion efforts on campus. One such effort is the common policy of having at least one diverse individual serve on job search committees. Explicit or implicit policies such as these disadvantage these students and faculty by asking them to do more service than their peers. Second, these scholars often have a "cultural tax," serving as guides and gateways to other students and colleagues with similar backgrounds and experiences, thus taking on additional emotional work to help mentor these individuals through structures that are not accommodating them. These extra efforts are also true for international scholars, who face these extra service burdens as well as structural barriers, such as financial barriers with visa paperwork.

International scholars and students are not homogeneous and thus may experience similar and different cultural and educational barriers. International scholars' challenges fall into two major areas: cultural adjustment and educational/academic adjustment (Kaya, 2020). First, cultural adjustment is a struggle that international scholars and students commonly face. Their home culture and norms are very different from those in the United States; thus, they first experience a lack of belongingness and community. Missing family and home sometimes induces stress among international scholars and impairs their concentration level in learning and research work. However, cultural adjustment also occurs within their academic department. Every college department has a unique environment. Sometimes it is hard for international scholars and students to adjust or fit into the department if it has no scholars and/or students of color. So, being the only foreign international student/scholar in the department can affect the learning more because here the student is dealing with the adjustment of the departmental culture and country culture. This "legs on two boats" experience induces stress levels, and many international scholars and students feel overwhelmed by these adjustments and face challenges in focusing on their studies. In this case, the college department can play a significant role in mitigating international students' challenges. Adequate support from the department and understanding of international scholars' and students' distinct needs and experiences can decrease the stress of international students and scholars. International scholars will feel more included and supported in an accessible learning environment if they find academic and emotional/mental health support from the department and campus.

The second is an academic adjustment (Kaya, 2020). Many international students come to the United States from a country where technology is not being used in educational institutions. Those kinds of international students face considerable academic challenges in the United States when using common software, such as using PowerPoint and Canvas. This primary struggle can make them feel incapable of succeeding and sometimes causes "imposter syndrome," a psychological occurrence in which an individual doubts their skills, talents, or accomplishments and has a persistent internalized fear of being exposed as a fraud. It is not only technical difficulties, but international students experience content-based challenges too. Language is one of the factors that cause content-based challenges. Many international students' fourth or fifth language is English. They take longer to read and write to process their thoughts and comprehend the content. Sometimes these additional efforts can cause burn out because they struggle with time management as they must give more time to one task.

Lack of resources is another factor that causes content-based challenges for international students/scholars. For instance, Bangladesh is a country where only a few universities have research-based studies. Most Bangladeshi educational institutions need more research resources (labs, training services, funding, etc.). So, international students and scholars who need more research experience due to the educational system they had in their country may experience enormous struggles in the research field.

Finally, international scholars and students prefer inclusive language. All international students face massive challenges but are as equally capable as American students. Therefore, they do not wish to be treated differently. They do not want to experience the "us and them" culture. So, they expect more inclusive language, "we" instead of "you and I." They expect support, assistance, and resources to progress their learning without receiving the impression of being outsiders and outcasts.

## CONCLUSION

Within academia, we are a part of many co-cultures. As scholars, one of our academic missions is connecting underrepresented individuals and communities to and within academia to make academia more inclusive and responsive to the concerns of people who may feel invisible and marginalized within larger social structures and policies. This is complex work with many institutional barriers; thus, we can often feel ineffective, despite working with very talented scholars and community members. We are nuanced, complex individuals with competing interests within academia, within communities, and between academia and communities (Palmer-Wackerly et al., 2021). To truly transform and diversify the ways of doing and being within academic research, we need to start with ourselves and examine "how" and "why" we do research in the first place, even if imperfectly. This is the story of our academic journeys and how they relate to two recent research studies examining culture, identity, and language in the rural Midwest. We connect theory to practice by centering our participants' voices through micro- to macro-sensemaking and advocating for the use of storytelling to influence structural change. We hope our sharing will inspire emerging scholars to share their stories too—*between* partnerships and *within* partnerships. At the very least, we are connecting our humanity to our research, which hopefully increases transparency and trust with each other and with our community partners, communicating that we want to co-create inspiring, inclusive, and innovative spaces with a strong sense of belongingness for all.

## REFERENCES


Ahn, S. J. (Grace), Cripe, E. T., Welles, B. F., McGregor, S. C., Pearce, K. E., Usher, N., & Vitak, J. (2021). Academic caregivers on organizational and community resilience in academia (fuck individual resilience). *Communication, Culture & Critique, 14*(2), 301–305. doi:10.1093/ccc/tcab027

Chaidez, V., Qiu, Y., Palmer-Wackerly, A. L., Tippens, J. A., Parra, G. R., Habecker, P., Gocchi Carasco, K., Soliz, J., Pytlik Zillig, L. M., & Dombrowski, K. (2021). Ethnic comparisons in perceptions of health, happiness, hope and related social determinants of health in a majority-minority midwest town. *The Journal of Sociology & Social Welfare, 48*(1). <https://scholarworks.wmich.edu/jssw/vol48/iss1/6>

Coemans, S., Wang, Q., Leysen, J., & Hannes, K. (2015). The use of arts-based methods in community-based research with vulnerable populations: Protocol for a scoping review. *International Journal of Educational Research, 71*, 33–39. <https://doi.org/10.1016/j.ijer.2015.02.008>

Dombrowski, K., Khan, B., Moses, J., Channell, E., & Misshula, E. (2013). Assessing respondent driven sampling for network studies in ethnographic contexts. *Advances in Anthropology, 3*, 1–9. doi:10.4236/aa.2013.31001.

Dunker, C. (2022, April 10). "It just came out of nowhere"—Mental health providers no longer receiving reimbursement for interpreters. *Lincoln Journal Star*. <https://journalstar.com/news/state-and-regional/govt-and-politics/it-just-came-out-of-nowhere-mental-health-providers-no-longer-receiving-reimbursement-for-interpreters/article_48a4d727-d7d6-592d-a51f-16616fc88b82.html>

Dutta. (2018). Culture-centered approach in addressing health disparities: Communication infrastructures for subaltern voices. *Communication Methods and Measures, 12*(4), 239–259. <https://doi.org/10.1080/19312458.2018.1453057>

Dutta, M. J. (2008). *Communicating health.* Polity Press.

Fine, G. A. (2002). The storied group: Social movements as "bundles of narratives". In J. E. Davis (Ed.), *Stories of change: Narrative and social movements* (pp. 229–246). State University of New York Press.

Foster, V. (2012). The pleasure principle: employing arts-based methods in social work research. *The European Journal of Social Work, 15*, 532–545. <http://dx.doi.org/10.1080/13691457.2012.702311>.

Harter, L. M. (Ed.). (2013). *Imagining new normals*. Kendall Hunt.

Harter, L. M., Broderick, M., Venable, S. & Quinlan, M. M. (2013). Organizing for social change: Personal stories and public health activism. In L. M. Harter (Ed.), *Imagining new normals* (pp. 149–169). Kendall Hunt.

Harter, L. M., Hamel-Lambert, J., & Millesen, J. L. (2011). *Participatory partnerships for social action and research.* Kendall Hunt.

Harter, L. M., Quinlan, M. M., & Ruhl, S. (2013). The storytelling capacities of arts programming in healthcare contexts. In L. M. Harter (Ed.), *Imagining new normals* (pp. 29–50). Kendall Hunt.

Horstman, H. K., & Holman, A. (2018). Communicated sense-making after miscarriage: A dyadic analysis of spousal communicated perspective-taking, well-being, and parenting role salience. *Health communication, 33*(10), 1317–1326. <https://doi.org/10.1080/10410236.2017.1351852>

Horstman, H. K., Holman, A., & McBride, C. M. (2020). Men's use of metaphors to make sense of their spouse's miscarriage: Expanding the communicated sense-making model. *Health Communication*, *35*(5), 538–547. doi:10.1080/10410236.2019.1570430

Jay, E-K., Moxham, L., & Patterson, C. (2021). Using an arts-based approach to explore the building of social capital at a therapeutic recreation camp. *International Journal of Mental Health Nursing.*, *30*(4), 1001–1009. <https://doi.org/10.1111/inm.12856>

Johnson, A. W. (2020, June 30). *Institutional mixed messaging.* Inside Higher Ed. <https://www.insidehighered.com/advice/2020/06/30/all-faculty-members-should-work-diversity-and-equity-initiatives-and-be-rewarded>

Kaya, J. (2020). Inside the international student world: Challenges, opportunities, and imagined communities. *Journal of International Students, 10*(1), 124–144. <https://doi.org/10.32674/jis.v10i1.1031>

Koenig Kellas, J. (2022). Communicated narrative sense-making theory. In D. O. Braithwaite & P. Schrodt (Eds), *Engaging theories in interpersonal communication: Multiple perspectives* (3rd ed.) (pp. 117–129). Routledge.

Koenig Kellas, J., & Kranstuber Horstman, H. (2015). Communicated narrative sense-making: Understanding family narratives, storytelling, and the construction of meaning through a communicative lens. In L. Turner, & R. West (Eds.), *Sage handbook of family communication* (pp. 76–90). Sage.

Koenig Kellas, J., Morgan, T., Taladay, C., Minton, M., Forte, J., & Husmann, E. (2020). Narrative connection: Applying CNSM theory's translational storytelling heuristic. *Journal of Family Communication*, *20*(4), 360–376. <https://doi.org/10.1080/15267431.2020.1826485>

Lu, L. & Yuen, F. (2012). Journey women: Art therapy in a decolonizing framework of practice. *The Arts in Psychotherapy*, *39*(3), 192–200. <https://doi.org/10.1016/j.aip.2011.12.007>

Mazak, C. (2020, September 22). Abundance vs. scarcity (No. 47) [Audio podcast episode]. In *Academic writing amplified.* Cathy Mazak. <https://scholarsvoice.org/podcast/abundance-vs-scarcity/>

McLeroy, K. R., Bibeau, D., Steckler, A., & Glanz, K. (1988). An ecological perspective on health promotion programs. *Health Education Quarterly, 15*(4), 351–377. <https://doi.org/10.1177/109019818801500401>

McNiff, S. (2007). Art-based research. In J. G. Knowles & A. L. Cole (Eds.) *Handbook of the Arts in Qualitative Research: Perspectives, Methodologies, Examples, and Issues* (pp. 29–41). Sage. <https://methods.sagepub.com/book/handbook-of-the-arts-in-qualitative-research/n3.xml>

Mulongo, P. McAndrew, S., & Ayodeji, E. (2021). Resettling into a new life: Exploring aspects of acculturation that could enhance the mental health of young refugees resettled under the humanitarian programme. *International Journal of Mental Health Nursing, 30*(1), 235–248. <https://doi.org/10.1111/inm.12777>

Nápoles, A. M., Santoyo-Olsson, J., Karliner, L. S., O'Brien, H., Gregorich, S. E., & Pérez-Stable, E. J. (2010). Clinician ratings of interpreter mediated visits in underserved primary care settings with ad hoc, in-person professional, and video conferencing modes. *Journal of Health Care for the Poor and Underserved, 21*(1), 301–317. <https://doi.org/10.1353/hpu.0.0269>

Nebraska Education Profile (n.d.). *Nebraska Education Profile.* <https://nep.education.ne.gov/>

Palmer-Wackerly, A. L., Chaidez, V., Wayment, C., Baker, J., Adams, A., & Wheeler, L. (2019). Listening to the voices of community health workers: A multilevel, culture-centered approach to overcoming structural barriers in U.S. Latinx communities. *Qualitative Health Research, 30*(3), 423–436. <https://doi.org/10.1177/1049732319855963>

Palmer-Wackerly, A. L., Coffey, J., Stefka, C., Gonzalez, L., Chaidez, V., Wheeler, L. A., Acosta, L., & Chai, W. (2022). *Using narrative mapping to center rural, Latinx adolescent voices in co-creating a research agenda.* Paper presented to the Applied Communication Division at the annual meeting of the National Communication Association, New Orleans, LA.

Palmer-Wackerly, A. L., Reyes, M. S., Ali, S. H., Carrasco, K. G., Habecker, P., Houska, K., Chaidez, V., Soliz, J., Tippens, J. A., Holland, K. J., Pytlik Zillig, L., Patterson, K. & Dombrowski, K. (2021). Examining and evaluating multilevel communication within a mixed-methods, community-based participatory research project in a rural, minority-majority town. *Journal of Applied Communication Research, 49*(2), 129–147. <https://doi.org/10.1080/00909882.2020.1851042>

Schlange, S. A., Palmer-Wackerly, A. L. & Chaidez, V. (2022). A narrative review of medical interpretation services and their effect on quality of healthcare. *Southern Medical Journal, 115*(5), 317–321. <https://doi.org/10.14423/SMJ.0000000000001392>

Thompson, M. (2021). Narrative mapping: Participant-generated visual methodology for health communication research and pedagogy. *Health Communication, 36*(5), 630–638. <https://doi.org/10.1080/10410236.2020.1733228>

Tippens, J. A., Parra, G., Habecker, P., Gocchi Carrasco, K., Andrews III, A. R., Palmer-Wackerly, A. L., Chaidez, V., Soliz, J., Pytlik Zillig, L. & Dombrowski, K. (2020). Emotional support and mental health among Somali men in a rural midwestern town. *Journal of Rural Mental Health, 44*(3), 170–183. <https://doi.org/10.1037/rmh0000136>

Toney, A. M., Martin T., Sanchez, S., Kelley, M. S., Palmer-Wackerly, A. L., & Chaidez, V. (2022). Examining the macrosystem level of influence on community health worker effectiveness in the state of Nebraska: A qualitative approach. *Journal of Community Health. 47*(3), 510–518. <https://doi.org/10.1007/s10900-022-01075-7>

U.S. Census Bureau. (2021a). *American community survey 5-year estimates.* Retrieved from Census Reporter Profile page for Lexington city, Dawson County, NE <http://censusreporter.org/profiles/06000US3104791728-lexington-city-dawson-county-ne/>

U.S. Census Bureau. (2021b). *American community survey 5-year estimates.* Retrieved from Census Reporter Profile page for Dawson County, NE <https://censusreporter.org/profiles/05000US31047-dawson-county-ne/>

U.S. Census Bureau. (2021c). *American community survey 5-year estimates.* Retrieved from Census Reporter Profile page for [rural town, NE].

U.S. Department of Health & Human Services (2020, November 20). *Civil rights: Limited english proficiency (LEP).* <https://www.hhs.gov/civil-rights/for-individuals/special-topics/limited-english-proficiency/index.html#:~:text=Title%20VI%20of%20the%20Civil,persons%20with%20limited%20English%20proficiency>

U.S. Department of Health & Human Services (n.d.). *Social Determinants of Health.* Office of Disease Prevention and Health Promotion. <https://health.gov/healthypeople/priority-areas/social-determinants-health>

Vacchelli, E. (2018). Embodiment in qualitative research: Collage making with migrant, refugee and asylum seeking women. *Qualitative Research, 18*(2), 171–190. <https://doi.org/10.1177/1468794117708008>

Van Lith, T. (2014). A meeting with "I-Thou": Exploring the intersection between mental health recovery and art making through a co-operative inquiry. *Action Research, 12*(3), 254–272. <https://doi-org.libproxy.unl.edu/10.1177/1476750314529599>

Wagner, P. E., Ellingson, L. L., & Kunkel, A. (2016). Pictures, patience, and practicalities: Lessons learned from using photovoice in applied communication contexts. *Journal of Applied Communication Research, 44*(3), 336–342. <https://doi.org/10.1080/00909882.2016.1192292>.

Wang, C., & Burris, M. A. (1997). Photovoice: Concept, methodology, and use for participatory needs assessment. *Health Education & Behavior, 24*(3), 369–387. doi: 10.1177/109019819702400309

Wang, C., Burris, M. A., & Ping, X. Y. (1996). Chinese village women as visual anthropologists: A participatory approach to reaching policymakers. *Social Science & Medicine, 42*(10), 1391–1400. https://doi.org/10.1016/0277-9536(95)00287-1

Warren, M. R., Calderón, J., Kupscznk, L. A., Squires, G., & Su, C. (2018). Is collaborative, community-engaged scholarship more rigorous than traditional scholarship? On advocacy, bias, and social science research. *Urban Education, 53*(4), 445–472. <https://doi.org/10.1177/0042085918763511>

PART FIVE

# Culturally Informed Health Promotion Campaigns

CHAPTER TWELVE

# Creating a Student-Led Healthy Aging Program for Diverse Older Adults in Alaska

## Using Persuasive Hope Theory

AMBER K. WORTHINGTON, BRITTENY M. HOWELL,
DALE M. GOLDEN AND ALLEX MAHANNA

The fifth and final part of this edited volume covers "Culturally Informed Health Communication Campaigns." The goal of this part is to examine culturally informed health campaigns in diverse communities in the arctic and subarctic regions of Alaska. This part begins with Chapter Twelve, which examines culturally appropriate language choices for older adults in Alaska. Chapter Thirteen focuses on moving beyond Eurocentric theories to explore culturally rooted Indigenous perspectives and Alaska Native health inequalities, and Chapter Fourteen discusses ways to integrate culture into public health campaigns with a specific focus on immigrant populations in Alaska.

Older adults in the United States do not obtain sufficient dietary intake of fruits and vegetables (Nicklett & Kadell, 2013) or engage in recommended levels of physical activity (Sparling et al., 2015; Watson et al., 2016). These trends are evident in Alaska, where older adults' low dietary quality and physical activity contribute to high rates of obesity, Alzheimer's Disease and Related Dementias, and other chronic conditions (Cobb et al., 2014; Garrett et al., 2015; Howell, 2020; Mayeda et al., 2016). Further, Alaska has the highest proportion of older adults in the United States (Administration on Aging, 2017; Alaska Commission on Aging, 2017) and also faces some of the greatest geriatric provider shortages per capita in the country (Kaiser Family Foundation, 2022; United Health Foundation, 2020), leading to an increased need for older adults to engage in preventative health behaviors.

Health campaigns designed to increase intake of fruits and vegetables and physical activity in diverse populations of older adults may be an effective way to increase preventative behaviors (Cress et al., 2005; Wood & Neal, 2016). Additionally, lifespan perspectives in message design suggest that positive, hopeful messages are likely an effective way to motivate older adults to engage in desired preventative health behavior changes (Notthoff & Carstensen, 2014; Nussbaum & Worthington, 2017). This chapter outlines the process of using Persuasive Hope Theory (Chadwick, 2015) and additional work on hope to create one such program. We first consider the need for healthy aging programs among diverse older adults and lifespan perspectives on message design. We then outline Persuasive Hope Theory (Chadwick, 2015) and additional work on hope to demonstrate how these can be used to create effective hope messages to increase fruit and vegetable intake and exercise patterns. We integrate this information and discuss the development of our 15-week healthy aging program for diverse older adults aged 55+ in Alaska using specific message features and curriculum components to evoke hope. Finally, we explore our rationale and training for student instructors to deliver this healthy aging program.

## HEALTH PROMOTION AMONG DIVERSE OLDER ADULTS

Health education has been shown to improve dietary and physical activity behaviors for older adults, which can increase quality of life (Notthoff & Carstensen, 2014; Romieu et al., 2017) and decrease risk of Alzheimer's Disease and Related Dementias (Jiang et al., 2017; Zhou et al., 2017); however, these changes are difficult for older adults to maintain over time due to a variety of social, emotional, environmental, and cognitive barriers (Schwarzer, 2008; Wood & Neal, 2016). For example, research shows that older adults are more likely to engage in behavior changes when others in their social networks, such as friends and family, are supportive of these changes (Howell & Bardach, 2018). Older adults may exhibit low intentions to change their diet and exercise levels due to lack of belief in their ability to make sustained changes (Bennett & Gaines, 2010), and they may believe that it is "too late" for them to make meaningful behavior changes (Bardach, Schoenberg, & Howell, 2016). Such beliefs contribute to older adults' perceptions that such health behavior changes will have little effect on their overall health (Williams et al., 2005). Older adults also do not accurately estimate their obesity and chronic illness risk and its connection to their current dietary and activity patterns (Bierbauer et al., 2017). Together, these factors negatively impact older adults' emotional states and decrease their motivation and intentions for behavior change.

Critical knowledge gaps exist concerning the most effective educational interventions to improve diet and physical activity behaviors among diverse, low-income older adults in Alaska. Studies suggest that interventions for adults should be limited to a small number of strategic messages; reinforce and personalize health messages; provide hands-on activities, incentives, and cues; promote diffusion and information-sharing among participants; and use appropriate persuasive theories to incite behavior change (Park et al., 2011); however, little is known about the factors that motivate healthy aging behaviors among diverse, urban Alaskan seniors, including Alaska Native Elders (Lewis, 2010).

Historically, Indigenous voices in healthy aging research have been missing (Pace & Grenier, 2017). Indigenous peoples in the United States have a long history of oppression and being forbidden to practice their language and cultural beliefs, which have long-standing effects on well-being throughout their lifespan (Langdon, 1987; Lewis, 2013). American Indian and Alaska Native peoples are more at risk than other groups for health conditions such as obesity, cardiovascular disease, and diabetes (Hutchinson & Shin, 2014). As American Indian and Alaska Native peoples are more likely than others to live in rural communities, there is also a discrepancy between the availability of health services and the higher risk for medical conditions (Towne et al., 2015).

There are also significant differences between Indigenous and Western perspectives on aging. Alaska Native Elders view aging as a holistic, dynamic process that includes spirituality and relationships, which significantly differs from the Western biomedical perspective (Lewis, 2013). Traditional ways of living, such as following a subsistence lifestyle, are related to how Alaska Native peoples define successful aging (Hopkins et al., 2007; Howell et al., 2023). Having a sense of purpose and role in one's family and community also positively impacts Alaska Native Elder health and well-being (Lewis, 2014). As such, American Indian and Alaska Native peoples believe aging contributes to experiences of resilience, well-being, connection to cultural values, and community engagement (Oré et al., 2016).

The relationships between Indigenous Elders and their communities are especially important in successful aging, as Indigenous communities highly respect their Elders (Lewis, 2013). As one ages, their role in the community changes as well. Experiences related to increased life satisfaction and changes in perspective with age include more emphasis on their culture, connection to the land, and enjoyment of daily activities (Wortman & Lewis, 2021). Additionally, research has demonstrated that to reach Eldership in Alaska Native communities, four elements must be present: emotional well-being, community engagement, spirituality, and physical health (Lewis, 2011). There is limited research on successful aging for Indigenous peoples; however, models related to healthy aging can be more inclusive of Indigenous communities and Elders by including domains related to health and wellness, empowerment and resilience, engagement and behavior, and connectedness (Pace & Grenier, 2017).

Some studies have been conducted that suggest that optimism, resilience, and hope may be salient for *rural* Alaska Native Elders (e.g., Lewis, 2013); however, there remains a gap regarding health behavior change factors for Indigenous and other diverse seniors in *urban* Subarctic environments. Some studies indicate that increasing motivation and intentions leads to sustained behavior change, while other research indicates such changes may only be short-term for older adults (Brawley et al., 2003; Nigg & Long, 2012). Additionally, much work with Alaska Native adults has focused on their negative health behaviors and histories of trauma rather than their capacity for resilience (Crouch et al., 2020), defined as the ability to recover from and adapt to difficulties (see Healey Akearok et al., 2019). To date, we have not been able to locate empirical research that examines the use of persuasive hope messages to motivate diverse older adults to improve fruit and vegetable intake and physical activity patterns. We therefore turn now to discussing lifespan perspectives on message design and persuasive hope messages.

## LIFESPAN PERSPECTIVES ON MESSAGE DESIGN

Theoretical frameworks used in message design can be adapted with a lifespan perspective to effectively target older adults (Nussbaum & Worthington, 2017). Substantial work within the communication discipline has examined the use of fear in strategic message design (e.g., de Hoog et al., 2007; Hovland et al., 1953; Janis, 1967; Rogers, 1975; Witte, 1992; Witte & Allen, 2000); however, as outlined by Nussbaum and Worthington (2017), fear may be an ineffective message design tool for older adults for several reasons. First, older adults preferentially process and better remember positive, hopeful information that aligns with their desire to enhance their emotional well-being (Carstensen et al., 1999). Second, older adults may have low self-efficacy in several health contexts, such as engaging in preventative health behaviors, and fear is ineffective under conditions of low self-efficacy (Peters et al., 2013). Theoretical developments in emotional appeals suggest that hope and efficacy, instead of fear, can be used to motivate positive changes in behavioral intentions and behaviors (Chadwick, 2015; Nabi & Myrick, 2019). Thus, instead of using fear to create a problem-focused vision of the future, messages can use hope to create an opportunity-focused vision that builds on older adults' excitement and enthusiasm for desired future health outcomes. Additionally, hope-based messaging is a timely strategy for older adults, many of whom may still be experiencing high rates of depression due to COVID-19 restrictions and isolation (Armitage & Nellums, 2020). These hopeful messages may be particularly successful for diverse older adults in Alaska since evidence suggests that hope, optimism, and resilience are salient for Alaska Native Elders (see Lewis, 2013). Next, we outline Persuasive Hope Theory (Chadwick, 2015) and additional work on hope and how these can be used to create effective hope messages.

## PERSUASIVE HOPE THEORY

Persuasive Hope Theory (PHT) defines hope as a discrete, future-oriented emotion that can motivate people to adopt various behaviors by directing their thoughts toward opportunities for action that will enable them to achieve future rewards (Chadwick, 2015). A hope appeal is a message that arouses hope in an attempt to persuade people to adopt a specific behavior. PHT describes specific message features needed for an effective hope appeal.

PHT (Chadwick, 2015) notes that a hope appeal contains message content about a specific opportunity for action and the efficacy of a specific recommended behavior to achieve a desired future outcome. The hope appeal content about the specific opportunity includes message features designed to evoke appraisals of importance, goal congruence, possibility, and future expectation. The hope appeal content about the efficacy of a specific recommended behavior to achieve a desired future outcome includes message features designed to evoke appraisals of response efficacy and self-efficacy.

After reading the hope appeal, the first thing someone does is appraise the opportunity using perceptions of importance, goal congruence, possibility, and future expectation. Perceived importance includes an appraisal of whether the future outcome is personally relevant. Perceived goal congruence includes an appraisal of whether the future outcome is consistent with someone's personal goals or motives. Perceived possibility includes an appraisal of whether the future outcome is likely to occur. Perceived future expectation includes an appraisal of whether the outcome would lead to a better future. If someone perceives the opportunity as low (i.e., low appraisals of importance, goal congruence, possibility, and/or future expectation), then they will not feel hope. Conversely, if someone perceives the opportunity as high (i.e., high appraisals of importance, goal congruence, possibility, and future expectation), then they will feel hope. According to PHT, these feelings of hope are motivational and can lead to increased attention to the message, interest in the topic, perceptions that the message is effective, and intentions to perform the recommended behavior (Chadwick, 2015).

The next thing someone does when reading the hope appeal is to appraise the efficacy. This includes an appraisal of response efficacy, which is an assessment of whether they believe that the recommended behavior will help them achieve the desired outcome. This also includes an appraisal of self-efficacy, which is an assessment of whether they believe they are capable of doing the recommended behavior. If someone perceives the efficacy as low (i.e., low response efficacy and/or low self-efficacy), then they will not feel hope. If someone perceives the efficacy as high (i.e., high response efficacy and high self-efficacy), then they will feel hope. Again, these feelings of hope are motivational and can lead to intentions to perform the behavior, as well as attention, interest, and perceived effectiveness (Chadwick, 2015).

## Message Features to Evoke Hope

In order to create an effective hope appeal, it is therefore important for the appeal to contain message features that lead to appraisals of importance, goal congruence, possibility, future expectation, response efficacy, and self-efficacy, which will, in turn, evoke feelings of hope. Message features to increase appraisals of importance include using the second person (e.g., "you") and focusing on how the behavior would impact the message receiver (Chadwick, 2010). Message features to increase appraisals of goal congruence also focus on how the opportunity would be consistent with the message receiver's goals. A hope appeal can increase appraisals of possibility through the inclusion of specific message features again including the second person (e.g., "we"), as well as information that states that it is possible for the message receiver to create a better future; additional modifiers like "very" can be used to create additional emphasis (Chadwick, 2010). Message features to increase appraisals of future expectation include explicitly stating that the future will be much better if the message receiver adopts the recommended action; additional modifiers like "many" and "much" can also be added to emphasize the future expectation. Chadwick (2010) provides examples of messages on climate change with high importance, goal congruence, possibility, and future expectation that are displayed in Table 12.1.

In addition to importance, goal congruence, possibility, and future expectation, PHT posits that to be effective a hope appeal should also contain message features that lead to appraisals of response efficacy and self-efficacy, which will contribute to the feeling of hope (Chadwick, 2010; Chadwick, 2015). There are several message strategies that can increase perceived response efficacy. The hope appeal could, for example, explicitly state that the recommended behavior has

Table 12.1: Examples of message features provided by Chadwick (2010) to evoke hope through appraisals of importance, goal congruence, possibility, and future expectation

| Message Feature | Example |
|---|---|
| Importance | "**The climate affects your well-being in many ways**... The climate will affect your health. Your health is affected by air quality...Protecting the climate is VERY important for your well-being" (p. 129). |
| Goal Congruence | "**Protecting the climate saves you A LOT of money**. You can make simple changes to protect the climate. You can use less energy, use less hot water, and make less trash. These changes are free or cheap. These small changes will directly save you at least $500 per year" (p. 130). |
| Possibility | "**It is very likely that we can make the climate better**. All over the world, people like you are taking action. They are using less energy, using less hot water, and making less trash. Billions of people are taking action to protect the environment. You can join the effort and make it even more likely that we will make the climate better" (p. 131). |
| Future Expectation | "**Protecting the climate will make the future much better**. Protecting our climate will bring a wonderful future. Our air will be much cleaner. Our weather will be much less extreme. Our summers will be beautiful and mild. We will experience many fewer diseases and will live much longer. Growing food will be easier and more productive. Protecting the climate will have By helping protect the climate, you can help create a wonderful future" (p. 130). |

previously been used successfully to achieve the desired future outcome (e.g., "This has been effective in the past!"). Several message strategies can also be used to increase perceived self-efficacy, including examples of others who have successfully performed the behavior or verbal encouragement (see O'Keefe, 2015). Additional message strategies to increase self-efficacy are explained below in more detail. We turn next to related research on hope that specifies additional message components that may be used to evoke hope.

## Additional Hope Research and Message Features

Convincing self-efficacy information can lead to feelings of hope given its association with behavioral confidence and situational control (see Nabi & Myrick, 2019). These self-efficacy messages may be particularly important for older adults, as self-efficacy among diverse older adults is associated with long-term maintenance of positive health behavior changes (Neupert et al., 2009), increased self-care (Kostka & Jachimowicz, 2010), overall satisfaction with life (Kostka &

Jachimowicz, 2010), and perceptions of healthy aging (Depp & Jeste, 2006). Self-Efficacy Theory (Bandura, 1977) posits four specific pathways that can be used to generate feelings of self-efficacy: enactive mastery experience, vicarious experience, verbal persuasion, and physiological or affective states.

Enactive mastery experience occurs when a person has successfully performed the recommended behavior. Vicarious experience occurs when a person is able to watch a similar other successfully perform the recommended behavior, and this leads to feelings of self-efficacy through an appraisal of one's own performance against that of the other (Bandura, 1977). Ashford and colleagues (2010) conducted a systematic review of interventions to increase physical activity self-efficacy and found that programs that included vicarious experience produced significantly higher levels of self-efficacy compared to programs that did not. Williams and French (2011) conducted a systematic review and also found that the inclusion of a vicarious experience technique to "facilitate social comparison" by drawing a person's attention to others' performance in physical activity interventions resulted in significantly higher self-efficacy than those that did not.

Verbal persuasion occurs when others express to a person that they are capable of performing a recommended behavior (Bandura, 1977). Ashford and colleagues (2010) also found that programs that included feedback on a person's past performance or feedback on others' past performance resulted in higher levels of self-efficacy compared to programs that did not. These results align with those of Williams and French (2011), who found that programs that included praising participants for their attempts to achieve a specific behavioral goal were associated with significantly higher self-efficacy than interventions that did not.

The final pathway noted in Self-Efficacy Theory is physiological or affective states. These states can increase self-efficacy by reducing negative emotional states and correcting misinterpretations of bodily states (Bandura, 1977). This also aligns with the information presented on PHT which notes that affective states associated with feelings of hope can lead to self-efficacy and intentions to perform a recommended behavior (see Chadwick, 2015).

There are several additional low-cost motivational and behavioral strategies that can be used to increase self-efficacy, a sense of control, and positive emotions such as hope (Lachman et al., 2018). For example, setting and committing to realistic goals can encourage participants to think about the future and thereby be motivated to change their behavior to achieve the desired future outcome (Lachman et al., 2018). It is also important for them to create an action plan for how to implement these goals (Lachman et al., 2018). This is further underscored in Hope Theory (Snyder, 2002), which notes that hopeful people pursue the realization of a positive or desired outcome. Hope Theory (Snyder, 2002) posits that pathways help people move from their current state to where they want to be in the future, and it is important for people to develop multiple pathways to prepare for potential obstacles that block a particular path. Some empirical work also supports these ideas, as Williams and French (2011) found that programs that included information on where, when, and how to perform a physical activity behavior (e.g., by providing information on local places where people can exercise) were associated with significantly higher self-efficacy and physical activity behaviors than programs that did not.

Lachman and colleagues (2018) note that self-efficacy can also be generated using positive, gain-framed messages with clear communication of the benefits of the program. This is related to substantial work in the communication field that has examined gain-framed messages (e.g., O'Keefe & Jensen, 2003). Gain-framed messages state that a recommended behavior will allow someone to attain a desirable outcome or avoid an undesirable outcome, whereas loss-framed messages indicate that a recommended behavior will allow someone to avoid a desirable outcome or attain an undesirable outcome (see Liu et al., 2019). Table 12.2 provides examples of gain-framed and loss-framed messages.

The message features outlined above can be incorporated into interventions designed to incite positive health behavior changes in order to make them more effective. We turn now to discussing the development of a 15-week healthy aging program for diverse older adults in Alaska using all of these strategies.

Table 12.2: Examples of gain- and loss-framed messages similar to those provided by Liu and colleagues (2019)

| Frame | Outcome | Message |
|---|---|---|
| Gain | Attain Desirable | Frequent exercising can lead to increased independence as you get older. |
| | Avoid Undesirable | Frequent exercising can prevent decreased independence as you get older. |
| Loss | Avoid Desirable | Infrequent exercising can hinder independence as you get older. |
| | Attain Undesirable | Infrequent exercising can lead to decreased independence as you get older. |

## CASE STUDY: HEALTHY AGING PROGRAM DEVELOPMENT

Researchers from communication, public health, health sciences, and dietetics collaborated to develop a 15-week healthy aging program to be delivered among community-dwelling older adults age 55+ in their subsidized housing complexes in Anchorage, Alaska. This 15-week program was an expansion of a previously developed 10-week community wellness pilot program for older adults in Alaska (see Howell et al., 2021). The process for the development of the 15-week healthy aging program is outlined below in Figure 12.1.

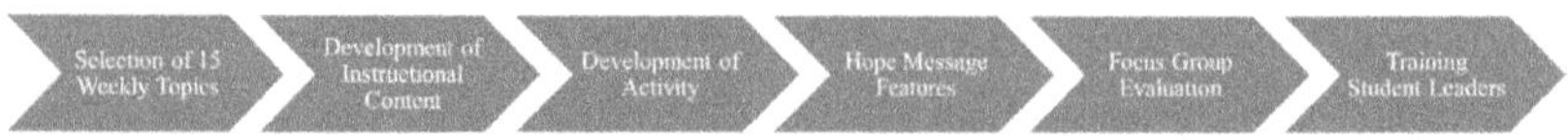
Selection of 15 Weekly Topics
Development of Instructional Content
Development of Activity
Hope Message Features
Focus Group Evaluation
Training Student Leaders

Figure 12.1: Process for the development of the 15-week healthy aging program

The weekly content of the program included (1) an introduction to healthy aging; (2) physical activity for older adults; (3) changing nutritional needs as we age; (4) goal setting; (5) evaluating internet health information; (6) stress reduction; (7) brain health for older adults; (8) mid-program and goal review; (9) grocery shopping on a budget; (10) social health for older adults; (11) safe physical activity and food storage at home; (12) positive attitudes for a healthy life; (13) staying engaged in the community; (14) program review and goal check-in; and (15) program "graduation" and celebration.

## Development of Instructional Content and Activities

Each weekly session was designed to last 45–60 minutes and included an evidence-based instructional component with discussion questions, as well as an activity related to the content followed by light physical activity instruction. The content in each instructional component was curated with information specific to diverse, lower-income, and community-dwelling older adults in Alaska.

Three of the 15 sessions were devoted to setting and reviewing goals and creating action plans using the S-M-A-R-T method (see University of California, 2016). The "S" stands for "Specific." For example, instead of "I want to eat healthier" a specific goal would be "I want to try one new recipe this week" or "I will fill half of my dinner plate with vegetables." The "M" stands for "Measurable." For example, instead of "I'd like to exercise more" a measurable goal would be "I will spend 20 minutes per day exercising." The "A" stands for "Attainable." For example, someone's goal may be to walk in the community 5K this year, but a more attainable goal might be to build the stamina to walk for 10 minutes, then 20 minutes, and so on. The "R" stands for "Relevant." This involves thinking about what makes the goal important and understanding how achieving the goal leads to a better future. The "T" stands for "Timely" and includes setting deadlines to meet goals. For example, instead of "exercise more," a goal with a deadline could be that "by the end of this week, I will have gone on three 20-minute walks." This method for setting goals has been used effectively for older adults and may be particularly useful in instances of low self-efficacy, such as with older adults engaging in preventative health behaviors (Beristain et al., 2020). After developing the initial curriculum content, the team added additional message features and curriculum components to increase participants' hope.

## Hope Message Features

After the initial development of the instructional content and activity for each weekly session, additional message features and curriculum components were added specifically designed to evoke hope using the aforementioned message features. Each weekly session contained an introduction statement and conclusion statement designed to evoke perceptions of importance, goal congruence, possibility, and future expectation. For example, Week 1: Introduction to Healthy Aging contained the following introduction statement:

> *Staying healthy as you get older positively impacts your well-being in many ways. Healthy aging will allow you to do the things that YOU want to do for many years to come, which is VERY important! It is possible for you to take small steps now to stay healthy that will make your future much better.*

In line with the message features and examples provided by Chadwick (2010; 2015) (see Table 1), this introduction statement contains message features to evoke appraisals of importance (i.e., "Staying healthy as you get older positively impacts your well-being" and " … which is VERY important"), goal congruence (i.e., " … do the things that YOU want to do … "), possibility (i.e., "It is possible for you to take small steps…"), and future expectation (i.e., " … that will make your future much better"). As an additional example, Week 2: Physical Activity for Older Adults contained the following conclusion statement:

> *Remember that staying physically active as you get older positively impacts your well-being in many ways. Staying physically active will allow you to do the things that YOU want to do for many years to come, which is VERY important! It is possible for you to take small steps now to increase your physical activity that will make your future much better.*

In line with the message features and examples provided by Chadwick (2010, 2015; see Table 1), this introduction statement contains message features to evoke appraisals of importance (i.e., " … staying physically active as you get older positively impacts your well being" and " … which is VERY important"), goal congruence (i.e., " … do the things that YOU want to do…"), possibility (i.e., "It is possible for you to take small steps…"), and future expectation (i.e., " … that will make your future much better").

In addition to the introduction and conclusion statements provided in each weekly session, additional message features were included to evoke appraisals of importance, goal congruence, possibility, and future expectation, as well as curriculum components designed to increase hope and self-efficacy through enactive

Table 12.3: Examples of curriculum components designed to incorporate message features to increase feelings of hope

| **Hope Features** | **Curriculum Components** |
|---|---|
| Importance | • Introduction & conclusion statements<br>• Statements that the recommended behavior would impact "you" (i.e., older adults) throughout the instructional content<br>• Statements that the desired outcome was "very important" throughout the instructional content |
| Goal Congruence | • Introduction & conclusion statements<br>• Statements that the recommended behavior would help "you" (i.e., older adults) achieve "your" goals throughout the instructional content |
| Possibility | • Introduction & conclusion statements<br>• Statements that the recommended behavior was likely to bring about the desired outcome throughout the instructional content<br>• Language that the recommended behavior and desired outcome was "possible" throughout the instructional content |
| Future Expectation | • Introduction & conclusion statements<br>• Statements that the recommended behavior would make the future much better throughout the instructional content |
| Enactive Mastery Experience | • Each week included light physical activity instruction and participation |
| Vicarious Experience | • Each week participants performed light physical activity in a group setting, where they were able to view others successfully performing the behaviors |
| Verbal Persuasion | • Each week, the student instructors provided verbal encouragement to participants regarding their abilities to make dietary and physical activity changes |
| Goals & Action Plans | • S-M-A-R-T goal setting and actions plans in Week 4, 8, and 14 (i.e, 20 % of the program) |
| Gain-Framed Messages | • Statements that show the participant they can *gain a desirable outcome* (e.g., "Improving your behaviors and overall health now can help make sure that you have the energy to do the things you love: like hobbies or spending time with family"; Week 1) or *avoid an undesirable outcome* (e.g., "Specific exercises can help balance to prevent falls"; Week 1). |

mastery experiences, vicarious experiences, verbal persuasion, goal setting / action planning, and the use of gain-framed messages. Examples of these curriculum components are displayed in Table 3.

## Focus Group Program Evaluation and Improvements

Before implementing the healthy aging program, focus groups were organized to gain feedback on the curricular content. Specifically, the researchers were seeking feedback on student presentation of the material, length of the material, and amount of information provided in each weekly session. The focus groups were conducted with two weeks' worth of program materials; there was a separate focus group for each week's content. Recruitment for the focus groups included calling housing community residents that had expressed interest in the healthy aging program, as well as informing housing community staff of the focus groups to inform residents. Each focus group included five participants of diverse ethnicities over the age of 55 years. Feedback from the focus groups included instructing student teachers to enunciate and project their voices loudly when speaking, to shorten the amount of material presented in a single session, and to improve the handouts with more information for participants. Updates to the curriculum thus included reducing the amount of material presented each week, adding more information to the slides given to participants, providing instruction to the student teachers on how to effectively project their voices and communicate with participants, and improving some handouts for participants.

## Student-Led Program and Training Student Instructors

The 15-week healthy aging program was designed to be delivered to older adults by interdisciplinary teams of undergraduate and graduate students. This program was therefore an example of an interprofessional education curriculum, where students learn to respectfully work with others, effectively communicate with participants and stakeholders, and appropriately assess the health needs of specific populations (in this case, older adults; see Interprofessional Education Collaborative, 2016). This type of program positively impacts students' career readiness (De Los Santos et al., 2014) and provides real-world experience with collaborative team-based practices (Goldberg et al., 2012). Further, undergraduate students rarely consider geriatrics or gerontology when making their career choices (Gorelik et al., 2000; Meiboom et al., 2015); however, working with older adults positively impacts students' attitudes toward aging (Gutheil et al., 2006) and their desire to work with a geriatric population (Tam, 2014). This is especially important in Alaska in light of the geriatric provider shortages (Kaiser Family Foundation, 2022; United Health Foundation, 2020), and our pilot project found that students who delivered a health program to older adults reported more interest in working with older populations (Howell et al., 2021).

In order to prepare the students to team-teach the healthy aging program, they participated in weekly training sessions led by the faculty research team in the academic semester prior to program implementation. These training sessions included background information and ethical practices in research, pedagogical techniques, and public speaking tips. The training sessions also taught students how to administer pre- and post-program surveys, as well as the Senior Fitness Test to measure fitness improvements over the course of the program. Finally, specific training sessions were held for students to practice teaching each of the 15-week sessions.

## CONCLUSIONS

In this chapter, we discussed the need to develop healthy aging programs for Alaska's diverse older adult population designed to increase fruit and vegetable intake and physical activity. We outlined our process of using Persuasive Hope Theory (Chadwick, 2015) and additional work on hope to develop our 15-week student-led healthy aging program for diverse older adults aged 55+ in Alaska using specific message features and curriculum components to evoke hope. We also summarized our focus group evaluation and improvements, as well as our training for student instructors to deliver this healthy aging program. The increased need for older adults in Alaska to engage in preventative health behaviors and lifespan perspectives in message design that suggest that positive, hopeful messages are likely effective in motivating desired preventative health behavior changes for older adults make this a promising approach.

*Research reported in this publication was supported by the National Institute on Aging of the National Institutes of Health under Award Number R15AG072369. The content is solely the responsibility of the authors and does not necessarily represent the official views of the National Institutes of Health.*

## REFERENCES

Administration on Aging. (2017). Profile of older Americans. *ACL Adm Community Living.* doi:10.1300/J369v06n01_06

Alaska Commission on Aging. (2015). Health aging in Alaska: Alaska's road map to successful aging. Retrieved from <http://dhss.alaska.gov/acoa/Documents/ACOA_AR2015.pdf>.

Armitage, R., & Nellums, L. B. (2020). COVID-19 and the consequences of isolating the elderly. *The Lancet Public Health*, *5*(5). <https://doi.org/10.1016/S2468-2667(20)30061-X>

Ashford, S., Edmunds, J., & French, D. P. (2010). What is the best way to change self-efficacy to promote lifestyle and recreational physical activity? A systematic review with meta-analysis. *British Journal of Health Psychology*, *15*(2), 265–288.

Bandura, A. (1977). Self-efficacy: Toward a unifying theory of behavioral change. *Psychological Review*, *84*(2), 191–215. <https://doi.org/10.1037/0033-295X.84.2.191>

Bardach, S. H., Schoenberg, N. E., & Howell B. M. (2016). What motivates older adults to improve diet and exercise patterns? *Journal of Community Health*, *41*(1). doi:10.1007/s10900-015-0058-5

Bennett, T., & Gaines J. (2010). Believing what you hear: The impact of aging stereotypes upon the old. *Educational Gerontology*, *36*(5), 435–445. doi:10.1080/03601270903212336

Beristain Iraola, A., Álvarez Sánchez, R., Petsani, D., Hors-Fraile, S., Bamidis, P., & Konstantinidis, E. (2020). Virtual coaching for older adults at home using SMART goal supported behavior change. *Companion Publication of the 2020 International Conference on Multimodal Interaction*, 251–255. <https://doi.org/10.1145/3395035.3425311>

Bierbauer, W., Inauen, J., Schaefer, S., Kleemeyer, M. M., Lüscher, J., König, C., Tobias, R., Kliegel, M., Ihle, A., Zimmerli, L., Holzer, B. M., Siebenhuener, K., Battegay, E., Schmied, C., & Scholz, U. (2017). Health behavior change in older adults: Testing the health action process approach at the inter- and intraindividual level. *Applied Psychology: Health and Well-Being*, *9*(3), 324–348. doi: <https://doi.org/10.1111/aphw.12094>

Brawley, L. R., Rejeski, W. J., & King A. C. (2003). Promoting physical activity for older adults: The challenges for changing behavior. *American Journal of Preventive Medicine*, *25*(3), 172–183. <https://doi.org/10.1016/s0749-3797(03)00182-x>

Carstensen, L. L., Isaacowitz, D. M., & Charles, S. T. (1999). Taking time seriously: A theory of socioemotional selectivity. *American Psychologist*, *54*(3), 165.

Chadwick, A. E. (2010). *Persuasive hope theory and hope appeals in messages about climate change mitigation and seasonal influenza prevention*. [Doctoral dissertation, The Pennsylvania State University]. Electronic Theses and Dissertations for Graduate School. <https://etda.libraries.psu.edu/catalog/10950>

Chadwick, A. E. (2015). Toward a theory of persuasive hope: Effects of cognitive appraisals, hope appeals, and hope in the context of climate change. *Health Communication*, *30*(6), 598–611. doi:10.1080/10410236.2014.916777

Cobb, N., Espey, D., & King, J. (2014). Health behaviors and risk factors among American Indians and Alaska Natives, 2000–2010. *American Journal of Public Health*, *104*(Suppl. 3), S481–S489. doi:10.2105/AJPH.2014.301879

Cress, M. E., Buchner, D. M., Prohaska, T., Rimmer, J., Brown, M., Macera, C., DiPietro, L., & Chodzko-Zajko, W. (2005). Best practices for physical activity programs and behavior counseling in older adult populations. *Journal of Aging and Physical Activity*, *13*(1), 61–74. doi:10.1123/japa.13.1.61.

Crouch, M. C., Skan, J., David, E. J. R., Lopez, E. D. S., & Prochaska, J. J. (2020). Indigenizing quality of life: The goodness of life for every Alaska Native research study. *Applied Research in Quality of Life*, *16*(3), 1123–1143. doi:10.1007/s11482-019-09782-5 de Hoog, N., Stroebe, W., & De Wit, J. B. (2007). The impact of vulnerability to and severity of a health risk on processing and acceptance of fear-arousing communications: A meta-analysis. *Review of General Psychology*, *11*(3), 258–285. <https://doi.org/10.1037/1089-2680.11.3.258>

De Los Santos, M., McFarlin, C. D., & Martin L. (2014). Interprofessional education and service learning: A model for the future of health professions education. *Journal of Interprofessional Care*, *28*(4), 374–375. doi:10.3109/13561820.2014.889102

Depp, C. A., & Jeste, D. V. (2006). Definitions and predictors of successful aging: A comprehensive review of larger quantitative studies. *The American Journal of Geriatric Psychiatry*, *14*(1), 6–20. doi:10.1097/01.JGP.0000192501.03069.bc

Garrett, M. D., Baldridge, D., Benson, W., Crowder, J., & Aldrich, N. (2015). Mental health disorders among an invisible minority: Depression and dementia among American Indian and Alaska Native elders. *The Gerontologist*, *55*(2), 227–236. doi:10.1093/geront/gnu181

Goldberg, L. R., Koontz, J. S., Rogers, N., & Brickell, J. (2012). Considering accreditation in gerontology: The importance of interprofessional collaborative competencies to ensure quality health care for older adults. *Gerontology & Geriatrics Education*, *33*(1), 95–110. doi:10.1080/02701960.2012.639101

Gorelik, Y., Damron-Rodriguez, J., Funderburk, B., Solomon, D. H. (2000). Undergraduate interest in aging: Is it affected by contact with older adults? *Educational Gerontology*, *26*(7), 623–638. doi:10.1080/036012700050200626

Gutheil, I. A., Chernesky, R. H., Sherratt, M. L. (2006) Influencing student attitudes toward older adults: Results of a service-learning collaboration. *Educational Gerontology*, *32*(9), 771–784. doi:10.1080/03601270600835470

Healey Akearok, G., Cueva, K., Stoor, J., Larsen, C., Rink, E., Kanayurak, N., Emelyanova, A., & Hiratsuka, V. (2019). Exploring the term "resilience" in Arctic Health and well-being using a sharing circle as a community-centered approach: Insights from a conference workshop. *Social Sciences*, *8*(2), 45. <https://doi.org/10.3390/socsci8020045>

Hopkins, S. E., Kwachka, P., Lardon, C., & Mohatt, G. V. (2007). Keeping busy: A Yup'ik/Cup'ik perspective on health and aging. *International Journal of Circumpolar Health*, *66*(1), 42–50. doi:10.3402/ijch.v66i1.18224

Hovland, C. I., Janis, I. L., & Kelley, H. H. (1953). *Communication and persuasion: Psychological studies of opinion change*. Yale University Press.

Howell, B. M. (2020). Interactions between diet, physical activity, and the sociocultural environment for older adult health in the urban Subarctic. *Journal of Community Health*, *45*(2), 252–263. doi:10.1007/s10900-019-00737-3

Howell, B. M., & Bardach, S. (2018). "It's a social thing": Sociocultural experiences with nutrition and exercise in Anchorage, Alaska. *Arctic Anthropology*, *55*(2), 1–16. doi: <https://doi.org/10.3368/aa.55.2.1>

Howell, B. M., Fried, R., & Hiratsuka, V. (2023). The importance of traditional foods and subsistence activities for healthy aging in Alaska Native communities. In B. M. Howell and R. Harrod (Eds.), *Anthropological Perspectives on Aging* (pp. 152–171). University of Florida Press.

Howell, B. M., Redmond, L. C., & Wanner, S. (2021). "I learned that I am loved": Older adults and undergraduate students mutually benefit from an interprofessional service-learning health promotion program. *Gerontology & Geriatrics Education*, *42*(2), 252–267. doi:10.1080/02701960.2020.1791104

Hutchinson, R. N., & Shin, S. (2014). Systematic review of health disparities for cardiovascular diseases and associated factors among American Indian and Alaska Native populations. *PLOS One, 9*(1), e80973. doi:10.1371/journal.pone.0080973

Interprofessional Education Collaborative. (2016). *Core Competencies for Interprofessional Collaborative Practice: 2016 Update*. Interprofessional Education Collaborative.

Janis, I. L. (1967). Effects of fear arousal on attitude change: Recent developments in theory and experimental research. *Advances in Experimental Social Psychology, 3*, 166–224. <https://doi.org/10.1016/S0065-2601(08)60344-5>

Jiang, X., Huang, J., Song, D., Deng, R., Wei, J., & Zhang, Z. (2017). Increased consumption of fruit and vegetables is related to a reduced risk of cognitive impairment and dementia: Meta-analysis. *Front Aging Neuroscience, 9*, 18. doi:10.3389/fnagi.2017.00018

Kaiser Family Foundation. (2022). Primary care health professional shortage areas. State Health Facts. Retrieved from <https://www.kff.org/other/state-indicator/primary-care-health-professional-shortage-areas-hpsas/?currentTimeframe=0&sortModel=%7B%22colId%22:%22Location%22,%22sort%22:%22asc%22%7D>.

Kostka, T., & Jachimowicz, V. (2010). Relationship of quality of life to dispositional optimism, health locus of control and self-efficacy in older subjects living in different environments. *Quality of Life Research, 19*(3), 351–361. doi:10.1007/s11136-010-9601-0

Lachman, M. E., Lipsitz, L., Lubben, J., Castaneda-Sceppa, C., & Jette, A. M. (2018). When adults don't exercise: Behavioral strategies to increase physical activity in sedentary middle-aged and older adults. *Innovation in Aging, 2*(1), 1–12. doi:10.1093/geroni/igy007

Langdon, S. J. (1987). *Native People of Alaska*. Greatland Graphics. ISBN 978-1-940381-00-8

Lewis, J. P. (2010). Successful aging through the eyes of Alaska Natives: Exploring generational differences among Alaska Natives. *Journal of Cross-Cultural Gerontology, 25*(4), 385–396. doi:10.1007/s10823-010-9124-8

Lewis, J. P. (2011). Successful aging through the eyes of Alaska Native Elders: What it means to be an Elder in Bristol Bay, AK. *Gerontologist, 51*(4), 540–549. doi:10.1093/geront/gnr006

Lewis, J. P. (2013). The importance of optimism in maintaining healthy aging in rural Alaska. *Qualitative Health Research, 23*(11), 1521–1527. doi:10.1177/1049732313508013

Lewis, J. P. (2014). What successful aging means to Alaska Natives: Exploring the reciprocal relationship between the health and well-being of Alaska Native Elders. *The International Journal of Aging and Society, 3*(1), 77–87. <https://doi.org/10.18848/2160-1909/CGP/v03i01/57722>

Liu, X., Shuster, M. M., Mikels, J. A., & Stine-Morrow, E. A. (2019). Doing what makes you happy: Health message framing for younger and older adults. *Experimental Aging Research, 45*(4), 293–305. doi:10.1080/0361073X.2019.1627491

Mayeda, E. R., Glymour, M. M., Quesenberry, C. P., & Whitmer, R. A. (2016). Inequalities in dementia incidence between six racial and ethnic groups over 14 years. *Alzheimer's & Dementia, 12*(3), 216–224. doi:10.1016/j.jalz.2015.12.007

Meiboom, A. A., de Vries, H., Hertogh, C. M. P. M., & Scheele, F. (2015). Why medical students do not choose a career in geriatrics: A systematic review. *BMC Medical Education, 15*(1), 101. doi:10.1186/s12909-015-0384-4

Nabi, R. L., & Myrick, J. G. (2019). Uplifting fear appeals: Considering the role of hope in fear-based persuasive messages. *Health Communication, 34*(4), 463–474. doi:10.1080/10410236.2017.1422847

Neupert, S. D., Lachman, M. E., & Whitbourne, S. B. (2009). Exercise self-efficacy and control beliefs: Effects on exercise behavior after an exercise intervention for older adults. *Journal of Aging and Physical Activity, 17*(1), 1–16. doi: 10.1123/japa.17.1.1

Nicklett, E. J., & Kadell, A. R. (2013). Fruit and vegetable intake among older adults: A scoping review. *Maturitas, 75*(4), 305–312. doi:10.1016/j.maturitas.2013.05.005

Nigg, C. R., & Long, C. R. (2012). A systematic review of single health behavior change interventions vs. multiple health behavior change interventions among older adults. *Translational Behavioral Medicine, 2*(2), 163–179. doi:10.1007/s13142-012-0130-y

Notthoff, N., & Carstensen, L. L. (2014). Positive messaging promotes walking in older adults. *Psychology and Aging, 29*(2), 329–341. doi:10.1037/a0036748

Nussbaum, J. F., & Worthington, A. K. (2017). Lifespan and developmental considerations in health and risk message design. In R. L. Parrott (Ed.), *Health and Risk Message Design and Processing, Communication: Oxford Research Encyclopedias.* Oxford University Press. doi: <https://doi.org/10.1093/acrefore/9780190228613.013.318>

O'Keefe, D. J. (2015). *Persuasion: Theory and research* (3rd ed.). Sage Publications.

O'Keefe, D. J., & Jensen, J. D. (2007). The relative persuasiveness of gain-framed loss-framed messages for encouraging disease prevention behaviors: A meta-analytic review. *Journal of Health Communication, 12*(7), 623–644. doi:10.1080/10810730701615198.

Oré, C. E., Teufel-Shone, N. I., & Chico-Jarillo, T. M. (2016). American Indian and Alaska Native resilience along the life course and across generations: A literature review. *American Indian and Alaska Native Mental Health Research, 23*(3), 134–157. doi:10.5820/aian.2303.2016.134

Pace, J. E., & Grenier, A. (2017). Expanding the circle of knowledge: Reconceptualizing successful aging among North American older Indigenous Peoples. *Journals of Gerontology – Series B Psychological Sciences and Social Sciences, 72*(2), 248–258. doi: 10.1093/geronb/gbw128

Park, Y. H., Song, M., Cho, B., Lim, J., Song, W., Kim, S. (2011). The effects of an integrated health education and exercise program in community-dwelling older adults with hypertension: a randomized controlled trial. *Patient Education and Counseling, 82*(1), 133–137. doi:10.1016/j.pec.2010.04.002

Peters, G. J. Y., Ruiter, R. A., & Kok, G. (2013). Threatening communication: A critical re-analysis and a revised meta-analytic test of fear appeal theory. *Health Psychology Review, 7*(Suppl. 1), S8–S31. doi:10.1080/17437199.2012.703527

Rogers, R. W. (1975). A protection motivation theory of fear appeals and attitude change. *Journal of Psychology, 91*(1), 93–114. doi:10.1080/00223980.1975.9915803

Romieu, I., Dossus, L., Barquera, S., Blottière, H. M., Franks, P. W., Gunter, M., Hwalla, N., Hursting, S. D., Leitzmann, M., Margetts, B., Nishida, C., Potischman, N., Seidell, J., Stepien, M., Wang, Y., Westerterp, K., Winichagoon, P., Wiseman, M., & Willett, W. C. (2017). Energy balance and obesity: What are the main drivers? *Cancer Causes & Control, 28*(3), 247–258. doi: <https://doi.org/10.1007/s10552-017-0869-z>

Schwarzer, R. (2008). Modeling health behavior change: How to predict and modify the adoption and maintenance of health behaviors. *Applied Psychology, 57*(1), 1–29. doi: <https://doi.org/10.1111/j.1464-0597.2007.00325.x>

Snyder, C. R. (2002). Hope theory: Rainbows in the mind. *Psychological Inquiry, 13*(4), 249–275. DOI: <https://www.jstor.org/stable/1448867>

Sparling, P. B., Howard, B. J., Dunstan, D. W., & Owen, N. (2015). Recommendations for physical activity in older adults. *BMJ (Clinical Research Ed.), 350*, h100. doi: <https://doi.org/10.1136/bmj.h100>

Tam, M. (2014). Intergenerational service learning between the old and young: What, why and how. *Educational Gerontology, 40*(6), 401–413. doi:10.1080/03601277.2013.822201

Towne Jr, S. D., Probst, J. C., Mitchell, J., & Chen, Z. (2015). Poorer quality outcomes of Medicare-certified home health care in areas with high levels of Native American/Alaska Native residents. *Journal of Aging and Health, 27*(8), 1339–1357. doi:10.1177/0898264315583051

United Health Foundation. (2020). 2019 Senior Report: Alaska. America's Health Rankings. Retrieved from <https://www.americashealthrankings.org/learn/reports/2019-senior-report/state-summaries-alaska>.

University of California. (2016). SMART goals: A how to guide. Retrieved from <https://www.ucop.edu/local-human-resources/_files/performance-appraisal/How%20to%20write%20SMART%20Goals%20v2.pdf>

Vandsberger, E., & Wakefield, M. (2006). Service learning with rural older adults. *Journal of Intergenerational Relationships, 3*(4), 83–97. doi:10.1300/J194v03n04_06

Watson, K. B., Carlson, S. A., Gunn, J. P., Galuska, D. A., O'Connor, A., Greenlund, K. J., & Fulton, J. E. (2016). Physical inactivity among adults aged 50 years and older—United States, 2014. *Morbidity and Mortality Weekly Report, 65*(36), 954–958. doi: <http://dx.doi.org/10.15585/mmwr.mm6536a3externalicon>

Williams, D. M., Anderson, E. S., & Winett, R. A. (2005). A review of the outcome expectancy construct in physical activity research. *Annals of Behavioral Medicine, 29*(1), 70–79. doi:10.1207/s15324796abm2901_10

Williams, S. L., & French, D. P. (2011). What are the most effective intervention techniques for changing physical activity self-efficacy and physical activity behaviour – and are they the same? *Health Education Research, 26*(2), 308–322. <https://doi.org/10.1093/her/cyr005>

Witte, K. (1992). Putting the fear back into fear appeals: The extended parallel process model. *Communication Monographs, 59*(4), 329–349. <https://doi.org/10.1080/03637759209376276>

Witte, K. & Allen, M. (2000). A meta-analysis of fear appeals: Implications for effective public health campaigns. *Health Education and Behavior, 27*(5), 591–615. doi:10.1177/109019810002700506

Wood, W., & Neal, D. T. (2016). Healthy through habit: Interventions for initiating & maintaining health behavior change. *Behavioral Science & Policy, 2*(1), 71–83. doi:10.1353/bsp.2016.0008

Wortman, E. S., & Lewis, J. P. (2021). Gerotranscendence and Alaska Native successful aging in the Aleutian Pribilof Islands, Alaska. *Journal of Cross-Cultural Gerontology, 36*, 43–67. <https://doi.org/10.1007/s10823-020-09421-9>

Zhou, Z., Fu, J., Hong, Y. A., Wang, P., & Fang, Y. (2017) Association between exercise and the risk of dementia: results from a nationwide longitudinal study in China. *BMJ Open*, 7(12), e017497. doi:10.1136/bmjopen-2017-017497

CHAPTER THIRTEEN

# An Alaska Native Integrated Lifecycle, Ecological, and Cultural Approach to Understanding Alzheimer's Disease, Caregiving, and Social Determinants of Health

ROSELLEN M. ROSICH, STEVEN J. HARRIS AND MARIA C. CROUCH

The current zeitgeist in lifespan human development is beginning to move past Eurocentric theories to explore culturally rooted perspectives (Misra & Babu, 2013) and focus on relationships and the ecological context in which people grow and develop (Osher et al., 2020). In addition, the focus on human functioning across the lifespan within an ever-changing world is moving beyond binary categories (i.e., stability vs. change, continuity vs. discontinuity, nature vs. nature) to describe and explain development. The fusion of these categories and the bidirectional influences which emanate from multiple levels of domains (i.e., biological, cognitive, psychosocial) now also include contextual influences, which include historical, socioeconomic, and ecological micro and macro factors. Utilization of metatheoretical perspectives (Overton, 2010), Developmental Systems Theorics (e.g., Ford & Lerner, 1992; Overton, 2015), sociocultural perspectives (e.g., Vygotsky, 1978), and ecological approaches (e.g., Bronfenbrenner, 1977, 2005) have set the stage to move beyond Eurocentric perspectives. This entails identifying and analyzing various culturally embedded phenomena and exploring specific contextual influences on development, thus moving scientific investigation to include the use of Indigenous concepts, methodological innovations, and choice of research issues and problems (Misra & Babu, 2013).

This chapter will provide support for how critical it is for one to move beyond Eurocentric perspectives when describing and explaining growth and development and in understanding perceptions of what constitutes health and health-related issues (i.e., social determinants of health [SDOH]; perceptions of dementia and caregiving). By providing a discussion of the sociocultural, ecological, and historical contextual factors which have impacted Alaska Native people's physical and psychological functioning over several different epochs, one will grasp the complexity of growth and development. In addition, one will also realize that people are impacted across the lifespan not only by biological forces internal to themselves but also by immediate micro-meso-ecosystem ecological factors (e.g., family, relational, local, community), as well as broader macroecological cultural forces (e.g., history, social class, values, customs). Embedded within these various systems are forces associated and directed at Alaska Native peoples' family of origin (e.g., colonialism, oppression, marginalization, racism, discrimination, separation from ancestral land), and these forces at various levels have influenced their views of memory functioning and aging. However, no matter what ecological forces were imposed upon Alaska Native peoples[1], they continued to grow, develop, and adapt. The chapter also provides a description of research on perceptions of memory and dementia and includes a description of the Alaska Native Lifecycle Theory—a theory which is ecologically and contextually relevant, strength-based, and exemplifies cultural/community resilience with respect to views on dementia and caregiving along with how the theory relates to SDOH. A discussion exploring culturally rooted Indigenous perspectives focusing upon relationships, ecological context relating to Alaska Native health inequalities as well as differences in social status and resilience across the lifespan, occurs next. The chapter concludes with recommendations on how Alaska Native theory, in collaboration with Alaska Native Elders and Alaska Native subject matter experts, can inform ADRD health promotion programming for Alaska Native peoples.

1 The plural is being utilized here and continues throughout the chapter (i.e., beliefs, communities, peoples, values), for it denotes the diversity of Alaska Native tribes and the multiple perspectives of their worldviews and belief systems.

## SOCIAL INEQUALITIES, HEALTH, AND THE LIFESPAN PERSPECTIVE

The connection between social inequality and health has been known for centuries. According to Mechanic (2000), the turning point occurred in the mid-19th century, when careful, detailed inquiries in England, France, Germany, and the United States on how the conditions of 'the poor' shortened the lifespan were beginning to take place. Much of this was an outcome of the Industrial Revolution when there were significant increases in disease and poverty. The scientific community during this period was now exploring not only the biological underpinnings of diseases but also the social roots of diseases (Mechanic, 2000). In contemporary times, reemergence of interest in focusing upon social and contextual conditions impacting health in the United States began with Healthy People 2010 SDOH objectives (Healthy People, 2022). SDOH are non-medical and focus on conditions in which people are born, grow, work, live, and age and incorporate the broader macro-level cultural and social factors that impact and shape the ecology in which people grow and develop. Issues regarding social inequalities and SDOH once again became predominant with the COVID-19 health pandemic (e.g., who was succumbing to it as well as accessibility of vaccinations for several different ethnic groups; Centers for Disease Control and Prevention, 2022).

With respect to lifespan and health inequalities, SDOH researchers have indicated that it is beneficial to distinguish between lifespan development and life-course to understand social status as it incorporates various aspects of the social environment and health status (Alwin & Wray, 2005; Braveman et al., 2011; Christensen & Damon, 2022; Singh et al., 2018). For example, Alwin and Wray (2005) argue that "…a life-course concept can be viewed as embedded in a more general [lifespan developmental] perspective" (p. 1). The more general lifespan developmental perspective deals with the length of life for an individual organism and, according to Alwin and Wray (2005), "… draws attention to the temporal scope of inquiry, and a [lifespan developmental] perspective focuses therefore on the effects of social status differences on health across the entire life span" (p. 9). From a lifespan development perspective, this is important as one of the basic tenets of this approach conceptualizes human development as multidimensional and multidirectional processes of growth involving both gains and losses (Baltes, 1987). Furthermore, human development can be viewed as being embedded in multiple social contexts and ecologies. Hence, development is conceived as a dynamic process in which the ontogeny of development interacts with the social environment and within interconnected social settings, which is embedded in a multilayered social and cultural context (Bronfenbrenner, 1977; Dannefer, 1984).

This ecological systems model provides a perspective by which multiple influences (i.e., within concentric and overlapping circles) impact human development and focuses upon larger social-ecological forces within the environment as important contributing factors (Bronfenbrenner, 1977). This theory is an appropriate framework for understanding how outcomes of broader sociocultural ecological non-controllable micro/macro-aggressions directed at one's family of origin (i.e., colonialism, oppression, marginalization, racism, discrimination, separation from ancestral land) can produce internal community psychological outcomes such as historical trauma, historical oppression, and postcolonial distress and how these factors can be interrelated, cumulative, and compounding across the lifespan (Gone et al., 2018; Kirmayer et al., 2014). Hence, the general lifespan developmental concept is the one associated with the study of health inequalities for it can be utilized to address health gains and losses from the moment of conception to death.

The life-course, or lifecycle, refers to the social pathways defined by events and transitions experienced by individuals or groups as exemplified in Alaska Native lives, and the sequences of roles and experiences followed by individuals over particular phases of their lives and over a specific history in which their development has taken place (e.g., Elder, 1974; Elder & Johnson, 2003; Elder et al., 2003). The role of history is important in understanding social inequalities and health disparities within Alaska Native populations. Like research with Indigenous peoples in other countries, forms of adversity that Indigenous communities have faced stem from the history of colonization, the unequal power and exploitative relationships that came with contact with Europeans, and the active suppression of their cultural traditions, community, and autonomy (Kirmayer et al., 2009). A study (Duran et al., 1998) looking at the disruption of Indigenous life in the United States found close parallels to Aboriginal disruptions that took place in Canada and generated a list of six interconnected sociocultural ecological factors which lead to these disruptions: (1) first contact; (2) economic competition; (3) invasion and war; (4) subjugation and reservation; (5) boarding school; and (6) forced relocation and termination. According to this study as well as others (e.g., Hill, 2006), these events produced drastic transformations in Indigenous[2] life, involving loss of identity, trust, and disrupted connection to land and community. This research (Hill, 2006) further supports an adapted and reconceptualized ecological theoretical systems model (Fish & Syed, 2018), which posits that environmental changes that occur across the lifespan reflect the historical factors that have shaped lived

2 Where appropriate, we use Indigenous throughout to represent cross Tribal research and identity inclusive of Alaska Native peoples in addition to Canadian Aboriginal and American Indian Tribes in the Lower 48 U.S.

experiences of both American Indian/Alaska Native (AI/AN) peoples. Moving toward the person and considering culture emphasizes AI/AN ways of being as a priority in identity development in a social environment. By positioning one's culture in the context of historical and contemporary stressors and inequities (i.e., historical oppression), a culturally relevant and holistic strength-based approach is required to understand growth and development and beliefs regarding disease (Crouch & Rosich, 2023).

Another key lifespan theoretical tenet deals with factors likely to place the person at developmental risk at specific "critical" periods of the lifespan. Current research in the area indicates that dimensions of health should be guided by a lifespan perspective, for one must remember that health at any given point in time is influenced by past experiences as well as present circumstances (Max Planck Institute, 2023). This approach "recognizes that poor health and premature death are preceded by the long-term accumulation of experiences that are harmful to health and that critical exposures in early life may have harmful effects many decades later. Accordingly, inequalities in mortality are partly attributable to differences in social status throughout the life course" (Max Planck Institute 2023, p. 1). Developmental risk is associated with the opposite—that of protective factors and the notion of resilience.

## SOCIAL ECOLOGICAL MODEL OF RESILIENCE

While a robust body of literature on resilience has developed over the past several decades, contributing to an understanding of individual and relational dimensions of resilience, the role of culture and context has remained on the sidelines of resilience research (Boyden & Mann, 2005). Most resilience studies have been conducted by researchers in Western contexts, focusing on outcomes deemed positive by members of dominant social groups (e.g., educational attainment) and failing to account for heterogeneous cultural and contextual differences in the expression and experience of resilience (Ungar, 2012). However, alternative perspectives (e.g., those of minorities as well as Indigenous peoples) must be included in the lifespan literature because there are multiple theoretical perspectives on resilience dominated by the majority group and hence not always applicable to those outside of the mainstream culture (Ungar, 2012).

The social-ecological model of resilience highlights the complexity of the construct. Resilience is not only a concept that lies at an individual developmental level but also one that operates at a group or community development level (Unger, 2012); a level of functioning that is not considered much within the resilience area and one that is pertinent to a discussion of Alaska Native peoples' cultural practices and healthcare beliefs. In addition, it can be utilized to discuss the process of navigating and negotiating for health-sustaining resources within a context of adversity. This process is embedded within the individual's social ecology (i.e., individual/group capacity, relationships, community resources, cultural values, and physical resources), and resilience is not considered a state of achievement but rather a process by which a state of well-being is regained or maintained despite adverse experiences (Unger, 2012). Hence, it is made up of gains as well as losses and supports the lifespan developmental approach.

An increasing body of recent work within lifespan development is approaching resilience from a "socioecological" perspective, in which individual risk and resilience (i.e., protective factors) are understood as being shaped by a dynamic environment. This includes the individual's biological and psychosocial experience, as well as the immediate ecological micro-environment of family, school, and neighborhoods and the broader or macro-level environment of social, economic, and political processes (Burnette 2015; Burnette & Figley, 2016; Kirmayer et.al, 2009; Kirmayer et al., 2011). This perspective is also becoming more prevalent among individuals who are studying Indigenous growth and development, as well as understanding perceptions of Alaska Native peoples regarding dementia and caregiving (Crouch & Rosich, 2023). Researchers (Fleming & Ledogar, 2008) have discussed how Indigenous researchers have added a relational, cultural dimension to resilience by focusing on "traditional" activities in people's lives, such as spirituality, healing practices, and language. Healy's (2006) definition of "cultural resilience" augments this addition and expands it to include "…the capacity of a distinct community or cultural system to absorb disturbance and reorganize while undergoing change, to retain key elements of its structure and identity that preserve its distinctiveness" (p. 10). This pattern can be seen in research that is presented later regarding Alaska Native peoples and their perceptions and beliefs on memory, dementia, and caregiving. The developmental trajectory of Alaska Native lives and healthcare beliefs reflect a balance of risks and protective factors (i.e., cultural/community resilience) that have assisted in their adaption but also show how these factors revolved around steadfast cultural beliefs and practices that reflected their view of the lifecycle. Like that suggested by others (e.g., Burnette & Figley, 2016), a culturally congruent view of an Indigenous nature reflects the importance of interconnections and holistic views regarding a balance between the physical, mental, emotional, spiritual, environmental, and community health, which indicates that resilience is multidetermined and occurs across various ecologies (i.e., family, local community, sociocultural). However, to further understand how multiple ecologies may dynamically interact, a discussion of SDOH, health inequalities, and their connections with the historical context of Alaska Native peoples needs to occur.

## SOCIAL DETERMINANTS OF HEALTH, HEALTH INEQUALITIES, AND THE ALASKA NATIVE HISTORICAL CONTEXT

Lifespan human development can be seen as the outcome of dynamic interactions between individuals and several nested environments (Bronfenbrenner, 1977; Bronfenbrenner, 2005; Halfon & Hochstein, 2002). Sociocultural environments impose social norms, establish patterns of social control, affect stress (positively or negatively), and impact environmental opportunities, thereby shaping specific behaviors which may be beneficial or detrimental to health (Pellmar et al., 2002). Consequently, prior research (Lipina, 2016; Singh et al., 2018) has indicated that many aspects of health, including neurocognitive, are affected by environmental factors throughout the lifespan. Namely, SDOH, which is defined as "the non-medical factors that influence health outcomes… the conditions in which people are born, grow, work, live, and age, and the wider set of forces and systems shaping the conditions of daily life" (World Health Organization, 2023, n.p.). These variables can be grouped into five broad categories: economic stability, education access and quality, healthcare access and quality, neighborhood and built environment, and social and community context (Healthy People, 2022). Inequalities in these dimensions play a salient role in enduring and perpetuating health disparities in the United States among certain groups by systematically limiting opportunities to be healthy and receive care (Christensen & Damon, 2022). This is especially apropos to Alaska Native communities.

When addressing health disparities in Alaska Native communities, it is critical to consider the historical context in which these disparities originate. While there are parallels between the history of Alaska Native and American Indian peoples, these are two conglomerate populations representing many diverse cultures, languages, and ways of life. Both groups' pasts, however, have been scarred by settler-colonialism, genocide, forced cultural assimilation, and territorial loss.

The speed at which colonization took place in Alaska is of noteworthy distinction. After landing in Alaska in 1741, Vitus Bering claimed the Alaskan country for the Russian Empire with no concern for the native peoples who had lived there for thousands of years (Carnegie Corporation of New York, 2019). In contrast to European invaders of other regions of the Americas, Russian hunter-traders generally stayed in Alaska just long enough to gather their quota of sea otters and fur seals (Postnikov, 2016). However, that does not mean that the land's Native peoples were not affected by the presence of these invaders. On the contrary, all Alaska Native peoples experienced Russian influence (often negative in character) in some form. Analogous to the American Indian population, Alaska Native peoples were also plagued by smallpox and syphilis upon unwanted contact with Russian settler colonizers. These diseases are suspected to have reduced some Alaska Native populations by as much as 20 %–50 % (Substance Abuse and Mental Health Services Administration, 2018). During early European colonization, private Russian companies conducted the fur trade principally throughout the Aleutian Islands and around Kodiak Island. As a result, the Unangan (Aleut, a term given by Russian colonizers) and Sugpiaq/Sugcestun (Alutiiq) peoples were the most impacted by the Russians' presence in Alaska (Houdek, n.d.). The Russian settlers also inflicted deep trauma by relocating Alaska Native people from smaller villages into a few sizable communities to facilitate convenient control and provision. The lives of many Alaska Native peoples were disturbed for almost a century as the Russian settlers pressured them to be loyal subjects and followers of the Russian Orthodox Church (Alaska Advisory Committee, 2002). Then, in 1867, the United States purchased Alaska from Russia, again with indifference for the Alaska Native peoples who had thrived there long before European arrival. Over the following 150 years, the United States displaced and oppressed Alaska Native peoples from 229 distinct tribes to gain access to natural resources such as oil, whaling, seal fur, salmon, and gold (McAbee, 2021).

While Alaska Native peoples continue to survive through their collective strengths, racism, discrimination, and systemic oppression have placed many Alaska Native communities in precarious situations. Recently, the Alaska Advisory Committee (2002) reported to the United States Commission on Civil Rights that because of factors such as historical discriminatory policies, insufficient resources, and inefficient federal program delivery, American Indian and Alaska Native populations experience poorer health outcomes, less education, and more unemployment compared to other racial and ethnic groups in the United States. For example, from 1819 to the 1970s, the United States embraced policies that established and supported American Indian boarding schools across the country (U.S. Department of the Interior Bureau of Indian Affairs, n.d.). Often, these schools were built in seasonal encampments unsuitable for annual residency. Today, many Native villages inhabit the exact precarious location where these federal government boarding schools had been established (U.S. Government Accountability Office, 2022).

Alaska Native villages face unique infrastructure challenges. The average Native village exists in very remote locations and consists only of a couple of hundred residents, the majority of whom are Alaska Native. Limited transportation has caused transportation expenses of goods and materials to be significantly higher in rural native villages than in most other communities in the contiguous 48 states. Additionally, few native villages have significant commercial activity, a traditional tax base, or a robust real estate market to provide funding for infrastructural development (Gladun et al., 2021; U.S. Government Accountability Office, 2022). Consequently, many Native villages (about 40 %) neither have piped water nor sewer systems (Estus, 2015; U.S. Government Accountability Office, 2022). Due to the confluence of these factors, when compared with the total population of the United States, AI/AN peoples have the highest poverty rate (23 %), among the lowest labor force participation (less than 60 % in 2018), and lower earnings compared with any other major racial group in the United States, resulting in cycles of generationally worsened SDOH, which has been exacerbated by decades-long underfunding and limited medical care access (Allard & Brundage, 2019; Pathak, 2021; Shrider et al., 2021; Smith-Kaprosy et al., 2012). This is very concerning for obvious reasons, but also regarding the risk of Alzheimer's Disease and Related Dementias (ADRD), as a substantial body of literature has highlighted the effects that SDOH has on neurocognitive health.

## ALZHEIMER'S DISEASE AND RELATED DEMENTIAS AND LIFESPAN ADVERSITY

Racial and ethnic minority groups and those with low socioeconomic status, as measured by education and lower income, are disproportionately affected by ADRD (Marden et al., 2017; Mayeda et al., 2016). Early-life food insecurity significantly increases the risk of cognitive impairment and ADRD later in life (Momtaz et al., 2014; Na et al., 2020; Tong et al., 2018). Moreover, a longitudinal study of cognitively unimpaired adults (*N*= 601) found that living in the most disadvantaged neighborhoods was associated with cognitive decline and cortical thinning in ADRD signature regions (Hunt et al., 2020). However, the interactions between chronic stressors and different SDOHs and their impact on health outcomes are complex and intricately interwoven (Braveman et al., 2011; Christensen & Damon, 2022). Recently, researchers have proposed that ADRD may not have a single origin but should be viewed as a spectrum of numerous chronic pathogenic modes converging on the continual stressing of central nervous system neurons (i.e., Theory of Multipathology Convergence, Decourt et al., 2022).

SDOH of Alaska Native peoples during early life may also increase their risk of developing ADRD later in life. Unfortunately, early neurodevelopmental stages are particularly vulnerable to environmental stressors such as abuse, substance misuse, mother separation, food insecurity, and neuroinflammation (Miller et.al., 2011). Early stressful events like poverty and racial discrimination can cause the release of cortisol, cytokines, and other chemicals that can harm the nervous system even within the perinatal period of life (Braveman et al., 2011; McEwen & Gianaros, 2010; Seeman et al., 2010; Williams & Mohammed, 2008). Moreover, a recent systematic review by Lemche (2018) proposed that early life stress may influence late-onset ADRD by interfering with the expression of tau protein (a major pathogenic factor of ADRD) in early ontogeny, which may, in turn, increase susceptibility. Considering that one in three AI/AN children live in poverty and that AI/AN people frequently experience geographic isolation, low income, low educational achievement, prejudice, stigma, and discrimination (Office of Minority Health, n.d.; Redbird, 2020), accumulating neural "insults" from adversity, especially during early life, may predispose AI/AN individuals to develop ADRD and dramatically increase the risk for other compounding diseases. Alaska Native peoples are disproportionately affected by obesity, diabetes, cardiovascular disease, metabolic syndrome, congenital heart disease, and stroke, which are all established as risk factors of ADRD (Benjamin et al., 2019; Breathett et al., 2020; Hutchinson & Shin, 2014; Mayo Clinic, 2022).

## ALASKA NATIVE LIFECYCLE AND CULTURAL PERSPECTIVES

When discussing the impact of SDOH in the context of health inequalities, it is crucial to analyze the long-lasting effects of colonization on Alaska Native communities. Traditional ways of life, culture, language, and beliefs have been the foundation of Alaska Native identities for centuries, but colonization has disrupted the transmission of these traditions (Kawagley et al., 1998; Napoleon, 2013). This cultural disconnection is a major factor in the high rates of mental health problems, substance use disorders, domestic violence, and suicide in AI/AN populations (Gone et al., 2019; Skewes & Blume, 2019). The lasting effects of colonization continue to affect SDOH today, as seen in the cultural and institutional systems that are often hostile to traditional ways of life. Postcolonial distress and chronic stressors, like poverty and food insecurity, also have a negative impact on SDOH across the lifespan (Kirmayer et al., 2014). Systemic racism exacerbates these challenges, leading to health disparities; barriers to accessing basic needs like healthcare, education, and clean water; and increased rates of age-related diseases, such as ADRD. To study the cultural beliefs and perceptions of Alaska

Native Elders[3] regarding memory and aging, the Alaska Native Elder Memory and Dementia Study sampled 12 Alaska Native Elders (4 males, 8 females) who were selected through a snowball method (Crouch & Rosich, 2023). Participants were recruited through personal connections of the researchers, colleagues with established ties to the Alaska Native Elder community, and referrals from previous participants. The average age of participants was 73, with tribal heritage from different Indigenous groups in Alaska such as Aleut, Athabascan, Inupiaq, Tsimshian, and Yup'ik. The participants were asked about topics such as their experiences with memory, ADRD, healthy aging practices, prevalence, assessment and management, caregiving, personal experiences with ADRD, utilization of healthcare services, and any additional questions they felt were important. As a result of this final question, one Elder emphasized the significance of Alaska Native peoples' spirituality, which was later incorporated into the study and became a central theme. Qualitative analysis in NVivo software revealed eight themes: (1) Traditional Knowledge and Values; (2) Caregiving Networks; (3) Memory Function; (4) Alaska Native Spirituality; (5) Stories, Generative Sharing, and Healing; (6) Historical Change; (7) Connection, Communication, and Compassion; and (8) Assisted Living. These themes were interrelated and portrayed a cultural viewpoint and story linked to colonization, societal change, health disparities, SDOH, and the healing power of culture on healthy aging, disease, and the lifecycle.

The participants emphasized that family and community relationships across their life play a crucial role in their health, well-being, and SDOH (Crouch et al., 2023a, 2023b; Crouch, & Rosich, 2023). While access to resources and opportunities is determined by larger systemic, structural, and political factors (i.e., macro-level), the participants recognized that the effectiveness and relevance of these resources are also tied to their cultural significance. They perceived that achieving a healthy balance between Western and Alaska Native cultures (living in both worlds) and decolonizing and incorporating Alaska Native values into Western contexts is essential for comprehensive health. The Alaska Native cultural perspective on aging and memory is deeply connected to a person's Indigenous identity, their coping mechanisms for historical and current traumas, and the ways in which they achieve success based on both Western and Indigenous standards of human development. Further, the Alaska Native Elder Memory and Dementia Study emphasizes the significance of Eldership within the Alaska Native lifecycle.

3 Elder/elder are descriptors of older Alaska Native people used by the culture and supported in its use by the Alaska Native Research Oversight Committee. The lowercase elder signifies all Alaska Natives between the ages of 54–60 and above, while the uppercase Elder signifies cultural bearers and holders of wisdom who are entrusted with the power to speak for the community in areas of cultural importance.

Elders symbolically (e.g., notion of ancestors watching over a person) and actively give love (e.g., listen, teach), pass on their culture and wisdom, and provide a sense of inclusion and recognition of ancestral wisdom and cultural practices. This research also recognizes the spiritual importance of Elders in their communities, as they hold valuable knowledge and are closer to the universe.

The beginning of life and the journey toward death are interconnected and inseparable, according to Alaska Native beliefs (Kawagley et al., 1998; Napoleon, 2013). The life-death cycle is closely tied to cultural rituals and ceremonies, which play a significant role in Alaska Native life and contribute to the quality and prosperity of the community. The end of one's lifespan is a crucial part of Alaska Native cultural practices, providing support and comfort to the community, and helping in the transition to the afterlife. This is especially important in the case of ADRD. An Alaska Native framework of the lifecycle can bring positive change and assist individuals in transitioning to the next life (Kawagley et al., 1998). Spirituality plays a central role in culturally relevant health equity, promoting growth, reflection, and connection (Crouch et al., 2023a, 2023b; Crouch, & Rosich, 2023). To understand the relationships between spirituality, ceremony, and successful lifespan development within the Alaska Native community, it is necessary to consider the underlying Alaska Native theories that shape these connections.

The Elluarrluteng Ilakutellriit is a Yupiit[4] theory of the Alaska Native lifecycle that emphasizes the importance of accessing one's inherent spiritual and cultural knowledge for success and critical consciousness (Orutsararmuit Native Council, 2008). The Elluarrluteng Ilakutellriit theory explains the spiritual and cultural development of a person as they move through different stages in life and their relationship with the universe, their physical body, community, and other relationships (Elizabeth Sunnyboy, Yup'ik, personal communication, 2015). It is divided into four quadrants: physical world, emotional world, mental world, and spiritual world. Each quadrant represents different aspects of life and their interconnectivity. The Elluarrluteng Ilakutellriit theory provides a holistic understanding of lifespan development and aging and consists of ceremonies and rituals that have been present since the beginning of recorded time and are reflective of significant milestones in life. It also sets the stage for a culturally informed discussion of SDOH across the lifespan.

The Alaska Native Lifecycle theory is a comprehensive representation of an Alaska Native framework of aging, reconciling historical and contemporary

4 There are 229 Federally recognized tribes living in Alaska with diverse belief systems; however, all the systems are grounded within respect, responsibility, kindness, empathy, generosity, and self-awareness. This EI theory reflects the most important spiritual and cultural factors in development through spiritual and cultural factors in development through different stages in life.

contexts (Crouch & Rosich, 2023). The model incorporates Western theories of development, the EI theory, and the Alaska Native Elder Memory and Dementia Study to show how community has been the foundation of successful development and aging across the lifespan. It takes into consideration the history of a people, SDOH, and epistemology that have been excluded from dominant theoretical and developmental paradigms. The model is divided into four quadrants: the physical world, emotional world, mental world, and spiritual world. Each quadrant reflects various aspects of development, such as cultural understandings of memory, caregiving, trauma, resilience, and spiritual views of death and dying. The themes in each quadrant are fluid throughout the model and represent key aspects of Alaska Native development and aging at different stages of life, all of which are understood through SDOH and the relationships to the Alaska Native Elder Memory and Dementia Study themes (see Figure 13.1).

The Physical World encompasses the start of one's physical existence and fundamental lessons about oneself and the community (Crouch & Rosich, 2023). This quadrant relates to cultural perspectives on memory function and ADRD, with

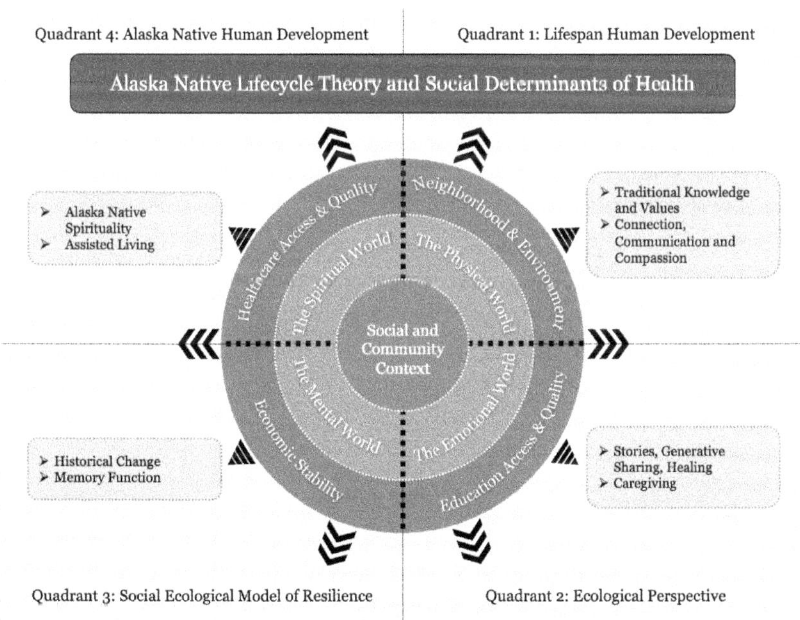


Figure 13.1: The Alaska Native Lifecycle Theory and Social Determinants of Health, adapted from Crouch & Rosich, 2023

the themes being (1) traditional knowledge and values and (2) connection, communication, and compassion. These themes play a crucial role in shaping a person's mental perspective on their self-identity, relationships, surroundings, and behavior as interdependent and independent beings in the world. Trauma during this crucial stage of development can have the most severe consequences, both in modern theory and in the Alaska Native worldview (Bowlby, 1988). This stage sets the foundation for successful aging or memory decline. This domain also aligns with sociocultural theory (Vygotsky, 1978) and Indigenous cultural identity development in numerous ways, but, most significantly, by emphasizing that culture plays the most crucial role in making connections and building a foundation for later life (Chandler, 2013; Cole et al., 1978). This quadrant states that a person begins their life, reaches important early developmental and cultural milestones, and learns how to care for themselves and others as part of their sociocultural community. This is reflected in the neighborhood and environment SDOH (Healthy People, 2022). This composes a person's environment where they live and work. For Alaska Native peoples this means safe neighborhoods, interconnected relationships, and transportation to name a few—all of which play a role in barriers and access to optimal early development and mitigation of parental and caregiver stressors that sets the stage for later life. The transition from this quadrant to the next is marked by learning and practicing communal helping and sharing, the fundamental principles of caregiving. Namely, roles within family, tribe, and community are changing and developing toward the advancement of the person and preservation of culture.

The Emotional World is an aspect of the lifecycle that is largely shaped by the interaction between a person's behavior within the tribe, their feelings toward others, and their self-perception (Crouch & Rosich, 2023). The key themes of (1) stories, generative sharing, and healing and (2) caregiving play a crucial role in helping Alaska Native individuals during their adolescence and early adulthood to develop the skills necessary to care for themselves, others, and the land. In this stage of life, individuals acquire important cultural skills, such as hunting, sewing, and gathering, which help them develop discipline, healthy nutrition, intergenerational connections and support, and a connection with the natural and spiritual world that promotes holistic health, memory and aging, and healing. Ecological theory is a useful framework to understand the impact of laws, dominant society, community norms, and tribal expectations on this stage of development (Bronfenbrenner, 1977). For example, during this time, young people learn about personal and political sovereignty, Western systems and expectations, and ceremony and rituals. Additionally, many grow up in multigenerational households or communities, where they take on caregiving roles for both young children and elders. The SDOH domain of "Education Access and Quality" is the most salient for Alaska Native peoples in this aspect of their lives (Healthy People, 2022). Colonial histories of segregation, traumas, and boarding schools have drastically impeded both educational quality, access, and achievement (Barnhardt, 2001). However, tribal sovereignty, prosperity, and resilience has been integral to mitigating barriers and improving SDOH (Tippeconnic, 1999).

The Mental World is a significant part of the lifespan where trauma and resilience can manifest (Crouch & Rosich, 2023). In accordance with Alaska Native beliefs, all Indigenous peoples have undergone trauma either through intergenerational transmission or contemporary events such as lateral violence and abuse (Gone et al., 2019; Napoleon, 2013). Addressing these traumas is considered a major milestone in adulthood. The themes of (1) historical change and (2) memory function are central to this quadrant. A healthy mind and body are crucial for a fulfilling life, and this quadrant provides opportunities for healing and promoting healing in others. Cultural survival and thriving also play a key role in resilience, as it is expressed through systems that impact the individual, community, and relationships (Ungar, 2012). Trauma and unhealed trauma can lead to memory decline and disrupt a successful lifecycle. The SDOH domain of economic stability is critical in this aspect of life, given that lower socioeconomic status, poverty, and limited resources impact one's holistic health and can create disparities therein (Healthy People, 2022; Hutchinson & Shin, 2014; Redbird, 2020). This quadrant leads to the next stage in life where one prepares for family caregiving responsibilities, becoming an Elder, and the physical death.

The Spiritual World deals with topics like death and dying, different religious beliefs about the afterlife, and the practicalities of end-of-life care (Crouch & Rosich, 2023). This includes themes of (1) Alaska Native spirituality and (2) assisted living. In traditional Alaska Native communities, care for loved ones was provided until their death, but Western practices have influenced this and often involve care outside of the home or community (e.g., hospital or nursing home; Anderson & Woticky, 2018; Racine et al., 2022). This final aspect brings together all the previous aspects and shows how they contribute to a person's overall health and wellbeing throughout their life, including reducing memory loss, forming close relationships between generations, and giving meaning to issues surrounding ADRD, death, and beyond. This model represents the continuous cycle of family life in Alaska Native communities, where caregiving (of self, others, younger generations) plays a crucial role in maintaining function and continuity (Crouch & Rosich, 2023; McGoldrick, 1992). The SDOH domain of healthcare access and quality becomes most salient in this aspect of the lifecycle (Anderson & Woticky, 2018; Healthy People, 2022). Not only does culture determine the process, ceremony, and meaning around dying, but it also can be best supported within the medical setting. Further, all SDOH's are embedded within the SDOH domain of social and community context (Healthy People, 2022; see center circle within Figure 13.1) for Alaska Native peoples believe everything is done in community and with ancestors, relatives, family, and friends to the betterment of one another (Kawagley et al., 1998). One does not develop independently of their sociocultural environment; rather, their development is a product of it.

## HEALTH COMMUNICATION AND DESIGNING ALASKA NATIVE HEALTH CAMPAIGNS

The work we have done has supported the planning of an ADRD health promotion program. This includes developing a rationale based on Alaska Native theory and in collaboration with Alaska Native Elders and Alaska Native subject matter experts (i.e., meetings and a subsequent survey supporting the teaching modules); conducting in-depth interviews with Alaska Native Elders about beliefs and perceptions of ADRD to inform assessment of patient and caregiver needs; and taking a public health and ecological perspective that is based in theory-driven intrapersonal and community level factors to understand and explain the data for optimal and culturally relevant health promotion (McKenzie, 2009). Next steps would include individual level and community level assessment to further understand and contextualize needs for patients, families, and caregivers at the intersection of prevention, treatment, and health promotion. Community level factors span institutional rules and regulations (e.g., tribal health systems, healthcare protocols); community systems and partners (e.g., local tribal organizations, senior centers); and state and federal policy (e.g., epidemiology, allocation of resources; Rimer & Glanz, 2005).

Recommendations for designing relevant health promotion programming include involvement of Alaska Native Elders and caregivers for they are integral to every phase of the programming from planning to implementation to evaluation (Crouch et al., 2023b; McKenzie, 2009). A recent review of health promotion programming for global Indigenous healthy aging observed that an intergenerational approach is salient for cultural responsivity and program sustainability (Oosman et al., 2021). Hence, designing health campaigns must focus on the following: (1) cultural stories; (2) Indigenous imagery; and (3) Indigenous language, words, and place. Designing health campaigns should also be followed up with continued evaluation of cultural salience and applicability. Recommended health promotion programming that is indigenized is critical to access and reach, and usability and must include: (1) health literacy interventions that support medical provider–patient relationship building, engagement, and knowledge sharing; (2) educational media campaigns for awareness raising and prevention; (3) website repository of health communication and health promotion resources; and, lastly, (4) community art events to promote dialogue, share culture, create collaboration, and promote health literacy.

From a broader provider perspective, mechanisms for reimbursement for traditional healers must be expanded for studies have demonstrated that traditional cultural healing practices and cultural teachings are essential in promoting AI/AN peoples' mental health, recovery, and healing (Buchwald et al., 2000; Garroutte et al., 2003). Additionally, a shift in emphasis from evidence-based practices to practice-based must occur if lawmakers and service providers genuinely want to be culturally appropriate. They must become more aware of what people are doing in their communities that are successful, and it is critical to support ongoing efforts and assist communities in developing or demonstrating evidence for their initiatives. Finally, to adequately address AI/AN peoples' health needs, it is important to integrate mechanisms and support within health systems that address the variety of stressors (e.g., SDOH, racism, discrimination, historical traumas) AI/AN experience and that acknowledges the current realities of AI/AN peoples.

## CONCLUSIONS

The Alaska Native Lifecycle theory presented in this chapter integrates historical and contemporary contexts into a comprehensive alternative framework regarding growth, development, and aging. The theory is ecologically and contextually relevant, strength based, and exemplifies community resilience with respect to views on memory, ADRD, and aging. Further this Alaska Native theory can be used to shed light on how development and socialization can be disrupted during each pathway of the lifecycle (i.e., physical, emotional, mental, spiritual) by external micro-macro ecological forces.

Ontogenetic development is complex; however, it appears clear that historical oppression, colonialism, discrimination, and racism can disrupt development and socialization at critical periods and lead to health inequalities and social status differences which persist across the lifespan. Health at any given time is influenced by past experiences as well as present circumstances, and in the case of Alaska Native peoples, there is an interdependence between the two. In this case it is important to understand that… "The past is not a burden. It is a scaffold which brought us to this day. We are free to be who we are—to create our own life out of our past and out of the present. We are our ancestors. When we heal ourselves, we also heal our ancestors, our grandmothers, our grandfathers, and our children. When we heal ourselves, we heal Mother Earth."—Rita Pitka Blumenstein (Alaska Native Elder/Tribal Doctor; AIANNH, 2021).

## ACKNOWLEDGMENTS

This chapter was directly influenced by the decolonizing work and the traditional knowledge of the Ancestors, Elders, and peoples of the Yukon-Kuskokwim region of Alaska. It was informed by the work of Elizabeth Sunnyboy (Yupik) through the Yukon-Kuskokwim Health Corporation. She and others recorded the words and wisdom of Elders, received their guidance on the content, and obtained their permission to use it for the purposes of indigenizing and teaching. We would like to recognize the following people who directly contributed:

| | | |
|---|---|---|
| Peter Jacobs, Sr. | Zacharia Stevens | William Lomack |
| William Lomack | Annabelle Olick | Esther Green |
| Jonathan Johnson | Winifred Beans | Nastasia Andrew |
| Lucy Beaver | Helen Seton | Bessie Alexie |
| Lena Long | Sophie Jenkins | Henry Guy |
| Peter Jacobs, Sr. | Zacharia Stevens | Elizabeth Sunnyboy |

We would like to thank all the Ancestors, Elders, and people involved not listed here.

## REFERENCES

AIANNH (2021, Aug 10). The passing of a legend: Rita Pitka Blumenstein (1936-August 6, 2021). <https://www.aiannhcaucus.com/post/the-passing-of-a-legend-rita-pitka-blumenstein-1936-august-6-2021>

Alaska Advisory Committee. (2002). *Racism's frontier: The untold story of discrimination and division in Alaska*. Retrieved Jan 5, 2023, from <https://www.usccr.gov/files/pubs/sac/ak0402/ak02.pdf>

Allard, D., & Brundage, V. (2019). American Indians and Alaska Natives in the U.S. labor force. *Monthly Labor Review*. <https://doi.org/10.21916/mlr.2019.24>

Alwin, D. F., & Wray, L. A. (2005). A life-span developmental perspective on social status and health. *The Journals of Gerontology: Series B: Psychological Sciences and Social Sciences, 60*(Suppl 2), 7–14. <https://doi.org/10.1093/geronb/60.Special_Issue_2.S7>

Anderson, M., & Woticky, G. (2018). The end of life is an auspicious opportunity for healing: Decolonizing death and dying for urban Indigenous people. *International Journal of Indigenous Health, 13*(2), 48–60. <https://doi.org/10.18357/ijih.v13i2.32062>

Baltes, P. (1987). Theoretical propositions of life-span developmental psychology: On the dynamics between growth and decline. *Developmental Psychology, 23*, 611–626. <http://dx.doi.org/10.1037/0012-1649.23.5.611>

Barnhardt, C. (2001). A history of schooling for Alaska Native people. *Journal of American Indian Education, 40*(1), 1–30. <https://www.jstor.org/stable/24398586>

Benjamin, E. J., Muntner, P., Alonso, A., Bittencourt, M. S., Callaway, C. W., Carson, A. P., Chamberlain, A. M., Chang, A. R., Cheng, S., Das, S. R., Delling, F. N., Djousse, L., Elkind, M. S., Ferguson, J. F., Fornage, M., Jordan, L. C., Khan, S. S., Kissela, B. M., Knutson, K. L., Virani, S. S. (2019). Heart disease and stroke statistics—2019 update: A Report from the American Heart Association. *Circulation,* 139(10). <https://doi.org/10.1161/cir.0000000000000659>

Bowlby, J. (1988). *A secure base: Parent-child attachment and healthy human development*. New York, NY: Basic Books.

Boyden, J., & Mann, G. (2005). Children's risk, resilience, and coping in extreme situations. In M. Ungar (Ed.), *Handbook for working with children and youth: Pathways to resilience across cultures and contexts*, pp. 3–25. Thousand Oaks, CA: Sage Publications.

Braveman, P., Egerter, S., & Williams, D. R. (2011). The social determinants of health: Coming of age. *Annual Review of Public Health, 32*(1), 381–398. <https://doi.org/10.1146/annurev-publhealth-031210-101218>

Breathett, K., Sims, M., Gross, M., Jackson, E. A., Jones, E. J., Navas-Acien, A., Taylor, H., Thomas, K. L., & Howard, B. V. (2020). Cardiovascular health in American Indians and Alaska Natives: A scientific statement from the American Heart Association. *Circulation, 141*(25). <https://doi.org/10.1161/cir.0000000000000773>

Bronfenbrenner, U. (1977). Toward an experimental ecology of human development. *The American Psychologist, 32*(7), 513–531. <https://doi.org/10.1037/0003-066X.32.7.513>

Bronfenbrenner, U. (2005). Ecological systems theory. In U. Bronfenbrenner (Ed.), *Making human beings human: Bioecological perspectives on human development*, pp. 106–173. Thousand Oaks, CA: Sage Publications.

Buchwald, D., Beals, J., & Manson, S. M. (2000). Use of traditional health practices among native Americans in a primary care setting. *Medical Care, 38*(12), 1191–1199. <http://www.jstor.org/stable/3767997>

Burnette, C. (2015). Historical oppression and intimate partner violence experienced by indigenous women in the United States: Understanding connections. *Social Service Review, 89* (3), 531–563. <https://doi.org/10.1086/683336>

Burnette, C. E., & Figley, C. R. (2016). Historical oppression, resilience, and transcendence: Can a holistic framework help explain violence experienced by indigenous people? *Social Work, 62*(1), 37–44. <https://doi.org/10.1093/sw/sww065>

Carnegie Corporation of New York. (2019). *The exploration of Alaska. U.S.-Russia relations: Quest for stability*. Retrieved January 29, 2023, from <https://usrussiarelations.org/2/timeline/first-contact/3>

Centers for Disease Control and Prevention, CDC. (2022). CDC COVID-19 Response Health Equity Strategy. Retrieved Feb 1, 2023, from <https://www.cdc.gov/coronavirus/2019-ncov/community/health-equity/cdc-strategy.html>

Christensen, L., & Damon, S. (2022). Social Determinants of Health and response to disease associated with health outcomes of American Indian and Alaska Native Patients. *JAMA Network Open,* 5(3), e224827. <https://doi.org/10.1001/jamanetworkopen.2022.4827>

Chandler, M. J. (2013). On being Indigenous: An essay on the hermeneutics of "cultural identity". *Human Development, 56*(2), 83–97. <https://doi.org/10.1159/000345775>

Cole, M., John-Steiner, V., Scribner, S., & Souberman, E. (Eds.). (1978). *Mind in society: The development of higher psychological processes.* L. S. Vygotsky. Harvard University Press.

Crouch, M. C., Cheromiah Salazar, M. B. R., Harris, S. J., & Rosich, R. M. (2023a). Dementia, substance misuse, and social determinants of health: American Indian and Alaska Native peoples' prevention, service, and care. *Chronic Stress, 7,* 1–9. <https://doi.org/10.1177/24705470 2211494>

Crouch, M. C., Kim, S. M., Asquith-Heinz, Z., Decker, E., Andrew, N. T., Lewis, J. P., & Rosich, R. M. (2023b). Indigenous Elder-centered methodology: Research that decolonizes and indigenizes *AlterNative: An International Journal of Indigenous Peoples, 19*(2), 1–10, <https://doi.org/10.1177/ 11771801231155437>

Crouch, M. C., & Rosich, R. (2023). Continuity, connectedness, and community: An Alaska Native lifecycle explanatory model of caregiving networks. In J. P. Lewis, & T. Heinonen (Eds.), *Social aspects of aging in Indigenous communities.* Oxford, UK: Oxford University Press.

Dannefer, D. (1984). Adult development and social theory: A paradigmatic reappraisal. *American Sociological Review, 49*(1), 100– 116. <https://doi.org/10.2307/2095560>

Decourt, B., D'Souza, G. X., Shi, J., Ritter, A., Suazo, J., & Sabbagh, M. N. (2022). The cause of Alzheimer's Disease: The theory of multipathology convergence to chronic neuronal stress. *Aging and Disease, 13*(1), 37. <https://doi.org/10.14336/ad.2021.0529>

Duran, E., Duran, B., Yellow Horse Brave Heart, M., & Yellow Horse-Davis, S. (1998). Healing the American Indian soul wound. In Danieli, Y. (Eds.), *International handbook of multigenerational legacies of trauma.* Plenum Press. <https://doi.10.1007/978-1-4757-5567-1>

Elder, G. H., Jr. (1974). *Children of the great depression: Social change in life experience.* Chicago, IL: University of Chicago Press.

Elder, G. H, Jr, & Johnson, M. K. (2003). The life course and aging: Challenges, lessons, and new directions. In R. A. Settersten (Ed.), *Invitation to the life course: Toward new understandings of later life,* pp. 49–81. Amityville, NY: Baywood.

Elder, G. H., Jr., Johnson, M. K., & Crosnoe, R. (2003). The *Emergence and development of life course theory.* In J. T. Mortimer & M. J. Shanahan (Eds.), *Handbook of the life course. Handbooks of sociology and social research.* Springer, Boston, MA. <https://doi.org/10.1007/978-0-306-48247-2_1>

Estus, J. (2015). For rural Alaskans, lack of running water and sewage a source of health problems. *USC Annenberg Center for Health Journalism.* Retrieved Jan 5, 2023, from <https://centerforhealthjournalism.org/2015/06/04/rural-alaskans-lack-running-water-and-sewage-results-health-problems>

Fleming J, & Ledogar RJ. (2008). Resilience, an evolving concept: A review of literature relevant to aboriginal research. *Pimatisiwin, 6*(2), 7–23.

Fish, J., & Syed, M. (2018). Native Americans in higher education: An ecological systems perspective. *Journal of College Student Development, 59*(4), 387–403.. <https://doi:10.1353/csd.2018.0038>

Ford, D. H., & Lerner, R. M. (1992). *Developmental Systems Theory: An Integrative Approach.* Thousand Oaks, CA: Sage Publications, Inc.

Garroutte, E. M., Goldberg, J., Beals, J., Herrell, R., & Manson, S. M. (2003). Spirituality and attempted suicide among American Indians. *Social Science & Medicine, 56*(7), 1571–1579. <https://doi.org/10.1016/s0277-9536(02)00157-0>

Gladun, E., Nysten-Haarala, S., & Tulaeva, S. (2021). Indigenous economies in the Arctic. *Elementa: Science of the Anthropocene,* 9(1). <https://doi.org/10.1525/elementa.2019.00088>

Gone, J. P., Hartmann, W. E., Pomerville, A., Wendt, D. C., Klem, S. H., & Burrage, R. L. (2019). The impact of historical trauma on health outcomes for indigenous populations in the USA and Canada: A systematic review. *The American Psychologist, 74*(1), 20–35. <https://doi.org/10.1037/amp0000338>

Halfon, N., & Hochstein, M. (2002). Life course health development: An integrated wframework for developing health, policy, and research. *Milbank Quarterly, 80*(3), 433–479. <https://doi.org/10.1111/1468-0009.00019>

Healy, P. (2006). Human rights and intercultural relations: A hermeneutico-dialogical an approach. *Philosophy & Social Criticism, 32*(4), 513–541. <https://doi.org/10.1177/0191453706064023>

Healthy People 2030. (2022). Social determinants of health. *U.S. Department of Health and Human Services.* Retrieved Jan 5, 2023, from <https://health.gov/healthypeople/priority-areas/social-determinants-health>

Hill, D. L. (2006). Sense of belonging as connectedness, American Indian worldview, and mental health. *Archives of Psychiatric Nursing*, 20(5), 210–216.

Houdek, J. (n.d.). *Russian America.* LitSite Alaska. Retrieved January 29, 2023, from <http://www.litsitealaska.org/index.cfm?section=digital-archives&page=Government&cat=Making-of-Alaska&viewpost=2&ContentId=2738>

Hunt, J. F. V., Buckingham, W., Kim, A. J., Oh, J., Vogt, N. M., Jonaitis, E. M., Hunt, T. K., Zuelsdorff, M., Powell, R., Norton, D., Rissman, R. A., Asthana, S., Okonkwo, O. C., Johnson, S. C., Kind, A. J. H., & Bendlin, B. B. (2020). Association of neighborhood-level disadvantage with cerebral and hippocampal volume. *JAMA Neurology, 77*(4), 451. <https://doi.org/10.1001/jamaneurol.2019.4501>

Hutchinson, R. N., & Shin, S. (2014). Systematic review of health disparities for cardiovascular diseases and associated factors among American Indian and Alaska Native populations. *PloS One, 9*(1), e80973–e80973. <https://doi.org/10.1371/journal.pone.0080973>

Kawagley, A. O., Norris-Tull, D., & Norris-Tull, R. A. (1998). The Indigenous worldview of Yupiaq culture: Its scientific nature and relevance to the practice and teaching of science. *Journal of Research in Science Teaching, 35*(2), 133–144. <https://doi.org/10.1002/(SICI)1098-2736(199802)35:2<133::AID-TEA4>3.0.CO;2-T>

Kirmayer, L. J., Sedhev, M., Whitley, R., Dandeneau, S., & Isaac, C. (2009). Community resilience: Models, metaphors, and measures. *Journal of Aboriginal Health*, 7(1), 62–117.

Kirmayer, L. J., Dandeneau, S., Marshall, E., Phillips, M. K., & Williamson, K. J. (2011). Rethinking resilience from indigenous perspectives. *The Canadian Journal of Psychiatry, 56*, 84–9. <https://doi:10.1177/070674371105600203>

Kirmayer, L. J., Gone, J. P., & Moses, J. (2014). Rethinking historical trauma. *Transcultural Psychiatry, 51*(3), 299–319. <https://doi.org/10.1177/1363461514536358>

Lemche, E. (2018). Early life stress and epigenetics in late-onset Alzheimer's Dementia: A systematic review. *Current Genomics, 19*(7), 522–602. <https://doi.org/10.2174/13892029196661712291 45156>

Lipina, S. J. (2016). The biological side of social determinants: Neural costs of childhood poverty. *PROSPECTS, 46*(2), 265–280. <https://doi.org/10.1007/s11125-017-9390-0>

Marden, J., Tchetgen, E., Kawachi, I., & Glymour, M. (2017). Contribution of socioeconomic status at 3 life-course periods to late-life memory function and decline: Early and late predictors of dementia risk. *American Journal of Epidemiology, 186*(7), 805–814. <https://doi.org/10.1093/aje/kwx155>

Max Planck Institute for Demographic Research. (2023). *Population Health: Social and Economic Determinants in Health and Life Expectancy.* Retrieved March 4, 2023, from <https://www.demogr.mpg.de/en/research_6120/department_myrskylae_11664/population_health_3922/social_and_economic_determinants_in_health_and_life_expectancy_5103>

Mayeda, E., Glymour, M., Quesenberry, C., & Whitmer, R. (2016). Inequalities in dementia incidence between six racial and ethnic groups over 14 years. *Alzheimer's & Dementia, 12*(3), 216–224. <https://doi.org/10.1016/j.jalz.2015.12.007>

Mayo Clinic. (2022). *Alzheimer's disease* (CON-20155101). Retrieved Jan 5, 2023, from <https://www.mayoclinic.org/diseases-conditions/alzheimers-disease/symptoms-causes/syc-20350447>.

McAbee, T. (2021). *Life after colonization.* Public Health Post. Retrieved Jan 5, 2023, from <https://www.publichealthpost.org/research/life-after-colonization/>

McEwen, B. S., & Gianaros, P. J. (2010). Central role of the brain in stress and adaptation: Links to socioeconomic status, health, and disease. *Annals of the New York Academy of Sciences, 1186*(1), 190–222. <https://doi.org/10.1111/j.1749-6632.2009.05331.x>

McGoldrick, M. (1992). Ethnicity and the family life cycle. *Family Business Review, 5*(4), 437–459. <https://doi.org/10.1111/j.1741-6248.1992.00437.x>

McKenzie, J. F. (2009). *Planning, implementing, and evaluating health promotion programs, a primer* (5th ed.). San Francisco, CA: Pearson/Benjamin Cummings.

Mechanic, D., (2000). Essay: Rediscovering the social determinants of health, *Health Affairs, 19*(3), 269–276. <https://doi/10.1377/hlthaff.19.3.269>

Miller, G. E., Chen, E., & Parker, K. J. (2011). Psychological stress in childhood and susceptibility to the chronic diseases of aging: Moving toward a model of behavioral and biological mechanisms. *Psychological Bulletin, 137*(6), 959–997. <https://doi.org/10.1037/a0024768>

Misra, G., & Babu, N. (2013). Emerging perspectives on human development research. *Psychological Studies, 58*, 349–352. <https://doi.org/10.1007/s12646-013-0234-6>

Momtaz, Y., Haron, S., Hamid, T., Ibrahim, R., & Masud, J. (2014). Does food insufficiency in childhood contribute to dementia in later life? *Clinical Interventions in Aging, 49*. <https://doi.org/10.2147/cia.s69220>

Na, M., Dou, N., Ji, N., Xie, D., Huang, J., Tucker, K. L., & Gao, X. (2020). Food insecurity and cognitive function in middle to older adulthood: A systematic review. *Advances in Nutrition, 11*(3), 667–676. <https://doi.org/10.1093/advances/nmz122>

Napoleon, H., (2013). *Yuuyaraq: The way of the human being.* Anchorage Public Library.

Office of Minority Health. (n.d.). Profile: American Indian/Alaska Native. U.S. Department of Health & Human Services. Retrieved February 1, 2023, from <https://minorityhealth.hhs.gov/omh/browse.aspx?lvl=3&lvlid=62>

Oosman, S., Nisbet, C., Smith, L., & Abonyi, S. (2021). Health promotion interventions supporting Indigenous healthy aging: A scoping review. *International Journal of Circumpolar Health, 80*(1), 1950391. <https://doi.org/10.1080/22423982.2021.1950391>

Orutsararmuit Native Council (2008). *Healthy families. Yupik style* [PowerPoint slides]. <https://peerta.acf.hhs.gov/sites/default/files/public/uploaded_files/Association%20of%20Village%20Council%20Presidents%20Healthy%20Families_-nh_15_md.pdf>

Osher, D., Cantor, P., Berg, J., Steyer, L., & Rose, T. (2020). Drivers of human development: How relationships and context shape learning and development. *Applied Developmental Science, 24*(1), 6–36. <https://doi.org/10.1080/10888691.2017.1398650>

Overton, W. F. (2010). Life-span development: Concepts and issues. In W. F. Overton (Ed.) *Cognition, biology, & methods across the lifespan (Volume 1)*, pp.1–29. Hoboken, NJ: John Wiley.

Overton, W. F. (2015). Processes, relations, and relational-Developmental-Systems. In W. F. Overton & P. C. M. Molenaar (Eds.) *Handbook of child psychology and developmental science (Volume 1, 7th Ed.)*, pp. 9–62. Hoboken, NJ: Wiley.

Pathak, A. (2021). *How the government can end poverty for Native American women.* Center for American Progress. Retrieved March 4, 2023, from <https://www.americanprogress.org/article/government-can-end-poverty-native-american-women/>

Pellmar, T. C., Brandt, E. N., & Baird, M. A. (2002). Health and behavior: The interplay of biological, behavioral, and social influences: Summary of an Institute of Medicine Report. *American Journal of Health Promotion, 16*(4), 206–219. <https://doi.org/10.4278/0890-1171-16.4.206>

Postnikov, A. (2016). Learning from Each Other: On a History of Russian-Native Contacts in the Exploration and Mapping of Alaska and the Aleutian Islands (Late Eighteenth- Early Nineteenth Centuries). The Library of Congress. <https://www.loc.gov/rr/european/mofc/postnikov.html>

Racine, L., Fowler-Kerry, S., & Aiyer, H. (2022). Integrative review of the needs and challenges of Indigenous palliative care in rural and remote settings. *Journal of Advanced Nursing, 78*(9), 2693–2712. <https://doi.org/10.1111/jan.15287>

Redbird, B. (2020). What drives Native American poverty? *Institute For Policy Research.* Retrieved March 4, 2023, from <https://www.ipr.northwestern.edu/news/2020/redbird-what-drives-native-american-poverty.html.>

Rimer, B. K., & Glanz, K. (2005). *Theory at a glance: A guide for health promotion practice.* (2nd ed.). (NIHPub. No. 05–3896). US Department of Health and Human Services, National Institutes of Health, National Cancer Institute.

Seeman, T., Epel, E., Gruenewald, T., Karlamangla, A., & McEwen, B. S. (2010). Socio-economic differentials in peripheral biology: Cumulative allostatic load. Annals of the New York Academy of Sciences, 1186(1), 223–239. <https://doi.org/10.1111/j.1749-6632.2009.05341.x>

Shrider, E. A., Kollar, M., Chen, F., & Semega, J. (2021). *Income and poverty in the United States: 2020.* U.S. Census Bureau. Retrieved March 4, 2023, from <https://www.census.gov/library/publications/2021/demo/p60-273.html>

Singh, G., Daus, G., Allender, M., Ramey, C., Martin, E., Perry, C., De Los Reyes, A., & Vedamuthu, I. (2018). Social Determinants of health in the United States: Addressing major health inequality trends for the nation, 1935–2016. *International Journal of Maternal and Child Health and AIDS* (IJMA), *6*(2), 139–164. <https://doi.org/10.21106/ijma.236>

Skewes, M. C., & Blume, A. W. (2019). Understanding the link between racial trauma and substance use among American Indians. *The American Psychologist, 74*(1), 88–100. <https://doi.org/10.1037/amp0000331>

Smith-Kaprosy, N., Martin, P. P., & Whitman, K. (2012). An overview of American Indians and Alaska Natives in the context of social security and supplemental security income. *Social Security Bulletin, 72*(1). <https://www.ssa.gov/policy/docs/ssb/v72n4/v72n4p1.html>

Substance Abuse and Mental Health Services Administration. Behavioral Health Services for American Indians and Alaska Natives. Treatment Improvement Protocol (TIP) Series 61. HHS Publication No. (SMA) 18- 5070EXSUMM. Rockville, MD: Substance Abuse and Mental Health Services Administration, 2018.

Tippeconnic III, J. W. (1999). Tribal control of American Indian education: Observations since the 1960s with implications for the future. In K. G. Swisher, J. W. & Tippeconnic III. (Eds.), *Next steps: Research and practice to advance Indian education*. Appalachia Educational Laboratory.

Tong, M., Tieu, L., Lee, C. T., Ponath, C., Guzman, D., & Kushel, M. (2018). Factors associated with food insecurity among older homeless adults: results from the HOPE HOME study. *Journal of Public Health*, 41(2), 240–249. <https://doi.org/10.1093/pubmed/fdy063>

U.S. Department of the Interior Bureau of Indian Affairs. (n.d.). *Federal Indian boarding school initiative*. Retrieved March 4, 2023, from <https://www.bia.gov/service/federal-indian-boarding-school-initiative>

U.S. Government Accountability Office. (2022). *Alaska Native issues: Federal agencies could enhance support for native village efforts to address environmental threats*. (GAO Publication No. 22-104241). Washington, D.C.: U.S. Government Printing Office. Retrieved March 4, 2023, from <https://www.gao.gov/products/gao-22-104241>

Ungar, M. (Ed.). (2012). *The social ecology of resilience: A handbook of theory and practice*. Springer Science & Business Media, LLC.

Vygotsky, L. S. (1978). *Mind in society: The development of higher psychological processes*. In M. Cole, V. John-Steiner, S. Scribner, & E. Souberman (Eds.). Cambridge, Massachusetts: Harvard University.

Williams, D. R., & Mohammed, S. A. (2008). Discrimination and racial disparities in health: Evidence and needed research. *Journal of Behavioral Medicine*, 32(1), 20–47. <https://doi.org/10.1007/s10865-008-9185-0>

World Health Organization (2023). Retrieved Jan 5, 2023, from <https://www.who.int/health-topics/social-determinants-of-health-tab=tab_1>

CHAPTER FOURTEEN

# Culturally Informed Health Promotion Campaigns in Alaska: Findings from "Untapped Talents"

TZU-CHIAO CHEN, SARA L. BUCKINGHAM, SHANNON KUHN, AMANA MBISE, NYABONY GAT AND SOFIA SYTNIAK

Creating an effective culturally informed health campaign is multifaceted and complex. As increasingly more health campaigns consider culture to be an important factor (e.g., Dutta, 2007; Schliemann et al, 2019), health campaign designers are faced with several challenges. First, culture is an incredibly complex concept, and it can be very difficult to define (Martin & Nakayama, 2013; Williams, 1983). The definition of culture is also heavily debated (e.g., Collier et al., 2001; Martin & Nakayama, 1999, 2013). Second, beliefs about the best way to incorporate culture into health campaigns also vary. Some scholars believe that culture should be included in health campaigns based on the cultural dimensions or the surface levels that categorize cultures based on several characteristics (e.g., individualism/collectivism), while others consider deeper connections or the deep structures within culture and behaviors to be more effective (Dutta, 2007; Resnicow et al., 1999). The surface levels relate to behaviors and communicative patterns in certain cultural groups, while deep structures focus on the core values, beliefs, and worldviews of the cultures (Wang-Schweig et. al., 2014). Third, there are a wide range of strategies used to incorporate culture into health campaigns. For example, some health campaign designers focus on linguistic choices while others dive into historical impacts on behaviors (e.g., Ioannides et al., 2022; Mangione-Smith et al., 2004). Historical impacts, for instance, may involve colonial history and individual behaviors affected by the history. One example is how alcohol use disorders among

American Indian and Alaska Native peoples are related to colonization. and cultural oppression (White, 2000).

In this chapter, we start with a discussion on theoretical approaches to designing culturally informed health campaigns. We then focus specifically on how to create culturally informed health campaigns in Alaska. Alaska is one of the most diverse regions in the United States with immigrants from all over the world, as well as a significant Alaska Native population. Health campaigns in Alaska therefore need to incorporate cultural sensitivity for an incredibly diverse population to be effective. Finally, we share our findings from our study "Untapped Talent" and propose suggestions on how to create culturally informed health campaigns in Alaska based on these results.

## THEORETICAL APPROACHES TO DESIGNING CULTURALLY INFORMED HEALTH CAMPAIGNS

In this chapter, we define culture based on Hays's (2001) *Addressing* model: "Culture includes traditions of thought and behavior, such as language and history, that can be socially acquired, shared, and passed on to new generations" (p. 14). The *Addressing* is short for age & generation, developmental disability, disability (acquired), religion, ethnicity & race, socioeconomic status, sexual orientation, indigeneity, national origin & language, and gender. According to Hays (2001), culture is not a fixed or static concept but rather a dynamic and ever-evolving aspect of human identity that is influenced by various social, historical, and political factors. Culture can inform the creation of health campaigns in a myriad of different ways. Several theoretical approaches have been proposed, including the cultural sensitivity approach, the deep structure sensitivity approach, and the culture-centered approach.

The cultural sensitivity approach is characterized as one in which culture is seen as an independent variable (Dutta, 2007). Health campaign designers use cultural traits to segment the intended audience and create messages that fit these different audience characteristics (Kreuter, & McClure, 2004). Kreuter and McClure (2004) identified five factors that are important to consider when designing a health campaign using this cultural sensitivity approach, including the source, message, channel, receiver, and destination. Together, this indicates that, for example, people may be more likely to accept a health message when the source of that message presents with a similar cultural background (e.g., ethnicity, gender, age, socioeconomic status). Indeed, Ioannides and colleagues (2022) found that immigrants prefer to receive health information about COVID-19 from others from the same country of origin. Research has consistently shown that people are more likely to accept and act on health messages when they come from sources that are perceived to be similar to themselves, including those who share a similar cultural background. For example, a study by Spence and colleagues (2013) found that African American participants were more likely to view African American avatars on social media as trustworthy. African American audiences reported that African American avatars, no matter if the owner is actually African American, are more trustworthy, caring, and competent (Spence et al., 2013). Likewise, people may prefer to receive health messages via specific channels that are frequently used by their cultural group. For instance, Lee (2010) conducted two focus groups, one with nine Korean elders and one with nine Asian Indian elders. She identified three major channels that both groups used for health information: interpersonal channels, mass media channels, and community-specific channels. Within those three channels, participants believed the sources that used their languages and culture were more trustworthy. The participants were also more likely to seek health information from ethnic media sources, such as Korean/Hindu-language newspapers and television programs, compared to mainstream media sources. This preference for ethnic media was attributed to the perceived relevance and credibility of information that is targeted to one's cultural context, as well as the ability to access information in one's native language. As for community-specific channels, Asian Indian participants would seek health-related information in Hindu temples, while Korean participants would seek that type of health information in churches. These findings underscore the importance of understanding cultural preferences when designing health communication campaigns and targeting messages to the channels that are most likely to reach and resonate with specific cultural groups.

Health campaign designers using the cultural sensitivity approach may also focus on the importance of various cultural dimensions or values (Dutta, 2007). Hofstede (2011) proposed six cultural dimensions: power distance, uncertainty avoidance, individualism/collectivism, masculinity/femininity, long/short-term orientation, and indulgence/restraint. According to Hofstede (2011), those six dimensions are defined as:

1. Power Distance, related to the different solutions to the basic problem of human inequality;
2. Uncertainty Avoidance, related to the level of stress in a society in the face of an unknown future;
3. Individualism versus Collectivism, related to the integration of individuals into primary groups;

4. Masculinity versus Femininity, related to the division of emotional roles between women and men;
5. Long-Term versus Short-Term Orientation, related to the choice of focus for people's efforts: the future or the present and past.
6. Indulgence versus Restraint, related to the gratification versus control of basic human desires related to enjoying life. (p. 8).

People may prefer health messages designed using their own cultural values, and indeed, these dimensions have been applied to a plethora of health campaigns. The linguistic preference, for instance, in a high collectivist culture may be to use "we" language instead of "I" language. Individuals from a masculinity culture may prefer language that promotes competition more than language that promotes co-operation. These guidelines can be used to create health campaigns based on these cultural dimensions. For instance, Han and Jo (2012) conducted a message design study based on the intended audience's cultural dimensions of individualism or collectivism. They created messages for audiences in the United States using strategies with high individualism, while they created messages for audiences in South Korea and Japan using strategies with high collectivism. Specifically, the message features they included for high individualism included personal gain and/or loss, whereas the message features they included for high collectivism included family and community gain/loss. For instance, for high individualism messages, the researchers created a message that focused on protecting "your health and happiness" to emphasize individual gain. For high collectivism messages, the researchers created a message that focused on protecting "your family's happiness" to emphasize the community aspect. The results indicated that U.S. participants favored individualistic messages, and Japanese participants favored collectivism messages as hypothesized. However, Korean participants did not show preference for either type of message. Even though Japanese culture and Korean culture are similar in tradition, the results indicated that "some segments of Korean society have been inclined towards more individualistic cultural values since the 1980s" (Han & Jo, 2012, p. 89), while Japanese culture still emphasizes collectivist values such as family and community. These results indicate that health campaign messages based on cultural dimensions can influence whether an audience believes the messages are effective.

One of the advantages of using the cultural sensitivity approach is that clear guidelines have been developed to aid health campaign designers. For example, Hofstede (2011) identified all of the cultural dimensions for different countries. Health campaign designers may visit the website (<https://www.hofstede-insights.com/fi/product/compare-countries/>) (Hofstede Insights Oy., *Country comparison tool* 2023) and view the cultural dimension indexes of any country. This method is also suitable for segmenting audiences based on their countries of origin. Health campaign designers can then create messages based on those cultural indexes and linguistic preferences to create effective health campaigns. However, we must be cautious that individual differences exist within each cultural group. As Martin and Nakayama (1999, 2013) point out, cultural/individual dialectic tensions exist while engaging in intercultural communication.

The cultural sensitivity approach can improve the receptivity or acceptance of messages; however, Resnicow and colleagues (1999) believe this method applies "superficial" cultural characteristics. The "superficial" or "surface levels" of culture are important to communicate effectively with various audiences. However, those cultural characteristics may simplify the complexity of cultural roots and mislead health campaign designers to focus only on the surface levels of culture. Instead of focusing only on these "superficial" cultural characteristics, Resnicow and colleagues (1999) proposed that "deep structure sensitivity requires understanding the cultural, social, historical, environmental and psychological forces that influence the target health behavior in the proposed target population" (p. 12). Deep structure sensitivity thus emphasizes the importance of understanding deeper influences on specific cultures rather than just focusing on their cultural dimension indexes.

In order to adopt this deep structure sensitivity approach, health campaign designers need to conduct more in-depth research on why certain cultural aspects (e.g., ethnicity, national origin) lead to certain values and how those values affect effective message design. For instance, on the whole, Hispanic and Latine individuals tend to highly value religion (Resnicow et al., 1999), and East Asian individuals tend to highly value family and community as integral parts of their lives (Han & Jo, 2012). The advantage of deep structure sensitivity is that it provides an opportunity for health campaign designers to build a meaningful connection with their intended audience and craft the health messages based on ethnic and racial cultural roots. Doing so may enable the audience to feel a positive emotional link to the health message (Resnicow et al., 1999). Nevertheless, this method is also incredibly time consuming, and health campaign designers may need to make significant adjustments to their campaigns for culturally diverse audiences. Even though this method considers culture along deeper dimensions, it still focuses on using culture to support behavioral change. Indeed, Resnicow and colleagues (1999) noted that deep cultural structures are still predictors of health behaviors.

Unlike the cultural sensitivity approach and the deep structure sensitivity approach that view culture as an independent variable that can be used to change behaviors, Dutta (2007) proposed the "culture-centered approach" for health campaign design which views culture as "intrinsically linked to the social structures that surround them because the way resources are allocated and controlled significantly influences how meanings are created in the context of the life experiences of cultural participants" (p. 319). The culture-centered approach focuses on underprivileged groups and is rooted in the critical paradigm, which focuses on power and advocates for change (Martin & Nakayama, 1999, 2013). The culture-centered approach starts with identifying current health problems from within the community. This method emphasizes the links between culture and structure, the notion of multiple and shifting contexts, as well as agency and voice, and spaces of resistance" (Dutta, 2007, p. 318). In other words, the culture-centered approach is grounded in understanding a culture from within the community itself, finding solutions from within the community, giving power to underprivileged community members, taking the community environment into consideration, and encouraging dialogue between community members and the spaces where they live.

A good example of using the culture-centered approach is Hensel, Haakenson, and Mohatt's (2003) "The People Awakening Project." The People Awakening Project focused on sobriety in Alaska Native communities. The researchers worked with Alaska Native community members to identify factors that may help them stay sober. They interviewed 252 Alaska Natives living in the Yukon-Kuskokwim Delta, mostly Yup'ik and Athabaskan people. They further adopted the culture-centered approach by seeking help from within the community, identifying the problems from historical and socioeconomic cultural components, and giving agency to the participants. For instance, they discovered that Alaska Native people who stayed sober were strong-willed and had clear goals. Most had seen the damage that alcohol misuse can cause as children. They also identified the importance of religion while remaining sober. The researchers identified five stages of recovery from alcohol misuse: *problem drinking*, *thinking it over*, *experimenting with sobriety*, *stage one sobriety*, *and stage two sobriety*. In order to help Alaska Native people recover from alcohol misuse, the research team found seven measures to apply: recovery factors from alcohol misuse, protective factors from alcohol use, the person's social network, Alaska Native cultural practices, and three measures of alcohol consequences (i.e., the negative effects of alcohol in a person's life). The research team put together an interactive computer CD for youth. The CD contained 20 audio stories from the life stories of sober individuals and included photographs of the storytellers. A booklet with 39 more stories was also attached to the interactive CD. The research team distributed the materials to their tribal partners to help youth gain awareness of alcohol misuse. This approach echoed the culture-centered approach since it put the Alaska Native culture at the core. The solutions are from the community within. It also applied the tradition of storytelling, which is extremely important in Alaska Native cultures. In their following project, Allen and colleagues (2014) generated the collaborative culturally grounded CBPR (community-based participatory research) logic model to address the importance of Yup'ik culture enhancing the previous People Awakening Project. Their project extended the scope to include suicide prevention. The researchers crafted their strategies by working closely with community members to identify and address the unique cultural, historical, and social factors that contribute to alcohol abuse and suicide risk in the Yup'ik youth population.

Taken together, the cultural sensitivity approach, deep structure sensitivity approach, and culture-centered approach demonstrate diverse ways of incorporating culture into health campaigns across three different levels. First, using the cultural sensitivity approach, health campaign designers can integrate cultural dimensions when creating health campaigns by segmenting audiences by their country of origin and using the relevant cultural dimension indexes. Doing so is easier to implement since the campaign can be crafted based on specific cultural dimensions; however, it may be superficial and ignore the deeper meanings of culture. Second, using the deep structure sensitivity approach, health campaign designers can take deeper cultural factors, specifically cultural elements, into consideration. Doing so requires a deeper dive into the cultural roots of the intended audience and requires the health campaign designer's desire to explore various socioeconomic and historical events that influence the culture. This is advantageous in that it can create a more effective health campaign that connects with the intended audience; however, health campaign designers would need to spend significant time creating an appropriate campaign that could not be used for different audiences. Third, using the culture-centered approach, health campaign designers can immerse themselves into the community to discover the relevant health problems and solutions from an insider perspective. The advantage in using this approach is that it will generate effective solutions for a specific cultural group and empower community members who are marginalized and/or have less power and privilege to address health issues with more culturally informed resources. At the same time, the disadvantage in using the culture-centered approach is rooted in the idea that power structures are difficult to change, and it takes significant time to uncover the relevant cultural and societal issues within the community.

## CULTURALLY INFORMED HEALTH CAMPAIGNS IN ANCHORAGE, ALASKA

Anchorage, Alaska is one of the most diverse cities in the United States (Farrell, 2018). Health campaign designers have to be creative and dynamic in order to design effective and culturally informed health campaigns for this culturally diverse audience. Health campaign designers working on these campaigns (and others) face several cultural challenges in creating effective messages for those in Anchorage. In this section, we discuss the cultural diversity within Anchorage and examine how this cultural diversity influences health campaign designers' choices for message features, message dissemination, and so on.

## Cultural Diversity in Anchorage, Alaska

The population of Anchorage, Alaska is incredibly diverse, and, indeed, Anchorage is one of the most diverse cities in the United States (Farrell, 2018). Anchorage is located within Dena'ina Ełnena, the traditional homelands of the Dena'ina Athabascan people and the Native Village of Eklutna. Anchorage is also home to Alaska Native people from all over the state of Alaska, including Alaska Native people from the five main groups today: Northwest Coast Indians (Tlingit, Haida, Tsimshian), Inupiaqs, Yupiks, Aleuts, and Athabascans (State of Alaska, n.d., *Alaska Natives*). The U.S. Census website revealed that 15.7 % of the population in Alaska were American Indian/Alaska Native in 2021 (US Census Bureau, *U.S. Census Bureau quickfacts: Alaska* 2023). In addition to Alaska Native people, Anchorage has seen increasing numbers of international immigrants in the past decades, growing from 13,000 in 1990 to 35,400 people (or 8.9 % of the population) in 2018 (U.S. Census Bureau, 2023). The Anchorage School District is also ranked 17th in the United States for its diversity (Niche, *2024 most diverse school districts in America* 2023). The population in Anchorage based on race/ethnicity in 2021 was 5.8 % Black or African American, 9.3 % Native American and Alaska Native, 10.1 % Asian, 3.2 % Native Hawaiian or other Pacific Islanders, 9.7 % Hispanic or Latine, and 8.8 % two races or more; 56 % White, without Hispanic or Latine ethnicity alone ((US Census Bureau, *U.S. Census Bureau quickfacts: Anchorage Municipality (County), Alaska* 2023).

## Diverse Cultures in Anchorage, Alaska

The Alaska Native and immigrant populations in Anchorage have led to a multitude of diverse cultural landscapes. Alaska Native culture plays an important role in this multicultural backdrop. In his article "Yuuyaraq: The Way of the Human Being," Napoleon (1991) describes "Yuuyaraq" as a philosophy and way of life that has been practiced by the Yup'ik people. It is a holistic approach to life that emphasizes the interconnectedness of all things and the importance of maintaining balance and harmony in all aspects of life, including the relationships between humans and the natural world. At the core of Yuuyaraq is the belief that everything in the world has a spirit and deserves respect. The philosophy emphasizes the importance of living in harmony with nature, being mindful of the impact of human actions on the environment, and taking only what is necessary to sustain oneself. Yuuyaraq also places great emphasis on community and the well-being of others. It encourages individuals to be respectful and caring toward others and to work together to ensure the survival and prosperity of the community as a whole. Overall, Yuuyaraq is a way of life that is grounded in respect, balance, and interconnectedness, and it continues to be an important part of the cultural heritage of the Yup'ik people.

Alaska Native cultures are very unique. According to Roderick (2010), there are several key characteristics of Alaska Native cultures: (1) Alaska Native people honor the land and water they live in upon which life depends; (2) Alaska Native people respect and share sources with each other; (3) Alaska Native Elders are respected in the community, and younger people should learn from them; (4) Alaska Native people highly appreciate the attitude of humility and patience; (5) Alaska Native people believe that everything in the world is interconnected; (6) Alaska Native people take verbal and written promises very seriously; and (7) Alaska Native people consider individuals within their own cultures, histories, and traditions, which emphasizes the roots of where an individual came from and how they grew up.

Immigrants from all over the world choose Anchorage as their new home. More than one in every 10 Anchorage residents were born outside of the United States. The number of immigrants in Anchorage increased by about 57 % in the past two decades, while its U.S.-born population only increased 14 % during the same time period (U.S. Census Bureau, 2023). The largest immigrant groups in Anchorage are from the Philippines, South Korea, Mexico, Canada, Thailand, Russia, Germany, and the Dominican Republic (U.S. Census Bureau, 2023). Anchorage also welcomed a large number of refugees and asylees for a city of its size, with the local resettlement agency currently serving people from 28 countries, including Somalia, Sudan, Iraq, Bhutan, Congo, Myanmar, Cuba, Laos, and Ukraine (Catholic Social Services, n.d.). The Anchorage School District is one of the most diverse in the United States; approximately 20 % of its students collectively speak a total of 110 languages aside from English, with Spanish, Hmong, Samoan, Tagalog, and Korean being the most widely spoken languages.

In 2014, the Municipality of Anchorage joined an initiative called Welcoming America to create an inclusive and welcoming city for immigrants. Welcoming America has proposed the "Welcoming Standard" or core guidelines for communities to adopt and implement policies, programs, and partnerships that "give communities the welcoming edge" (Welcoming America, 2016, p. 4). While these guidelines reflect the evidence for immigrant integration and inclusion for policy makers and community members, it is not clear how the process of inclusion and acceptance is manifested.

With the diversity of cultures brought by Alaska Native people and immigrants, health campaign designers in Anchorage need to be more culturally informed. Creating culturally informed health campaigns has become vital in this region. We will use a COVID-19 campaign as an example of how culture can be integrated into health campaigns in Anchorage.

## Culturally Informed Health Campaigns in Anchorage: The Example of COVID-19

Anchorage, Alaska has a specific website dedicated to COVID-19 where Anchorage residents can find information needed about the pandemic (<https://covid-response-moa-muniorg.hub.arcgis.com/>) (Municipality of Anchorage, *Coronavirus response anchorage,* n.d.). On the website, information can be found in different languages. This part of the website links to the Centers for Disease Control and Prevention (CDC) website with multilingual content. Similar content can be found on the Alaska Department of Health website (<https://health.alaska.gov/dph/Epi/id/Pages/COVID-19/default.aspx>) (Alaska Department of Health, *Covid-19 in Alaska* 2022) as well. However, both websites present information primarily in English. Most of the information regarding vaccination, testing, and prevention has links to CDC websites with multilingual content. On the Alaska Department of Health YouTube Channel(<https://www.youtube.com/@alaskadhss/videos>) (Alaska Department of Health, *Alaska Department of Health YouTube* 2023), they offer several video clips in nine languages that are most spoken in Alaska related to COVID-19 information (Tagalog, Russian, Vietnamese, Chinese Mandarin, Japanese, Spanish, Samoan, Hmong, and Korean). Although it required significant resources to translate those video clips into those nine different languages, it does not appear they reached their target audience as well as they had hoped. For example, there were only 54 views on the Korean version (as of Jan 26, 2023). A successful health campaign should reach larger audiences and spread related information more widely.

These previous examples focus mostly on the language level. The campaign materials were focusing on linguistic aspects of cultures and did not address the deeper aspects of cultures. Campaigns can also work on reaching out widely to spread critical information. The following section will cover how several COVID-19 campaigns used a more integrative cultural-centered level.

A policy brief published in December 2020 titled "Building Trust in and Access to a COVID-19 Vaccine Among People of Color and Tribal Nations," (Trust for America's Health, *Building Trust in and access to a COVID-19 vaccine among people of color and tribal nations a framework for action convening: Technical resources* 2020) was co-authored by the Trust for America's Health, the National Medical Association, and UnidosUS. Two key communications recommendations were: (1) Equip trusted community organizations and networks within communities of color and tribal communities to participate in vaccination education. Ensure their meaningful engagement and participation by providing funding; and (2) Vaccine education messaging must be culturally and linguistically appropriate. Messaging campaigns must feature trusted messengers.

According to the CDC, Alaska Native/American Indian people experienced disproportionate rates of infection and mortality throughout the COVID-19 pandemic, rooted in historic health inequities (Arrazola et al., 2021). It was acknowledged that governmental outreach efforts to Alaska Native communities around the COVID-19 vaccine would need to overcome complex issues of vaccine hesitancy and generational mistrust. As trusted community-based organizations, Native Peoples Action Community Fund (NPACF) and Alaska Public Interest Research Group (AKPIRG) served as the lead project coordinators, in partnership with Alaska Department of Health and Social Services and the Alaska Native Tribal Health Consortium. NPACF and AKPIRG convened virtual Alaska Native Language panels to develop culturally relevant messages about COVID-19 vaccines in eight languages (Alaska Native Tribal Health Consortium, *Covid-19 vaccine materials in Alaska native languages* 2022). The language panels were multigenerational, with language learners, Elders, teachers, and other language experts. Each panelist contributed their own unique talents from orthography expertise and technology skills to artistic vision and traditional knowledge-all with the intent of translating important information to be communicated effectively and in a trustworthy manner with care for their communities (The Alaska Public Interest Research Group, *Akpirg* 2021). By uplifting Indigenous languages, facts, encouragement, and science through Indigenous knowledge systems, the panelists hoped to provide people with trustworthy information needed to make informed decisions. In particular, providing Elders and first-language speakers with information in their language was crucial to ensuring equitable access (ANTHC, 2021). The message development, coordination, and material printing and dissemination were funded by a grant from the Alaska Immunization Program to AKPIRG, who subcontracted NPACF and the language panelists.

The Alaska Literacy Program (ALP) is a well-established community-based organization that serves English Language Learners (ELL) and has built strong relationships with many different immigrant communities throughout Anchorage (Alaska Literacy Program, *Alp* n.d.). ALP's Peer Leader Navigator program is a health education and outreach initiative designed to improve the well-being of Anchorage's ELL residents, by helping to bridge the linguistic and cultural divides that prevent residents from accessing essential health services. This is implemented through a peer model where the multicultural, multilingual Peer Leader Navigators are trained as community health navigators to develop the necessary skills and knowledge to provide health promotion and disease prevention activities within their established communities (Alaska Literacy Program, *Covid-19* n.d.). During the COVID-19 pandemic, the local and state governments relied heavily on ALP to help build trust in the COVID-19 vaccine within immigrant communities. Initially, there was considerable fear, distrust, and misinformation around the vaccines, including among the Peer Leader Navigators. ALP hosted a series of educational meetings between the Peer Leader Navigators and health representatives, including the State's Chief Medical Officer, local public health nurses, and trusted pharmacists. After 2–3 months, the majority of Peer Leader Navigators chose to receive a COVID-19 vaccine and became advocates for being vaccinated against COVID-19. Advising government officials that the overly burdensome online appointment system was a barrier to vaccination, the Peer Leader Navigators agreed to have their vaccine experience documented and helped record audio messages for those videos to be shared across the state in different languages. In addition to vaccine advocacy and information dissemination, ALP hosted community vaccine clinics where Peer Leader Navigators provided cultural navigation and language support service, serving as both a trusted location and messenger of information.

The COVID-19 pandemic has presented significant challenges to healthcare systems and governments worldwide. Anchorage, Alaska, which is one of the most diverse cities in the United States, has demonstrated an exemplary approach to incorporating cultural diversity into health campaigns. Understanding the experiences of cultural minorities in the area is of utmost importance given the city's diverse population. To this end, Untapped Talent researchers conducted multiple studies to uncover the experiences of immigrants in Anchorage. The ensuing section will provide an overview of the findings of these studies.

## Findings from Untapped Talent

In order to achieve its goal of identifying factors that promote or hinder integration and inclusion in the municipality of Anchorage, Welcoming Anchorage and the Southcentral Alaska's Area Health Education Center investigated how other communities collected similar information. They then collaborated with researchers from the University of Alaska Anchorage to develop the study design, with a focus on community-engaged research principles (see Balls-Berry & Acosta-Pérez, 2017). This type of research involves working with partners who have unique skills and experiences, which can help build trust between marginalized community members and researchers. It can also improve the quality and usefulness of the data collected (Mikesell et al., 2013). The research partnership established the project "Untapped Talent." The study "Untapped Talent" examines the integration and inclusion of immigrants in Anchorage in various areas such as education, employment, healthcare, access to public spaces, interactions with government agencies, social networks, and fostering a sense of home.

Given the goals of the community organizations, the university-government-community partnership decided to use a sequential explanatory mixed-method design (Ivankova et al., 2006). This involved conducting a survey of immigrant residents to gather quantitative data, followed by focus groups with community members to better understand the survey results. This approach helped the team to identify barriers and facilitators to integration and inclusion, as well as any differences across various groups (e.g., age, time in Anchorage, English proficiency, culture), which could be useful in developing effective strategies for change.

The research team conducted two stages of studies to investigate the treatments of immigrants in Anchorage, Alaska. The first stage adopted quantitative methods, and the second stage adopted qualitative methods. The research team conducted ten focus groups with 85 participants in seven languages to investigate their experiences in Anchorage.

The scope of the study covered a wide range of topics that affect the integration of immigrants in the city of Anchorage. The research team investigated the immigrants' experiences with job hunting, accessing public spaces, interacting with law enforcement and government agencies, housing, using public transportation, accessing education, and so on. Healthcare is one of the important parts of this project. In this next section, we share our findings regarding healthcare and the difficulties of navigating health information. We specifically focus on barriers related to health campaigns, including language barriers, difficulties navigating the health system, and lack of trust between providers and patients.

## Language Barriers

Language barriers affect every aspect of immigrants' lives. Such challenges are not unique to immigrants in Anchorage; language barriers have been identified as a primary challenge of immigrants around the world (Allen, 2006; Resnyansky, 2016;

Suwinyattichaiporn, Chen, & Generous, 2016). For immigrants in Anchorage, language barriers play a significant role in feeling isolated and alone after moving to the area. Language is also essential for immigrants to seek out resources, find critical information, and contribute to the community. Language barriers influence immigrants' lives in many ways, including in areas related to healthcare and health campaigns. Participants pointed out that it is difficult to access the most up-to-date health information in their own languages. This is crucial for immigrants to feel safe and worry-free about health issues. The situation was particularly critical during our project period, as this research was conducted mostly during the COVID-19 pandemic. Our participants also reported experiencing confusion while accessing healthcare services due to language barriers. However, most healthcare organizations do offer interpretation services as long as patients request them.

For health campaign designers, these findings revealed two-fold recommendations. First, offering health campaigns that fulfill multilingual requirements is important, especially if the information is time-sensitive. Second, health campaign designers have to inform the audiences that multilingual services are available to them. Working with community leaders to disseminate this information is a good place to start since minorities may be more likely to trust information providers with similar cultural backgrounds (Lee, 2010; Spence et al., 2013). Those community leaders can also communicate with the minority audiences in their own languages. Language-related issues are also mentioned in the following sections since language is the key component for immigrants feeling integrated.

## Difficulties Navigating the Health System

Participants expressed their concerns regarding healthcare in Anchorage in a few ways:

1. Participants reported that it was difficult to find suitable insurance services. They found it challenging to determine the best health insurance plan and ways to make annual changes to plans.
2. Language barriers again deeply influenced participants' access to health information and healthcare. The participants reported that there was no medical service provided in their languages, which can be detrimental to their ability to receive appropriate care. Participants articulated the need for more interpreters in all healthcare settings and a need for more information about accessing interpretation and translation services. Many of them also did not realize that those services are provided free of charge for them.

3. Participants also mentioned that many constraints hinder timely healthcare. Medical providers do not coordinate well with each other, which results in the difficulties of transfer and getting referrals in a timely manner. Many participants also mentioned that they need to travel out of the state to be treated properly since there are not enough qualified health providers in the area.
4. Participants expressed their concerns about being misunderstood and not cared for. Some participants even mentioned that some health providers show some potential biases and assumptions about them.

The findings reflect the cultural-centered approach to creating health campaigns. Firstly, healthcare systems vary across different countries. These systems include health insurance, sharing health information with other healthcare providers, medical specialties, and so on. Health campaign designers may not realize that several practices are normal in the United States but are foreign to immigrants. For instance, Taiwan has National Health Insurance, which allows Taiwanese citizens to pay a comparatively small amount of money and receive healthcare nationwide. The system also allows healthcare providers to access patients' health-related information while providing treatments (Wu et al., 2010). These differences may not be recognized by health campaign designers. Secondly, language barriers are still a main concern for immigrants. From accessing health information to seeking healthcare providers, language plays a central role in healthcare accessibility for immigrants. Health campaign designers have to craft their health campaigns by considering the cultural roots of immigrants. In other words, they should be able to effectively explain the differences between the current healthcare systems and their home cultures in ways they can understand (e.g., language, ways of communicating, and nonverbal cues)

## Lack of Trust between Providers and Patients

Participants mentioned the discomfort interacting with and sometimes mistrust of the healthcare system. These issues directly link to the dissatisfactory healthcare system in the area. The following are some results from Untapped Talent:

1. Participants expressed that when they had access to healthcare providers from their cultural backgrounds and who spoke their languages, their care experience was transformed for the better.
2. Participants also mentioned that advocates, interpreters, healthcare outreach, and patient education connected to the healthcare system were seen

as ways of supporting patients to effectively communicate and advocate for their needs.

3. Asking questions and doing research helped participants inform themselves and contributed to a more positive interaction with the healthcare system.

These results echo information presented previously in this chapter. Namely, individuals tend to trust healthcare providers who can speak their languages and are from within their communities (see Ioannides et al., 2022; Lee, 2010; Spence et al., 2013). Since U.S. culture emphasizes personal choices and personal responsibilities (Hook & Rose Markus, 2020), immigrants from high power distance cultures may find it confusing when visiting healthcare providers and may consider those providers untrustworthy. Cultural-centered health campaign designers should be careful while creating health campaigns targeting culturally diverse audiences.

Gat and colleagues (2022) provide additional information on this topic. According to the findings, we may suggest several solutions for health campaign designers to create better health campaigns in Anchorage: (1) Language barriers need to be addressed while creating health campaigns; (2) Health campaign designers should reach out to audiences who need interpreters and articulate current policies; (3) Healthcare providers should provide readily accessible information regarding interpreters; (4) To improve the trust between patients and healthcare providers, cultural sensitivity training is necessary; and (5) Health campaign designers can also provide health-related information to immigrants with cultural adaptations.

## CONCLUSIONS

It is unwise to neglect culture when creating health campaigns for a myriad of reasons. First, the campaign may be inappropriate or offensive to its target demographic if culture is not considered in every step of the process of designing the campaign. Second, health campaign designers may not understand the roots of certain health issues within specific cultures if they do not understand their histories and contemporary cultural contexts. By understanding the roots of the issues, health campaign designers can create targeted campaigns to address the issues and provide proper guidance to the target demographic. Third, health strategies may not be as effective in reaching their target demographic and in promoting behavior change if they are not responsive to culture.

Since culture itself is a complex concept, how to incorporate culture into health campaigns can be very diverse, too. It is important to consider the goals of the campaign and choose the right methods to incorporate culture into health campaigns. Culture is part of society, and a good health campaign should never neglect the cultural influences on individuals' perceptions on health issues.

## REFERENCES

*2024 most diverse school districts in America.* Niche. (2023a). <https://www.niche.com/k12/search/most-diverse-school-districts/>

Alaska Department of Health. (2022). *Covid-19 in Alaska.* COVID-19 in Alaska, Department of Health and Social Services. <https://health.alaska.gov/dph/Epi/id/Pages/COVID-19/default.aspx>

Alaska Department of Health. (n.d.). *Alaska Department of Health.* Alaska Department of Health YouTube. <https://www.youtube.com/@alaskadhss/videos>

Alaska Literacy Program. (n.d.). *Alp.* ALP – Alaska Literacy Program. <https://www.alaskaliteracyprogram.org/>

Alaska Literacy Program. (n.d.). *Covid-19.* Anchorage PLNs. <https://sites.google.com/alaskaliteracyprogram.org/anchorageplns/health/covid?authuser=0>

Alaska Native Tribal Health Consortium. (2022, July 26). *Covid-19 vaccine materials in Alaska native languages.* Alaska Native Tribal Health Consortium. <https://www.anthc.org/covid-19-vaccine-materials-in-alaska-native-languages/>

Alaska Public Interest Research Group. (2021). *Akpirg.* AKPIRG 2.0. <https://www.akpirg.org/language-access>

Allen, D. (2006). Who's in and who's out? Language and the integration of new immigrant youth in Quebec. *International Journal of Inclusive Education, 10*(02–03), 251–263. <https://doi.org/10.1080/13603110500256103>

Allen, J., Mohatt, G. V., Beehler, S., & Rowe, H. L. (2014). People awakening: Collaborative research to develop cultural strategies for prevention in community intervention. *American Journal of Community Psychology, 54*, 100–111. <https://doi.org/10.1007/s10464-014-9647-1>

Arrazola, J., Masiello, M. M., Joshi, S., Dominguez, A. E., Poel, A., Wilkie, C. M., Bressler, J. M., McLaughlin, J., Kraszewski, J., Komatsu, K. K., Peterson Pompa, X., Jespersen, M., Richardson, G., Lehnertz, N., LeMaster, P., Rust, B., Keyser Metobo, A., Doman, B., Casey, D., … Landen, M. (2021, January 7). *Covid-19 mortality among American Indian and Alaska native persons – 14 states, January–June 2020.* Centers for Disease Control and Prevention. <https://www.cdc.gov/mmwr/volumes/69/wr/mm6949a3.htm>

Balls-Berry, J. E., & Acosta-Pérez, E. (2017). The use of community engaged research principles to improve health: Community academic partnerships for research. *Puerto Rico Health Sciences Journal, 36*(2), 84–85. <https://www.ncbi.nlm.nih.gov/pubmed/28622404>

*Catholic Social Services.* (n.d.). Refugee assistance and immigration services. Retreieved from <https://www.cssalaska.org/our-programs/refugee-assistance-immigration-services/>

Collier, J., Hegde, R., Lee, W., Nakayama, T., & Yep, G. (2001). Dialogue on the edges: Ferment in communication and culture. In M. J. Collier (Ed), *Transforming Communication about Culture: Critical New Directions*, (pp. 219–280). <https://doi.org/10.4135/9781452233208.n9>

Dutta, M. J. (2007). Communicating about culture and health: Theorizing culture-centered and cultural sensitivity approaches. *Communication Theory*, *17*(3), 304–328. <https://doi.org/10.1111/j.1468-2885.2007.00297.x>

Farrell, C. R. (2018). The Anchorage mosaic: Racial and ethnic diversity in the urban North. In J. K. Barnett, & I. C. Hartman (Eds.), *Imagining Anchorage: The making of America's northernmost metropolis* (pp. 374–391). University of Alaska Press. <https://doi.org/10.3138/9781442676015-toc>

Gat, N., Kuhn, S., Buckingham, S. L., Mbise, A., Chen, T.-C., & Sytniak, S. (2022). (rep.). *Untapped Talent: Immigrant Integration and Inclusion in Anchorage, Alaska* (pp. 1–65). Anchorage, AK: University of Alaska Anchorage.

Han, K. H., & Jo, S. (2012). Does culture matter?: A cross-national investigation of women's responses to cancer prevention campaigns. *Health Care for Women International*, *33*(1), 75–94. <https://doi.org/10.1080/07399332.2011.630117>

Hays, P. A. (2001). Addressing cultural complexities in practice. *Washington, DC: American Psychological Association*. <https://doi.org/10.1037/10411-000>

Hensel, C., Haakenson, S., & Mohatt, G. (2003). "It's been good, not drinking": Alaska Native narratives of lifetime sobriety. *Arctic Anthropology*, *40*(2), 75–82. <https://doi.org/10.1353/arc.2011.0032>

Hofstede, G. (2011). Dimensionalizing cultures: The Hofstede model in context. *Online Readings in Psychology and Culture*, *2*(1), 2307–0919.

Hofstede Insights Oy. (2023). *Country comparison tool*. Hofstede Insights. <https://www.hofstede-insights.com/fi/product/compare-countries/>

Hook, C. J., & Rose Markus, H. (2020). Health in the United States: are appeals to choice and personal responsibility making Americans sick?. *Perspectives on Psychological Science, 15*(3), 643–664. <https://doi.org/10.1177/1745691619896252>

Ioannides, S., Hess, I., Lamberton, C., Luisi, B., & Gupta, L. (2022). Engaging with culturally and linguistically diverse communities during a COVID-19 outbreak: A NSW Health interagency public health campaign. *Public Health Research and Practice*, *e32342215*. <https://doi.org/10.17061/phrp32342215>.

Ivankova, N. V., Creswell, J. W., & Stick, S. L. (2006). Using mixed-methods sequential explanatory design: From theory to practice. *Field Methods, 18*(1), 3–20. <https://doi.org/10.1177/1525822X05282260>

Kreuter, M. W., & McClure, S. M. (2004). The role of culture in health communication. *Annual Review of Public Health*, *25*, 439–455. <https://doi.org/10.1891/9780826161734.0007>

Lee, J. S. (2010). Channels of health communications used among Korean and Asian Indian older adults. *Social Work in Health Care, 49*(2), 165–175. <https://doi.org/10.1080/00981380903157997>

Mangione-Smith, R., Elliott, M. N., Stivers, T., McDonald, L., Heritage, J., & McGlynn, E. A. (2004). Racial/ethnic variation in parent expectations for antibiotics: Implications for public health campaigns. *Pediatrics*, *113*(5), e385–e394. <https://doi.org/10.1542/peds.113.5.e385>

Martin, J. N., & Nakayama, T. K. (1999). Thinking dialectically about culture and communication. *Communication Theory*, 1–25. <https://doi.org/10.1111/j.1468-2885.1999.tb00160.x>

Martin, J. N., & Nakayama, T. K. (2013). Thinking dialectically about culture and communication. In M. K. Asante, Y. Miike, J. Yin (Eds.), *The global intercultural communication reader*, (pp. 204–222). <https://doi.org/10.4324/9780203934982-15>

Mikesell, L., Bromley, E., & Khodyakov, D. (2013). Ethical community-engaged research: A literature review. *American Journal of Public Health, 103*(12), 7–14. <https://doi.org/10.2105/AJPH.2013.301605>

Municipality of Anchorage. (n.d.). *Coronavirus response anchorage*. Coronavirus Response Anchorage. <https://covid-response-moa-muniorg.hub.arcgis.com/>

Napoleon, H. (1991). *Yuuyaraq: The way of the human being*. Publications Centre, Centre for Cross-Cultural Studies, College of Rural Alaska, University of Alaska Fairbanks. <https://doi.org/10.1515/9780822390831-014>

Resnicow, K., Baranowski, T., Ahluwalia, J. S., & Braithwaite, R. L. (1999). Cultural sensitivity in public health: defined and demystified. *Ethnicity & disease*, *9*(1), 10–21. <https://www.jstor.org/stable/45410142>

Resnyansky, L. (2016). Scientific justification of social policies: concepts of language and immigrant integration. *Journal of Ethnic and Migration Studies*, *42*(12), 2049–2066. <https://doi.org/10.1080/1369183x.2016.1158645>

Roderick, L. (Ed.). (2010). *Alaska Native cultures and issues: Responses to frequently asked questions*. Fairbanks, AK: University of Alaska Press. <https://doi.org/10.5860/choice.48-3613>

Schliemann, D., Su, T. T., Paramasivam, D., Somasundaram, S., Ibrahim Tamin, N. S. B., Dahlui, M., … & Donnelly, M. (2019). The systematic cultural adaptation of a UK public health cancer awareness raising programme for Malaysia: the Be Cancer Alert Campaign. *Translational behavioral medicine, 9*(6), 1087–1099.

Spence, P. R., Lachlan, K. A., Westerman, D., & Spates, S. A. (2013). Where the gates matter less: Ethnicity and perceived source credibility in social media health messages. *Howard Journal of Communications, 24*(1), 1–16. <https://doi.org/10.1080/10646175.2013.748593>

State of Alaska. (2023). Alaska Natives. <https://alaska.gov/kids/learn/nativeculture.htm>

Suwinyattichaiporn, T., Chen, T. C., & Generous, M. A. (2016). Intercultural friendship initiation in the American classroom: Barriers, influencers, and pedagogical strategies. *Pennsylvania Communication Annual*, *72*(1), 59–80.

Trust for America's Health. (2020). *Building Trust in and access to a COVID-19 vaccine among people of color and tribal nations a framework for action convening: Technical resources*. ASPR TRACIE. <https://asprtracie.hhs.gov/technical-resources/resource/10242/building-trust-in-and-access-to-a-covid-19-vaccine-among-people-of-color-and-tribal-nations-a-framework-for-action-convening>

Wang-Schweig, M., Kviz, F. J., Altfeld, S. J., Miller, A. M., & Miller, B. A. (2014). *Building a conceptual framework to culturally adapt health promotion and prevention programs at the Deep Structural Level*. Health promotion practice. Retrieved March 23, 2023, from <https://www.ncbi.nlm.nih.gov/pmc/articles/PMC4184993/>

Welcoming America. (2016). *The welcoming standard & certified welcoming*. Retrieved from <https://www.welcomingamerica.org/sites/default/files/Welcoming%20Standard%20%2B%20Certified%20Welcoming.pdf>

White, W. L. (2000). The history of recovered people as wounded healers: I. From Native America to the rise of the modern alcoholism movement. *Alcoholism Treatment Quarterly*, *18*(1), 1–23. <https://doi.org/10.1300/j020v18n01_01>

Williams, R. (1983). *Culture and society, 1780–1950*. New York, NY: Columbia University Press.

Wu, T. Y., Majeed, A., & Kuo, K. N. (2010). An overview of the healthcare system in Taiwan. *London journal of primary care, 3*(2), 115–119. <https://doi.org/10.1080/17571472.2010.11493315>

U.S. Census Bureau (2023). QuickFacts: Anchorage Municipality, Alaska (County). Retrieved March 7, 2023, from <https://www.census.gov/quickfacts/fact/table/AK/PST045221>

# Epilogue: A Road Map for Health Communication Research That Makes a Difference

MARY LEE HUMMERT

As I read the chapters in this book, I reflected not only on the value of considering the ways in which the language we use in interaction influences the health status (physical, psychological, emotional) of individuals across the lifespan but also on the ways in which the chapters reveal the defining characteristics of health communication research that makes a difference in healthcare practice. Such research (1) brings a theory-rich, methodologically varied, social action/positive communication orientation to the study of health communication across the lifespan, attending to (2) interpersonal relationships, (3) the social environment, and (4) culture, in order to (5) develop beneficial communication practices for healthcare professionals, individuals, families, and communities. Each of these characteristics could be viewed as corresponding to one of the five parts of this book, but that conclusion would "miss the forest for the trees": It is in their interrelationship and foundation in the lifespan developmental perspective that these characteristics constitute effective health communication research. Each chapter shows an allegiance to that view.

The first part of this chapter provides an integrative view of this volume, exploring the shared commitments to effective health communication research across the chapters, and the second highlights the strategies that successfully integrate research into practice. Together, I believe they provide a road map for health communication research that makes a difference. The chapter concludes with a consideration of the importance of the lifespan developmental perspective as the foundation for this road map.

## THE TERRAIN: GUIDING PRINCIPLES FOR HEALTH COMMUNICATION RESEARCH

Effective communication research, whether focused on the health context or any other, must be guided by clear principles regarding the nature of communication, the importance of theory, the intimate relationship between theory and method, and an appreciation of the intrapersonal, interpersonal, and social forces woven into every interaction. The authors of the chapters in this volume clearly share such guiding principles for health communication research across the lifespan. Three statements summarize those principles: (1) A social action/positive communication orientation is essential; (2) Research must be grounded in theory and employ targeted methods to achieve its goals; and (3) Research must attend to culture writ small and large to be useful in theory development and in practice.

### A Social Action/Positive Communication Orientation

The relationship between language and social action has been acknowledged for centuries. Aristotle's *Rhetoric* is the prime example with its guidance on language as the means of persuasion. However, it was only in the last century that philosophers of language saw communication not simply as the means to social action but as constitutive of social action, as exemplified in Speech Act Theory (Austin, 1960; Searle, 1962). That is, every utterance is an action—whether we intend so or not. The language as social action perspective has been the dominant view within communication from that period as evident from this book series and in influential communication theories such as Communication Accommodation Theory (Giles et al., 2023). The chapters in this volume hold to this perspective but couple it with a positive communication focus.

The first part of this volume addresses the social action/positive communication orientation. Pitts (Chapter One, this volume) provides an overview that both contrasts it with traditional approaches to communication science (i.e., those emphasizing objectivity and rationality) and addresses its particular appropriateness for health communication research. Pitts points to the roots of positive communication in positive psychology and defines positive communication research as "scholarship [that] centers on conditions and (communication) processes that cultivate human flourishing and resilience" (p. 6). This definition speaks directly to the benefits of the positive communication perspective as a guiding principle for health communication research. The chapter includes a typology of positive communication acts (Mirivel, 2014), with an extended focus on compassionate communication and communication savoring. Mirivel and Blackburn (Chapter Three, this volume) further develop an understanding of the positive communication typology in their exploration of what constitutes peak communication experiences for adults. That is, those *memorable* interactions in which we *savored* every detail and *felt* happiness and joy.

Lest we confuse positive communication with easy and carefree interactions that only involve positive emotions, Pitts (Chapter One, this volume) reminds us "that human flourishing . . . means experiencing and managing the negative alongside the positive" (p. 8). Therefore, positive communication "can also be a force for social action through disruption" (p. 9). Harwood and Cooper (Chapter Two, this volume) address the disruptive aspect of positive communication in their call for humanizing and personalizing communication to members of negatively stereotyped groups such as those with Alzheimer's and related dementias. Such communication, they argue, is necessary to counter the consequences of stereotype-driven communication (e.g., patronizing speech) which acts to dehumanize and rob these individuals of personhood.

Although the social action/positive communication orientation is not the primary topic in the chapters in the remaining parts of the book, it is the guiding perspective in each of them as evident in their goals. Consider these examples: Building resilience is a goal articulated by Fisher (Chapter Four, this volume), Worthington and colleagues (Chapter Twelve, this volume), and Rosich and colleagues (Chapter Thirteen, this volume); Using positive communication to disrupt topic avoidance and unwillingness to communicate about health is a goal for Wright and Canzona (Chapter Five, this volume) and Campbell-Salome (Chapter Six, this volume); Anderson and McDermott (Chapter Nine, this volume) hope to use positive communication to reduce reliance on age stereotypes in the public relations arena; And Fowler (Chapter Seven, this volume) has the goal of outlining the communicative parameters that constitute successful aging.

## Theoretically Grounded with Targeted Research Methods

An important tenet of the social action/positive communication orientation holds that research must be grounded in theory, but that no singular theory can serve as a sufficient basis for all health communication research given the variation in research goals and the complexity of the health communication process. The same can be said of research methods. As Fisher (Chapter Four, p. 75, this volume) states, "*theoretically grounded targeted approaches*" are required (italics in original). Interpersonal communication, mediated communication, and health theories are most widely represented in the chapters, but those from psychology, public relations, and campaign design fields are featured in individual chapters.

The chapters in this volume illustrate how health communication researchers engage theory from a variety of disciplines and select targeted methods in alignment with their research goals. For instance, Gettings (Chapter Eight, this volume) wished to explore how the differing (i.e., gendered) work trajectories of women and men intersected with their transition to and experience of retirement. She chose the Communicated Narrative Sensemaking theory (Koenig-Kellas, 2017) as a guide given the equivocal nature of retirement as a life transition and evidence that "[s]ensemaking is of particular importance . . . to overall well-being . . ." (p. 168, this volume). Consistent with that theory and her goals, she interviewed recently retired women and men individually to gather their personal narratives. In general, authors with goals that required understanding the interplay of intrapersonal, interpersonal, and cultural forces on health communication practices and experiences relied on biopsychosocial, social-ecological and systems, cultural, and communicated sensemaking theories, and, in turn, employed qualitative research methods.

On the other hand, when research goals involved assessing the effectiveness of a health intervention, the validity of a model, or beliefs/preferences of a community or specific population, authors were guided by theories that generated testable hypotheses and employed surveys or experiments to collect data suitable for statistical analysis (See Chen et al., Chapter Fourteen, this volume; Wright & Canzona, Chapter Five, this volume; Fowler, Chapter Seven, this volume). Fowler (Chapter Seven, this volume), for example, described how the Theory of Motivated Information Management (TMIM: Afifi & Weiner, 2004) informed the initial Communication Ecology of Successful Aging Model (CEMSA). The hypothesized relationships in the model were then tested in large scale survey studies. In other cases, authors who engaged in multi-stage research relied on two or more theories and varied the methods across stages accordingly (e.g., Palmer-Wackerly & Wahed, Chapter Eleven, Study 1, this volume; Wright & Canzona, Chapter Five, Study 2, this volume).

Although a strong commitment to theory characterizes all the chapters in this volume, four provide particularly informative reviews of theory development in the health communication arena along with insights regarding how those theories inform methods. In the first chapter, Pitts outlines the distinguishing features of positive communication theory, addressing its roots in positive psychology as well as clarifying how its metatheoretical positions differ from traditional social science. Similarly, Fisher (Chapter Four, this volume) describes the historical development of the biopsychosocial, ecological, and systems theories of health that are so influential today, including how those theories link to and complement communication theories. In Chapter Ten (this volume), Krieger and Raisa show how

Social Identity (Tajfel & Turner, 1986), Self-Categorization (Turner, 1987), and Communication Accommodation (Giles et al., 2023) theories provide essential insights for enacting dialogic translational communication that is culturally sensitive and inclusive. While Pitts, Fisher, and Krieger and Raisa discuss theories that have reached a certain equilibrium so that they serve as guiding frameworks, Fowler (Chapter Seven, this volume) provides readers with a rare insider's view of the development of a theoretical model: the Communication Ecology Model of Successful Aging or CEMSA (Fowler et al., 2015). He shares with readers the various theories guiding the selection of model components and hypotheses regarding their relationships, problems encountered, adjustments made, components added, and so forth, providing a model of theory development that others might follow.

## Culture Writ Small and Large

Culture is commonly used to refer to the shared beliefs, values, norms, and so forth, of citizens of a country (e.g., Chinese culture, U.S. culture) or to all people from a region of the world (e.g., European culture, East Asian culture). However, culture is also applied to describe the shared beliefs, values, and norms of smaller groups within a country such as racial and ethnic groups, professional groups and communities, as well as those of even smaller groups such as families or work groups. From a sociological analysis perspective (Street, 2007), these three conceptions can be viewed as hierarchically organized and labeled macro-, meso-, and microcultures, with microcultures (e.g., families) embedded within mesocultures (e.g., Black American) which, in turn, exist within macrocultures (e.g., U.S. society). Pertinent to this volume, the beliefs, values, and norms within cultures at all levels include those for communication and health. Individuals stand at the center, with each person's identity and beliefs, values, and norms around communication and health reflecting to some degree the micro-, meso-, and macro-cultures within which they exist. The chapters in this volume provide examples of why considering culture, from micro- to macro-, is essential if effective health communication research is the goal.

### Microcultures: Families and Provider–Patient Interactions

Fisher (Chapter Four, this volume), Wright and Canzona (Chapter Five, this volume), and Campbell-Salome (Chapter Six, this volume) focus on interpersonal health communication between family members and/or between medical practitioners and patients. That is, they consider the influence of *microcultures* on those interactions. For example, Fisher (Chapter Four) and Campbell-Salome (Chapter Six) point to the role of long-term family communication patterns

(Koerner & Fitzpatrick, 2002) in the openness of communication between mothers and daughters about breast cancer (Fisher, Chapter Four) and between family members about genetic risk (Campbell-Salome, Chapter Six). Wright and Canzona (Chapter Five) explore how individuals' openness to or avoidance of discussing health topics with relational partners can affect their access to needed social support, as well as how their willingness to discuss those topics with their medical team affects their access to treatment.

### Mesocultures: Communities and Ethnic/Racial Groups

Several chapters examine the health communication experiences and preferences of individuals within specific communities and racial/ethnic groups, focusing on *mesocultures*. Palmer-Wackerly and Wahed's (Chapter11, this volume) research in two rural Nebraska communities illustrates the importance of considering mesocultures. In one community, they wished to gather the views of Hispanic and Somali immigrants on access to healthcare and communication with providers. Recognizing the need to accommodate the language backgrounds and cultural norms of the two immigrant groups, they used an arts-based project in the first stage of the research rather than more traditional methods. This approach enabled participants, as non-native English speakers, to share their perspectives in an affirming way that facilitated dialogue between members of the two immigrant groups and the healthcare providers in the community.

Krieger and Raisa (Chapter Ten, this volume) describe creating culturally sensitive eHealth interventions using Virtual Health Assistants (VHAs). The VHAs can be tailored to patients in gender, appearance, language, literacy, etc., to bring cancer education to those in underrepresented groups, immigrant populations, and rural communities. VHAs may be used alone or in tandem with Community Health Educators (CHEs) from the patients' communities.

Two chapters address culture in community health campaigns in Anchorage, Alaska. Worthington, Howell, Golden, and Mahanna (Chapter Twelve, this volume) describe the development of a student-administered Healthy Aging Program for residents of subsidized housing complexes. The goal of the program was to encourage residents to adopt healthy eating and exercise behaviors. A key consideration in developing the program was the diversity of the residents, many of whom are Alaska Natives. Based on the value placed on resilience, optimism, and hope within Alaska Native culture and a preference for positive emotions by older persons, the research team selected Persuasive Hope Theory (Chadwick, 2015) as the framework for the program. Chen and colleagues (Chapter Fourteen, this volume) examine both unsuccessful and successful health campaigns in Anchorage, a city with a widely diverse population that includes Alaska Natives from several Alaska

Native communities and a large number of immigrants from countries around the world. The authors offer guidance on constructing successful campaigns for large populations of high language diversity, emphasizing that translation of materials into multiple languages is important but does not guarantee a successful campaign if the materials are not culturally sensitive at a deeper level.

Alaska Native culture is the focus of Rosich and colleagues (Chapter Thirteen). These authors direct our attention to Alaska Native people's views on Alzheimer's disease and related dementias. However, their goal is not to identify individual perspectives on the disease but to build, through dialogue with Alaska Native elders, an understanding of how this disease and access to the social determinants of health fit into the cultural view of life, health, illness, and death for Native Alaskans. The discussion in the chapter and the resulting Alaska Native Life Cycle and Social Determinants of Health Model (Rosich et al., this volume, Figure 13.1, p. 287) provide an example of how researchers can develop insights into the deeper aspects of cultures that Chen and colleagues (Chapter Fourteen, this volume) view as essential for successful health campaigns.

### Macrocultures: Stereotypes, Age, and Gender in Western Cultures

Harwood and Cooper (Chapter Two, this volume) and Anderson and McDermott (Chapter Nine, this volume) draw attention to the influence of cultural age stereotypes in health communication. Harwood and Cooper (Chapter Two, this volume) discuss how age and other negative stereotypes can lead to interpersonal communication in healthcare settings that functions to dehumanize individuals and rob them of personhood. The chapter devotes special attention to communication with persons with Alzheimer's disease and related dementias, a group at high risk of the negative consequences of dehumanization. The chapter contrasts dehumanizing with humanizing communication and puts these concepts within the context of stereotyping, and communication and aging theories. Anderson and McDermott (Chapter Nine, this volume) direct attention to the ways in which negative age stereotypes are endemic in public relations materials. They outline and argue for employing the public relations concepts of legitimacy, dialogue, and advocacy in public relations campaigns to promote healthy aging and counter negative stereotyping.

Gettings (Chapter Eight) also looks to the ways in which the larger culture affects health and communication, but although her chapter focuses on retired men and women, gendered experiences and stereotypes, rather than age, are her concern. Gettings shows how the career and personal lives of men and women are inevitably gendered in U.S. society, with implications not only for their health during their working life but also for how they experience the transition to retirement.

### The Intersection of Micro-, Meso-, and Macrocultures in Human Experience

Although my discussion here has addressed the three levels of culture separately to reflect the emphasis in individual chapters, they are inextricably linked in the lived experience and cognitions of individuals. Fowler (Chapter Seven, this volume) captures this intersection in his discussion of the Revised Communication Ecology Model of Successful Aging Model (CEMSA; Fowler, Figure 7.2, this volume, p. 152) and its inclusion of "environmental chatter". That model illustrates how, through environmental chatter, each individual's experience of aging is subject to communicative influence from all cultural levels: Microculture (e.g., explicit messages about aging from friends and others, intergenerational communication that makes age salient in either positive or negative ways, family role models), mesoculture (e.g., explicit messages about aging at the organizational or community level, community role models), and macroculture (e.g., mediated messages that reinforce negative or positive age stereotypes). In turn, these cultural influences play out in the individual's own communication about aging, affecting the extent to which successful aging is achieved.

## THE DIRECTIONS: MOVING RESEARCH INTO PRACTICE

In 2001, Jon Nussbaum and I published an edited volume that focused on the ways in which communication in healthcare settings and within families affected the health of older individuals. Contributors included practitioners and communication scholars, reflecting a goal of the volume captured in its subtitle: *Linking Research and Practice for Successful Aging* (Hummert & Nussbaum, 2001). In their epilogue to that volume, Ryan and Norris (2001) noted the difficulty in achieving this goal given the institutional, professional, and interpersonal challenges to communication between researchers and practitioners, as well as between those professionals and the people they serve. For example, at the institutional level, universities and hospitals have different staff evaluation standards and institutional goals that can create conflicts between academic researchers and medical staff around study design and definitions of success. Use of professional or disciplinary terminology can result in misunderstandings between medical practitioners and communication researchers. Stereotypes about academics or medical staff, perhaps in conjunction with other group stereotypes, can lead to over- or underaccommodative interpersonal communication between a social scientist and a medical professional. These challenges also exist in the communication of medical practitioners and communication researchers with those they serve and the larger community, who come with their own goals and standards for success, professional backgrounds, and stereotypes.

Considering these challenges, Ryan and Norris proposed two strategies to enhance and support collaboration among communication researchers, practitioners, and community members that would facilitate moving research into practice: (1) Embed communication researchers in interdisciplinary teams and (2) involve cultural brokers. The research reported in this volume models these strategies in practice.

## Embed Communication Researchers in Interdisciplinary Teams

Interdisciplinary or multidisciplinary teams composed of practitioners from different specialties and/or professions are quite common today in response to the complexities of the healthcare system and the benefits to patient care (Schmutz et al., 2019). For example, for a person diagnosed with melanoma, a serious skin cancer, a cancer center team might include a dermatologist/oncologist, surgeon, plastic surgeon, nurse practitioner, psychologist/counselor, and social worker. These individuals would meet regularly to discuss the individual's response to treatment, the treatment program, any necessary modifications to that program, psychological state, and need for assistance with insurance or care at home. A team such as this is not immune to communication challenges due to professional stereotypes, differences in professional status, profession-specific terminology, and so forth (Dinh et al., 2020; Fisher & Canzona, 2014; Nussbaum et al., 2001). However, as employees of the same institution, the team members benefit from a similar understanding of institutional goals and their roles on the team. In addition, their regular meetings allow them to develop common understandings and a team identity (Dinh et al., 2020; Nussbaum et al., 2001).

Ryan and Norris (2001) pointed out that academic communication researchers who wish to work on interdisciplinary medical or community teams to bring their research into practice have neither the advantage of a shared understanding of goals and roles nor the ongoing regular contact necessary to develop a team identity. Their ability to bring research into practice is hampered by their outsider status. Accordingly, Ryan and Norris (2001) argued that communication researchers must be embedded in interdisciplinary teams to succeed in bringing research into practice. Several chapters in this volume provide evidence supporting this statement.

Communication researchers who are employed in healthcare organizations have the greatest opportunity to serve on interdisciplinary teams that lead to improved communication. For example, Fisher (Chapter Four, this volume) speaks about the importance of her position and that of her co-investigator Dr. Carma

Bylund within medical institutions—University of Florida Cancer Center and formerly Memorial Sloan Kettering Cancer Center, respectively—to their ability to conduct formative research and use the results in clinical practice. Their intervention to provide resources for family caregivers of those with blood cancers was conducted in collaboration with The Leukemia and Lymphoma Society and a multidisciplinary research team. The willingness of The Leukemia and Lymphoma Society to collaborate with the project was likely facilitated by the investigators' affiliation with a cancer center.

Campbell-Salome (Chapter Six, this volume) also discusses the importance of her position within the genomic health and population science departments at Geisinger Health System in Pennsylvania, which enables her to collaborate with "experts in implementation science, public health, and genomic medicine" (p. 125) on her research as well as with clinicians and genetic counselors who can incorporate that research into care. Krieger (Krieger & Raisa, Chapter Ten, this volume) and Canzona (Wright & Canzona, Chapter Five, this volume) are other contributors whose faculty positions at medical schools (University of Florida and Wake Forest University, respectively) and major clinics (Mayo Clinic, Krieger) facilitate interdisciplinary collaborations that can influence healthcare practice.

However, employment within a healthcare organization is not the only route to being embedded in an interdisciplinary research team that moves health communication research into practice. Grant-funded translational projects can also provide the necessary shared goals and support for communication scholars on interdisciplinary teams. For example, Worthington and colleagues' (Chapter Twelve, this volume) successful development of a 15-week healthy aging program for older Alaskans involved an interdisciplinary team of researchers from communication, public health, health sciences, and dietetics. Palmer-Wackerly and Wahed's (Chapter Eleven, this volume) two-year project assessing the health needs of the Hispanic/LatinX and Somali population of Lexington, Nebraska was also a long-term interdisciplinary grant-funded project. Members of the interdisciplinary team included university researchers, representatives of the local hospital, and community members. Likewise, Wright (Wright & Canzona, Chapter Five, this volume) has a long history of collaboration on grant-funded interdisciplinary research exploring computer-mediated communication in health promotion.

The benefits of these interdisciplinary collaborations to moving communication research into practice include the publications and presentations by team members in not only their own but also in other team members' professional journals and at their professional meetings. For instance, Campbell-Salome's publications (Chapter Six, this volume) appear in both communication journals and medical journals such as *The Journal of Genetic Counseling* and *Translational*

*Behavioral Medicine*. She argues that this practice extends the "reach and impact of health communication research . . . and its contributions outside of academia" (p. 125), making it more likely that it will reach audiences who can incorporate its results into practice.

## Involve Cultural Brokers

Cultural brokers bridge the gaps in understanding between two (or more) groups such as communication researchers and practitioners or research teams and community members (Ryan & Norris, 2001). They play many important roles in health research today (National Center for Cultural Competence, 2004). Several chapters in this volume describe how cultural brokers provided the research team with the insider insights, assessments, and outreach necessary to design and conduct acceptable, culturally appropriate research. They served as informants and evaluators during formative research, facilitated access to research participants during data collection, and, in some cases, served as co-investigators.

### Cultural Brokers and Formative Research

References to cultural brokers in this volume showed that they were important in many ways in formative research. Fisher (Chapter Four, this volume) conducted interviews and surveys of family caregivers of those with blood cancer to identify caregivers' needs as the first step in developing a targeted communication training program that would meet the unique needs of that population. Fisher credits the input of family caregivers at this early stage with alerting the team of the need to focus the training program on adult child caregivers for parents with blood cancers. Similarly, Campbell-Salome (Chapter Six, this volume) gathered information from patients with Familial Hypercholesterolemia (FH) to help develop chatbots (i.e., digital conversation agents) that would be used in a program to facilitate family communication about FH to at-risk relatives.

Worthington and colleagues (Chapter Twelve, this volume) described the importance of gathering insights from members of the target population at later stages of formative research. Prior to launching their student-led Healthy Aging program for a residential housing community, they asked several of the residents to review the program and provide feedback on it. That feedback was important in fine-tuning program content, as well as in providing guidance on presentational style for the student leaders.

Other individuals with expert knowledge or experience, but who were not members of the target population, also served as cultural brokers. For instance, genetic counselors used their experiences in counseling sessions to assist

Campbell-Salome (Chapter Six, this volume) in developing chatbots to facilitate communication within families about genetic results, as well as chatbots to prepare patients for what to expect at their appointment with a genetic counselor. And Fisher (Chapter Four, this volume) had an expert advisory board of family caregivers, physicians, oncology social workers, psychologists, behavioral scientists, and instructional design experts that provided feedback from the formative stage through the completion of the research. These experts serve as cultural brokers for their individual professional groups, helping the research team to avoid missteps and acknowledging the essential interdisciplinary nature of healthcare.

### Cultural Brokers, Access to Participants, and Data Collection

Wright and Canzona (Chapter Five, this volume) provide an example of a creative use of popular "mommy bloggers" as cultural brokers to reach and deliver information to mothers about environmental breast cancer risks. Results indicated the potential of trusted opinion leaders on social media as cultural brokers who can increase diffusion and acceptance of health information.

Cultural brokers were also integral to participant access and data collection for Palmer-Wackerly and Wahed's (Chapter Eleven, this volume) research with the Hispanic and Somali immigrant residents of Lexington, Nebraska. Community health workers who spoke Spanish and Somali led focus groups in Phase 1 and provided information about participants' wishes and concerns that was critical to the successful completion of the research: The community health workers alerted the research team that participants, many of whom were undocumented immigrants, were fearful about completing the written survey planned for the second phase of the study. As a result, the research team changed the survey recruitment design from random spatial sampling to respondent-driven sampling with the community health workers as sole recruiters and interviewers. This adjustment was successful in securing a survey sample of over 300 respondents, whereas the original plans may have resulted in a low response rate and survey data of limited utility.

### Cultural Brokers as Co-investigators

The deep involvement of the community health workers in the Palmer-Wackerly and Wahed (Chapter Eleven, this volume) community health study in Lexington, Nebraska, suggests that their role evolved from that of liaisons between the research team and the community to that of co-investigators. In other cases, cultural brokers served as co-investigators from the beginning of the research. In Palmer-Wackerly and Wahed's (Chapter Eleven, this volume) research with Hispanic/LatinX adolescents in rural Nebraska, the director of the youth group functioned as a cultural broker and co-investigator: He initiated the research by inviting the research team to start the project, guided them to narrow the research focus, and assumed a significant role in participant recruitment.

However, Rosich et al.'s research (Chapter Thirteen, this volume) provides the most complex example of cultural brokers as co-investigators: The 12 Alaska Native Elders who participated in the Alaska Native Elder Memory and Dementia study discussed in the chapter were simultaneously cultural brokers, co-investigators, and participants. They were participants in relating their own life experiences with the social determinants of health, cultural brokers in revealing to the research team the ways in which Native Alaskan culture was woven into their interpretation of their experiences, and co-investigators in contributing to the development of the Alaska Native Lifecycle Theory and Social Determinants of Health Model (Rosich et al., Figure 13.1, this volume, p. 287). Their critical role is implicated in Rosich et al.'s (Chapter Thirteen, this volume) recommendations for an ADRD public health campaign in Alaska Native communities and acknowledged explicitly in a special note at the end of the chapter.

## CONCLUSION: THE FOUNDATIONAL ROLE OF THE LIFESPAN DEVELOPMENTAL PERSPECTIVE

The chapters in this volume illustrate best practices in health communication research across the lifespan: (1) embrace of a social action/positive communication orientation; (2) use of a theoretically grounded and targeted methods approach; (3) attention to culture from micro- to macro-; and (4) adoption of strategies that move research into practice. Critically, a foundation in the lifespan developmental perspective ensures that these practices produce research that is effective in improving the health of individuals of all ages.

As Jon Nussbaum notes in the Introduction to this volume, because "the very nature of human interaction is constantly changing as we as individuals develop throughout our lives, . . . [a]n essential ingredient to our full understanding of the possible consequences for language and social interaction within the health context is the age and relational history of the interactants" (p. XXII, this volume). For example, Fisher (Chapter Four, this volume) describes how considering stage of life (i.e., young, middle, or older adulthood) as well as relational role (i.e., mother or daughter) emerged as critical factors in communication between mothers and daughters around breast cancer diagnoses and treatment, factors equally as important as disease stage. Other authors (Wright & Canzona, Chapter Five, this volume; Worthington et al., Chapter Twelve, this volume) point out how developmental life stage affects preferences for close versus new communication partners and positive emotions. The lifespan developmental perspective is woven into every chapter in this book and distinguishes this volume from others on health communication.

The foundational role of the lifespan developmental perspective in this volume is no accident: The editors of the five parts of this volume all completed their doctoral work with Jon Nussbaum, who has been the strongest advocate for this perspective in the communication discipline in general, and in the health context in particular, from the earliest stages of his career. Many other authors and coauthors are former or current students of the five editors, and so also appreciative of the value of the lifespan developmental perspective. This volume is both the "road map to effective health communication research that makes a difference" that I have outlined in this epilogue and a tribute to the work of Jon Nussbaum in bringing the lifespan developmental perspective to prominence within the discipline. Further, thanks to his research, teaching, mentorship, and the ongoing scholarship of the authors of this volume, we can be assured that the lifespan developmental perspective will continue to guide health communication research long into the future.

## REFERENCES

Afifi, W. A., & Weiner, J. L. (2004). Toward a theory of motivated information management. *Communication Theory, 14*(2), 167–190. <https://doi.org/10.1111/j.14682885.2004.tb00310.x>

Austin, J. L. (1962). *How to do things with words.* Oxford University Press.

Baltes, M. M., & Wahl, H. W. (1996). Patterns of communication in old age: The dependence-support and independence-ignore script. *Health Communication, 8(3)*, 217–231. <https://doi.org/10.1207/s15327027hc0803_3>

Brown, P., & Levinson, S.C. (1987). *Politeness: Some universals in language usage.* Cambridge University Press.

Chadwick, A. E. (2015). Toward a theory of persuasive hope: Effects of cognitive appraisals, hope appeals, and hope in the context of climate change. *Health Communication, 30*(6), 598–611. <https://doi.org/10.1080/10410236.2014.91677>

Dinh, J. V., Traylor, A. M., Kilcullen, M. P., Perez, J. A., Schweissing, E. J., Venkatesh, A., & Salas, E. (2020). Cross-disciplinary care: A systematic review on teamwork processes in health care. *Small Group Research, 51*(1), 125–166. <https://doi:10.1177/1046496419872002>

Fisher, C. L., & Canzona, M. R. (2014). Healthcare interactions in older adulthood. In J. F. Nussbaum (Ed.), *The handbook of lifespan communication* (pp. 387–404). Peter Lang.

Fowler, C. A., Gasiorek, J., & Giles, H. (2015). The role of communication in aging well: Introducing the Communicative ecology model of successful aging. *Communication Monographs, 82*(4), 431–457. <https://doi.org/10.1080/03637751.2015.1024701>

Giles, H., Edwards, A. L., & Walther, J. B. (2023). Communication Accommodation Theory: Past accomplishments, current trends, and future prospects. *Language Sciences, 99*,, 101571. <https://authors.elsevier.com/a/1hUV31OE9HWHOe>

Hummert, M. L., & Nussbaum, J. F. (Eds.). (2001). *Aging, communication, and health: Linking research and practice for successful aging*. Lawrence Erlbaum.

Koenig Kellas, J. K. (2017). Communicated narrative sense-making theory: Linking storytelling and well-being. In D. O. Braithwaite, E. A. Suter, & K. Floyd (Eds.), *Engaging theories in family communication* (pp. 62-74). Routledge.

Koerner, A. F., & Fitzpatrick, M.A. (2002). Toward a theory of family communication. *Communication Theory, 12*(1), 70–91.

Mirivel, J. C. (2014). *The art of positive communication: Theory and practice*. Peter Lang.

National Center for Cultural Competence (Spring/Summer, 2004). *Bridging the cultural divide in health care settings: The essential role of cultural broker programs.* Georgetown University Center for Child and Human Development <https://nccc.georgetown.edu/culturalbroker/index.html>

Nussbaum, J. F., Pecchioni, L., & Crowell, T. (2001). The older patient-healthcare provider relationship in a managed care environment. In M. L. Hummert & J. F. Nussbaum (Eds.), *Aging, communication, and health: Linking research and practice for successful aging* (pp. 23–42). Lawrence Erlbaum.

Ryan, E. B., & Norris, J. E. (2001). Communication, aging, and health: The interface between research and practice. In M. L. Hummert & J. F. Nussbaum (Eds.), *Aging, communication, and health: Linking research and practice for successful aging* (pp. 279–297). Lawrence Erlbaum.

Schmutz, J. B., Meier, L. L., & Manser T. (2019). How effective is teamwork really? The relationship between teamwork and performance in healthcare teams: a systematic review and meta-analysis. *BMJ Open, 9*:e028280. <https://doi:10.1136/bmjopen-2018-028280>

Street, Debra A. (2007). Sociological approaches to understanding age and ageing. In J. A. Blackburn & C. N. Dulmus (Eds.), *Handbook of gerontology: Evidence-based approaches to theory, practice, and policy* (pp. 143–168). John Wiley & Sons. <https://doi:10.1002/9781118269640.ch6>

Searle, J.R. (1965). What is a speech act? In M. Black (Ed.), *Philosophy in America* (pp. 221–239). Allen & Unwin and Cornell University Press.

Tajfel, H., & Turner, J. C. (1986). The social identity theory of intergroup behavior. In S. Worchel & G. Austin (Eds.), *Psychology of intergroup relations* (pp. 7–24). Nelson-Hall.

Turner, J. C. (1987). A self-categorization theory. In J. C. Turner, M. A. Hogg, P. J. Oakes, S. D. Reicher, & M. S. Wetherell (Eds.), *Rediscovering the social group: A self-categorization theory* (pp. 42–67). Blackwell.

# Index

# Language as SOCIAL ACTION

Howard Giles and David M. Markowitz
GENERAL EDITORS

This series explores new and exciting advances in the ways in which language both reflects and fashions social reality—and thereby constitutes critical means of social action. As well as these being central foci in face-to-face interactions across different cultures, they also assume significance in the ways that language functions in the mass media, new technologies, organizations, and social institutions. Language as Social Action does not uphold apartheid against any particular methodological and/or ideological position, but, rather, promotes (wherever possible) cross-fertilization of ideas and empirical data across the many, all-too-contrastive, social scientific approaches to language and communication. Contributors to the series will also accord due attention to the historical, political, and economic forces that contextually bound the ways in which language patterns are analyzed, produced, and received. The series will also provide an important platform for theory-driven works that have profound, and often times provocative, implications for social policy.

For further information about the series and submitting manuscripts, please contact:

Howard Giles
Department of Communication University of California at Santa Barbara Santa Barbara, CA 93106-4020
HowieG iles@cox.net

To order other books in this series, please contact our Customer Service Department at:

peterlang@presswarehouse.com (within the U.S.)
orders@peterlang.com (outside the U.S.)

Or browse online by series at:

www.peterlang.com

www.ingramcontent.com/pod-product-compliance
Ingram Content Group UK Ltd.
Pitfield, Milton Keynes, MK11 3LW, UK
UKHW020201290926
15471UKWH00005B/1006

9 781433 197550